Nutrition and Immunity

Nutrition and Immunity

M. ERIC GERSHWIN
Division of Clinical Immunology
Department of Internal Medicine
University of California
Davis, California

RICHARD S. BEACH
Departments of Nutrition and Internal Medicine
University of California
Davis, California

LUCILLE S. HURLEY
Department of Nutrition
University of California
Davis, California

1985

ACADEMIC PRESS, INC.

(Harcourt Brace Jovanovich, Publishers)

Orlando   San Diego   New York   London
Toronto   Montreal   Sydney   Tokyo

ACADEMIC PRESS, INC.
Orlando, Florida 32887

United Kingdom Edition published by
ACADEMIC PRESS INC. (LONDON) LTD.
24–28 Oval Road, London NW1 7DX

LIBRARY OF CONGRESS CATALOGING IN PUBLICATION DATA

Gershwin, M. Eric, Date
    Nutrition and immunity.

    Bibliography: p.
    Includes index.
    1. Immunity—Nutritional aspects.   2. Nutrition.
I. Beach, Richard S.   II. Hurley, Lucille S.   III. Title.
[DNLM: 1. Immunity.   2. Nutrition.   3. Nutrition Disorders
—immunology.   WD 100 G381n]
QR185.2.G47   1985   616.07'9   84-18582
ISBN 0-12-281450-9   (alk. paper)

PRINTED IN THE UNITED STATES OF AMERICA

85 86 87 88   9 8 7 6 5 4 3 2 1

From M.E.G., with love and gratitude, to
his mother and father,
        and
From R.S.B. and L.S.H., with affection, to
their children

Contents

3. Nutritional Assessment

4. Malnutrition and Infectious Disease: Studies from the Field

5. Nutritional Factors and Immune Ontogeny

6. Caloric Intake

7. Protein

8. Trace Elements

9. Vitamins

10. Lipids

11. Immunological Considerations of Breast Milk

12. Alcohol and Immune Function

13. Nutritional Modulation of Autoimmune Disease

14. Future Directions

Preface

The relationship between nutrition and immune function is gaining increased prominence and reflects a major expansion of both field and wet bench research. There is a growing realization that nutrition may influence immune function not only in populations with severe malnutrition and a high incidence of infectious disease, but more importantly in populations with relatively mild or single nutrient deficiencies. Furthermore, the function of nutrients in immune function is important for etiological and therapeutic considerations in chronic diseases. Fifteen years ago virtually every publication on nutrition–immunity dealt with the impact of nutritional factors in Third World nations. In the past ten years there has been a dramatic shift toward the study and recognition of single nutrient deficiencies in human subpopulations worldwide. Of particular interest is the role of nutrition in chronic diseases of Western populations, especially in neonatal development.

To help understand and put into perspective the interdisciplinary interaction between nutritional scientists and immunologists, the authors have reviewed more than a thousand publications dealing with this subject and have prepared a book of fourteen chapters containing a number of unique features. First, it is hoped that the book is highly readable, with each section having a large number of annotated references. Second, the perspective is not that of clinical observation but is rather a combination of empirical observations and epidemiology. The book begins with an introduction explaining the potential impact of nutritional factors on immune responsiveness. It then presents several chapters that deal with the evaluation of immune function and a chapter on nutritional assessment. Classic observations on malnutrition and infectious disease, involving field studies as well as studies on the effect of nutritional factors on immune ontogeny, are then presented. Then, there are separate chapters that deal with caloric intake, proteins, minerals, vitamins, lipids, breast milk, and alcohol. Chapters are also included that speculate on future directions and on the potential role of nutritional modulation in immune dysfunction. Special attention is paid to experimental studies on laboratory animals, including animal models, in an attempt to isolate specific factors in the interaction between nutrition and immunity.

Each author brings a unique perspective to the volume. Dr. Gershwin is a cellular and clinical immunologist whose major interests are autoimmune disease and the role of nutrition in modulating such disease. Dr. Beach is both a nutrition scientist and immunologist whose training has combined both fields. Dr. Hurley is a nutrition scientist with a major interest in developmental nutrition. Each chapter is meant to be an authoritative review presenting the current state of the art as well as providing key illustrations from classic papers in a given field.

It is hoped that the reader will gain an understanding of the synergism between nutritional factors and immunocompetence, and of the new methodologies and sensitive analytical techniques currently being used. It is apparent from this volume that nutrition and immunology are both relatively young disciplines that are developing at a rapid pace. While a considerable amount of information has already already been obtained, this volume also attempts to explore those areas that must still be studied. The large number of malnourished individuals in the world makes rapid application of these findings extremely important. Indeed, a major conclusion of the volume is that even if mortality is not the ultimate outcome of undernutrition, afflicted children may be irreversibly altered in structural and/or functional terms, leading to permanently stunted growth, learning deficits, and compromised immune function. This finding has serious implications for productive capacity.

Many people contributed in major and minor ways to the completion of this book. Foremost among these were Mark and Judy Van der Water, who painstakingly served in many editorial and technical capacities, and Nikki Rojo, a true "girl Friday."

1

The Potential Impact of Nutritional Factors on Immunological Responsiveness

INTRODUCTION

It has long been recognized that famine and pestilence frequently occur together. In part, their coincidence is related to the same types of factors; for example, both natural disasters and wars tend to precipitate these phenomena. Even a cursory review of history shows that these two major scourges have together frequently altered the course of world events. Scrimshaw *et al.* (1959) were the first to review numerous scientific findings and to present the concept of a synergistic interaction between nutrition and the immune response to infectious challenge. The interaction is profound because it is bidirectional: nutritional status influences host immunological function and the response to pathogenic challenge; conversely, infectious disease, whether acute or chronic, has a detrimental influence on the nutritional state. In an ecological milieu characterized by frequent contact with a wealth of pathogens as well as by diets deficient in a wide range of nutrients, the frequent result is a high infant and child mortality rate, often with half of the children dying before the age of 5 years.

During the past decade, it has become increasingly apparent that the synergistic interrelationship between nutritional factors and immunocompetence is of importance not only to populations in less developed countries but in developed ones as well. Fundamental to this new appreciation are studies underscoring a number of basic similarities between protein-energy malnourished children in developing countries and poorly nourished hospitalized patients in affluent ones, both groups having a similarly compromised immune function that often responded favorably to nutritional repletion. Moreover, new methodologies and more sensitive analytical techniques have enabled investigators in recent years to correlate aberrations in a variety of specific and nonspecific immune responses with marginal deficiencies of a variety of essential nutrients. Such deficits are being recognized as occurring more frequently in Western nations than was previously surmised, especially in certain population groups with high nutrient requirements. Moreover, there has been an increasing awareness that conditions associated with chronic overnutrition, e.g., obesity and diabetes, also significantly modulate immunological responsiveness. In addition, the diets frequently used to treat these afflictions, and their concomitant nutritional limitations, may also have a far-ranging influence on the host defense against infectious challenge. The impact on immunocompetence of diets markedly restricted for cultural or religious reasons has only recently begun to attract serious attention. As we learn more about what constitutes an optimal diet and what constitutes marginal deficiency, these findings will take on greater importance.

THE INFLUENCE OF NUTRITIONAL FACTORS ON IMMUNOLOGICAL PARAMETERS

There are many ways in which nutritional factors can influence the mobilization of an effective host response to pathogenic challenge (McGregor, 1982; Beisel, 1982). A wide variety of nutrients essential for survival and good health have now been demonstrated to have an impact on the immunocompetence of the host. The precise nature of this influence varies with individual nutrients. The effects of nutritional manipulation on immunocompetence may be qualitative, e.g., the absence of a delayed hypersensitivity response to specific skin test antigens, or quantitative, e.g., decreased titers of circulating antibodies in response to pathogenic challenge or vaccination precedures. Moreover, the dietary intake of both experimental animals and humans has been shown to affect both specific and nonspecific aspects of immunity. Some nutrients act directly on the lymphoid system and immune cell function, thereby altering the host immune response, whether cell mediated or humoral, to invasion by various pathogens. Nutritional factors acting directly on cells of the immune system may change the capacity of such cells to recognize a foreign stimulus. Some nutrients may exert a direct influence by altering the proliferative responses of these cells. Accessory cells may also be affected by the availability of essential nutrients, resulting in altered antigen presentation by macrophages. The activity of phagocytic cells may be modified either by impaired uptake of foreign material or by defective intracellular killing of ingested organisms. Cooperation between the various types of cells in the immune system may also be affected, thereby disrupting the immunological circuits necessary for selective potentiation and inhibition of specific subpopulations of lymphocytes. The organism's nutritional status may also affect nonspecific factors such as complement, natural killer (NK) cell activity, certain types of interferon, and acute-phase reactants, all of which are integral to the development of an intact host immunological function.

Nutrient availability may also have a substantial indirect impact on immunological responsiveness, for instance, by altering metabolic, neurological, or endocrine parameters, which also influence immunological function. The concerted interaction of amino acids, vitamins, and minerals, all of which must originate in the diet, is required for the synthesis of those proteins, e.g., immunoglobulins, enzymes, and lymphokines, which participate in immune responses. Insufficient availability of any of these nutrients involved in protein synthesis may result in a cessation or a sharp decline in the production of proteins. Furthermore, those factors actually produced under conditions of deficiency may be defective, resulting in aberrant antigen–antibody affinity. Similarly, nucleic acid synthesis requires the participation of a variety of nutrients; an inability to synthesize appropriate amounts of DNA and RNA could impose severe limitations on the proliferative capacity of cell populations in response to appropriate stimuli.

Other nutrients may be involved in the stability of the plasma membrane and the differentiation and expression of cell surface characteristics. If the deficiency of a nutrient alters the physiological function of immune cell types, it is certain to alter the expression of immunity; in such cases, it is important to determine whether the cells of lymphoid origin are more severely affected than other cell types. A number of hormones are known to have a notable impact on immunocompetence, and endocrine parameters can be affected by the nutritional state. Prostaglandins also seem to have a substantial effect on immunological function, and preliminary indications are that a wide range of essential and nonessential nutrients may influence their synthesis. There is increasing evidence that neuroendocrine factors can regulate immune responsiveness; nutritional influences may, at least in part, influence the immune response via such means. It is most likely that nutritional factors affect the development and maintenance of immunocompetence through multiple pathways and mechanisms.

NUTRITIONAL SEQUELAE OF INFECTIOUS DISEASE

The influence of nutritional intake on immunological function is only part of the reason why this synergistic interaction has such a profound effect on the host organism. Most forms of disease, whether acute or chronic, infectious or degenerative, result in alterations in many nutritional and metabolic parameters. The influence of the disease process on the intake, assimilation, and utilization of essential nutrients is the second major interactive force in the synergism between malnutrition and infection. The precise nature of the influence of infectious disease on the nutritional status of the host depends largely on the nature of the invasive pathogen. The impact on the host organism varies with the species of bacteria, viruses, fungi, or parasites; in addition, the number of pathogenic organisms, their virulence, and the immunocompetence of the host all play important roles in determining the severity of the outcome.

While the nature and severity of the nutritional and metabolic consequences may vary considerably, there are certain generalized sequelae associated with most forms of disease that have a well-established effect on the host's nutritional state. Perhaps the two most obvious are fever and anorexia, which are considered hallmark symptoms of the infected host; nonetheless, the specific purpose and nature of these two processes remain controversial. The nutritional consequences of a loss of appetite are readily apparent. However, if the diseased individual has only very limited stores of nutrients because of preexistent malnutrition or increased requirements, even a short period of decreased food intake may provide a severe nutritional insult. While estimates of the catabolic cost of fever vary, it is certain that the febrile period of an infectious episode is characterized by a hypermetabolic state, with a negative balance of many essential constituents of host metabolism such as vitamins and minerals. Altered metabolism of nearly all major classes of nutrients is seen in most infectious processes, including that of carbohydrates, lipids, protein, intracellular and extracellular electrolytes, trace elements, and both water-soluble and fat-soluble vitamins. While fever and anorexia usually peak early in the acute stages of pathology, metabolic and nutritional aberrations may continue well into the convalescent phase of the disease process, resulting in elevated requirements for a variety of nutrients for a prolonged period. In children living in less developed countries, the required increase in essential dietary constituents is seldom forthcoming; the result is often a cessation of growth and severe complications, with repeated episodes often leading to early mortality. Hospitalized patients in developed nations require progressive monitoring of nutritional indices throughout the disease process, with aggressive dietary-parenteral therapy when indicated during the acute or convalescent phase.

MEANS OF INVESTIGATING THE INTERACTIONS
BETWEEN NUTRITION, IMMUNITY, AND
INFECTIOUS DISEASE

Studies on the interaction between nutritional factors and immunological function fall into two categories: those using human subjects and those using animal models. Both systems offer distinct advantages. Carefully controlled laboratory experiments with a variety of animal species allow the investigator to manipulate a single variable, the intake of a specific nutrient, and assess its impact on a range of host defense mechanisms. Such studies provide knowledge of the basic biological role of various nutrients in the development and maintenance of immunological function. The limitations of such investigations lie in the fact that interspecies comparisons may not prove valid, and the metabolism of the specific nutrient may be influenced by multiple interactions of biochemical, nutritional, endocrine, and neurological factors. On the other hand, studies using malnourished populations in less developed nations and hospital patients in Western nations have assessed the interaction of all of these parameters in the whole organism in its customary ecological context. However, their major limitation lies therein, since it is impossible to quantify the relative importance of any single variable when it proves impossible to control the influence of multiple factors. Thus, the ability to understand the nature of the interaction between nutritional factors and immunological responses must be based on appropriately designed studies using human populations actually subjected to various forms of nutritional stress, as well as carefully controlled experiments using a variety of animal models.

The most common means of monitoring immunological function are discussed in Chapter 2; many of these assays will be referred to repeatedly throughout this volume. The assays have been devised to measure the functional ability of selective aspects of the immune response. Sophisticated testing procedures have been devised to assess specific aspects of both humoral and cell-mediated immunity, as well as nonspecific aspects of the overall immune response to pathogenic challenge. As discussed in Chapter 2, some tests are performed *in vitro,* some in the whole animal, and some either way. The precise nature of the test, using either the experimental animal or the human patient, takes on additional importance in the study of nutritional—immunological interactions. Many *in vitro* assays of immunological function involve the addition of fetal calf serum or another type of serum (rather than autologous plasma or serum). Fetal calf serum should have a normal complement of all of the nutrients and factors normally present in nutritionally replete animals. The use of such serum, particularly in the case of micronutrients, may introduce amounts of the nutrient in question at a level high enough to counteract the nutritional deficiency of the animal or patient being studied. In other cases, as in the investigation of nutritional factors in the development of immunocompetence, the use of such a complete serum may allow investigators to distinguish the effects due to developmental disability from those due to a short-term nutritional deficit in an adult animal or patient. Unfortunately, too frequently, little attention has been paid to variations in results as a function of these parameters.

At present, the impact of nutritional factors on immunological responsiveness has been substantiated to the extent that measurements of immunocompetence have been suggested as indicators of nutritional status. Indices of immunological function should prove even more useful when the exact influences of specific nutrient deficiencies on immunological responsiveness have been catalogued. While such information alone usually cannot provide a sound basis for the diagnosis of a specific nutrient deficiency, it may, along with other data on the biochemical and endocrine parameters related to the metabolism of the nutrient in question, allow the confirmation of the diagnosis. Moreover, the degree to which immunological function is compromised may provide an indication of the severity of the nutritional deficiency. Therefore, the measurement of immunological parameters may find particular utility in the delineation of marginal deficiency states.

THE SPECTRUM OF INTERACTIONS BETWEEN NUTRITION AND IMMUNOLOGY

It is important to emphasize that the interactions between nutritional and immunological factors represent a broad spectrum in terms of their aggregate influence on the whole organism. When the influence of a given nutrient on immunological responsiveness is being assessed, the degree to which dietary intake is either deficient or excessive is important. Moreover, the level of all nutrients in the diet must be considered, since there are complex interactions between many of them. Thus, while intake of the nutrient in question may be adequate, inadequate intake of another nutrient may affect its digestion, absorption, or metabolic utilization.

Another important factor to consider is the timing of the nutritional deficiency. Most investigations using experimental animals are designed to study the influence of nutrient deficiencies on either the development (including prenatal and postnatal) or the maintenance of immunocompetence in adult animals. However, many discussions on the interaction of nutrition and immunocompetence fail to consider the effects of timing. Moreover, in human studies, such as those conducted among children in Third World countries, very little attention has been given to establishing the timing and duration of the nutritional insult, e.g., the nutritional status of the mother during gestation or lactation. The nature of the infectious agent, whether bacterial, viral, fungal, or parasitic, must be considered. The impact of nutritional status on the host's immunological response to these organisms varies greatly with the nutrient deficiency in question, as well as with the pathogenic potential of the infectious agent being studied. Moreover, these organisms vary greatly in their ability to influence immunological responsivenss. Far too often, many of these components are not monitored closely enough, leaving the significance of the results open to question.

Finally, it must be realized that nutrition and immunology are both relatively young disciplines that are developing rapidly. While a considerable amount of information has already been obtained, vast areas remain virtually unexplored; these will become clear in the chapters that follow. The large number of malnourished individuals in the world makes rapid application of the findings in these two fields and their synergistic interplay imperative. In addition, it is becoming increasingly evident that the interaction between nutritional and immunological factors may have a role in the evolution of treatment regimes for many of the diseases that plague those living in the developed nations.

Despite our extensive experience with the two scourges of malnutrition and infectious disease, they continue to plague a large part of humanity and contribute to the majority of deaths in the world. As has been the case throughout history, those living on the margins of society, the poverty-stricken, must shoulder most of this burden; because they are generally ill-equipped to handle it, high levels of morbidity and mortality are the result. Rapidly growing infants and children are most likely to be caught up in the cyclical interactions between malnutrition and infectious disease. If outright mortality is not the ultimate outcome, the development of such children may be irreversibly altered in structural and/or functional terms; permanently stunted growth, learning deficits, and compromised immunological function may be the long-term results. Moreover, in adults, the synergistic impact of malnutrition and infectious diseases may result in compromised physical activity, and productive capacity may be significantly altered. So pervasive is the influence of malnutrition and infectious disease on all aspects of life in Third World countries that indices of nutritional status and infant mortality rates have been suggested with increasing frequency as the most reliable indicators of national development and the general quality of life in such countries.

2

Evaluation of Immunological Function

INTRODUCTION

The well-known observations by Jenner, Pasteur, and von Pirquet of natural and iatrogenic induced pathology are the basis of our knowledge of immune mechanisms, the development of vaccines, isolation of antibodies, and use of both immunostimulatory and immunosuppressive agents in efforts to achieve an optimal balance between immunological status and acquired disease. Indeed, the majority of immunological therapies currently employed in clinical medicine have long been idiomatic, e.g., smallpox vaccine, before mechanistic issues could be addressed. In fact, many elementary studies of immune mechanisms could not be seriously undertaken until a series of cascading fortuitous observations were made in mice, chickens, and human congenital immune deficiency states. These investigations led to the realization that the immune system can be subdivided and characterized into two major components, a thymic-derived (T cell) and a bursa-derived (B cell) pathway. This classification, although quite accurate, has been further refined by the use of monoclonal antibodies directed at subpopulations of lymphoid cells.

This dual-component concept, in which thymic-derived or cell-mediated immunity is distinguished from bursa-derived or humoral immunity, has gained widespread usage throughout all phases of developmental and comparative immunology, and it is now in vogue to study and classify qualitative alterations of these two major compartments in genetic, immunologic, and neoplastic diseases.

EXPERIMENTAL WORK IN ANIMALS

Although there have been many critical observations relative to the discovery that the immune system of vertebrates can be separated into a cell-mediated and a humoral component, the earliest serious experiments were derived from an accidental discovery in chickens. In 1956, Glick and his co-workers at the University of Wisconsin, studying the role of the bursa of Fabricius, an organ located just anterior to the cloaca of the chicken at the distal end of the gastrointestinal tract, discovered that bursectomy did not alter subsequent growth and weight gain. During the course of these studies, several of these neonatally bursectomized chickens were accidentally provided to Chang, another investigator. Chang used these birds, as well as normal chickens, in a student demonstration attempting to elicit an antibody response to the antigen *Salmonella typhimurium.* A number of the neonatally bursectomized chickens were unable to develop significant antibody titers following immunization. This relationship between neonatal bursectomy and absence of antibody production was quickly grasped by Glick *et al.* (1956).

This observation formed the vanguard of many studies that ultimately demonstrated the critical role of the bursa in the development of antibody formation. Specifically, it was shown that removal of the bursa immediately after hatching virtually eliminated the production of specific antibodies. In contrast, removal of the bursa later in life did not significantly impair antibody production. Neonatally bursectomized chickens, although having markedly reduced serum immunoglobulins and no plasma cells, had relatively normal numbers of small lymphocytes in both peripheral blood and spleen and were capable of normal allograft rejection. Even repeated antigenic stimulation of neonatally bursectomized chickens failed to elicit antibody production. Similarly, neonatal bursectomy blocked the development of splenic germinal centers (Cooper *et al.,* 1968).

This paradox of bursectomy and the failure of antibody production but retention of normal cell-mediated immunity (ability to reject allografts) was resolved by Cooper and co-workers. They found that thymectomized, irradiated, newly hatched chickens failed to develop cell-mediated immunity but that plasma cells, germinal centers, immunoglobulin levels, and circulating antibody responses all developed normally. On the other hand, bursectomy and irradiation in newly hatched chickens blocked the development of larger lymphocytes, germinal centers, and plasma cells and resulted in agammaglobulinemia and a deficiency of circulating antibodies. It became apparent that the thymus is necessary for differentiation of the small lymphocytes responsible for cell-mediated immunity and the bursa for the development of humoral immunity (Cooper *et al.,* 1968; Gatti *et al.,* 1970).

Study of the association of bursa development and B-cell ontogeny continues to be useful in understanding lymphocyte maturation. Bursectomy of chickens at serial ages after hatching has revealed an age-dependent relationship in the development of specific classes of immunoglobulins. For example, while neonatal bursectomy results in total inhibition of antibody production of all immunoglobulin classes, bursectomy performed shortly after hatching selectively inhibits IgG and IgA but not IgM antibody responses. This influence of the bursa on immunoglobulin appearance suggests that the ontogenesis of IgM precedes that of IgG and IgA, and the IgM-bearing B cells precede IgG- and IgA-bearing B cells. This progression of B-cell maturation has been demonstrated in other animals; the proposed order is IgM, IgG, and finally IgA. As might be predicted from these observations, a B cell–derived antibody can be produced by continued treatment of newborn animals with anti-antibody (antibody against the heavy chain components of IgM).

At approximately the same time that bursectomies were arousing interest, it was discovered that neonatal thymectomy of mice and rabbits resulted in severe impairment of allograft rejection. In contrast to neonatal bursectomy, neonatal thymectomy of mice depletes both small and medium-sized lymphocytes and markedly diminishes delayed hypersensitivity; however, adequate plasma cells and total immunoglobulin levels remain essentially at presurgical values. This dichotomy between the effects of thymectomy and the effects of bursectomy contributed enormously to the appreciation that each controlled a separate limb of the immune system. Thus, the concept of cell-mediated versus humoral immunity was established (Fig. 1).

It was also apparent that in addition to its influence on cell-mediated immunity, thymectomy resulted in defective antibody responses when experimentally manipulated animals were exposed to antigens such as sheep red blood cells (SRBC) and certain bacterial antigens. However, antibody responses to other antigens (e.g., pneumococcal polysaccharide) remained normal in thymectomized animals. Subsequent work demonstrated that the T-cell system frequently "cooperates" with cells of bursa origin to produce normal antibody formation. Thus, T cells are necessary for a normal B-cell response to certain antigens known as *thymic-dependent antigens* but not for other (thymic-independent) antigens. This latter group of antigens, which include pneumococcal polysaccharide, levan, lipopolysaccharide, DNP-Ficoll, polyvinyl, pyrolidone, and polyinosinic-polycytidylic (polyI · polyC), are unique and interesting because of their polymeric structures. While they elicit antibody responses without T-Cell help, only IgM is pro-

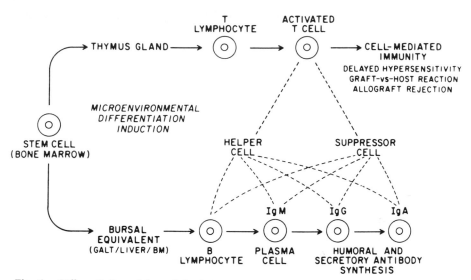

Fig. 1. Differentiation of the cellular immune system.

duced, and the immunocompetent cells stimulated develop no immunological memory and can be easily tolerized (Aaskov and Halliday, 1971; Abdou and Richter, 1970).

Further support for the contrasting influences of the thymus and bursa is derived from experiments illustrating that the deep cortical regions of the lymph node are most profoundly affected by neonatal thymectomy, whereas germinal centers, outlying cortical areas, plasma cells, and medullary cords are affected by bursectomy. Similarly, neonatal thymectomy of mice, much as in untreated patients with the DiGeorge Syndrome, results in characteristic wasting and runting phenomena. Moreover, the wasting seems to be directly related to the degree of development of the peripheral lymphoid tissue at the time of birth. Mice kept in germ-free environments develop less runting and wasting than animals that undergo neonatal thymectomy and are then exposed to pathogens. Finally, as might be predicted, thymectomy performed at 2–4 weeks of age is much less detrimental than when done at birth (Gutman and Weissman, 1972; DeSousa *et al.,* 1969; Good *et al.,* 1962).

Further experiments demonstrated that the ability to reject allografts or initiate graft-versus-host reactions, both abrogated by neonatal thymectomy, can be restored by thymus grafting. Syngeneic tissue was more effective than an allogeneic transplant in reconstituting immune function; transplants mismatched at the *H-2* locus usually failed to reconstitute. Moreover, in many instances, allogeneic grafts mismatched at the *H-2* locus induced lethal reactions. These observations held true when peripheral lymphoid tissue such as lymph node and spleen was used to reconstitute neonatally thymectomized mice (Davis, 1969; Dement, 1970).

Continued study of the inability of neonatally thymectomized mice to participate in cell-mediated immunity and of neonatally bursectomized chickens to produce immunoglobulins has led to the identification of the origin, site of differentiation, and recirculation patterns of lymphocytes. Hemopoietic stem cells arising from the yolk sac, liver, or bone marrow migrate, possibly under the influence of a humoral factor, to the primary lymphoid organs, the thymus or bursa. These stem cells differentiate within a local epithelial-reticular structure to form populations having specific surface marker characteristics of T or B cells (Gelfand and Pyke, 1974). Thymus-derived cells then circulate to populate the thymus-dependent areas of lymphoid tissues, whereas bursa-derived cells populate the thymus-independent areas of lymph nodes (Fig. 1).

Although the majority of experimental data used to separate cell-mediated from humoral immunity are derived from work on chickens and mammals, the two-component concept of immunity, i.e., cell-mediated and humoral immunity, can be illustrated using phylogenetic pathways (Table I) (Cooper, 1970; Burnet, 1974). Responsiveness to foreign material is one of the most fundamental and basic processes of life and can be demonstrated even in that primitive one-cell organism, the amoeba. However, the development of specialized immune apparatus appears to begin with the inverte-

Table I

Phylogeny of Immunity

Species	Cell-mediated immunity	Antibody response	Thymus	Plasma cells	Two-component lymph nodes
Earthworm	+ (limited)	−	−	−	−
Hagfish	+ (limited)	−	Primitive lymphoid hemoblast in anterior kidney	−	−
Horned shark	+ (more extensive than the above)	+ (weak but present)	Primitive pharyngeal epithelial structure	+	−
Leopard shark	+ (distinct thymus)	+	+	+	−
Frog	+	+	+	+	−
Alligator	+	+	+	+	−
Chicken	+	+	+	+	−
Mice	+	+	+	+	+

brates. Earthworms and caterpillars, for example, demonstrate the capacity to recognize specific antigenic determinants and can be induced to show immunologic memory. Moreover, although they do not possess central lymphoid organs, there is evidence of both rudimentary cell-mediated and humoral components of immunity. For example, earthworms within their coelomic fluid and hemolymph contain broadly reacting agglutinins to foreign erythrocytes and bacteria. Although these agglutinins are broadly reactive and do not migrate electrophoretically in the same region as γ globulins, they are nonetheless bacteriostatic and occasionally bactericidal. Although earthworms do not possess a thymus gland, they are capable of slowly rejecting allografts. Although the interrelationships of these primitive systems are not thoroughly understood, it is apparent that they are independent but interrelated systems.

Primitive separation of cell-mediated and humoral pathways exist far below the level of bird or mammalian phyla. The division of immunologic responsiveness into cell-mediated and humoral components has obviously been successful because nature has continued to conserve and differentiate within this major division, and the two-component concept of immunity can be illustrated in all higher forms of life. The separation of cell-mediated from humoral immunity is noted even in the marsupial mammals of Australia and New Zealand, animals long separated from the mainstream of evolution.

As one ascends the animal kingdom from invertebrates to the true vertebrates, anatomically distinct thymus gland and specific immunoglobulin-like proteins appear (Lcmmi *et al.,* 1974; Ruben and Balls, 1967) (Table I). Both T- and B-cell responses can be induced in the lowest vertebrate studied, the California hagfish (cyclostome). Moreover, probably secondary to the appearance of a thymus gland, cellular immunity, immunologic memory, and delayed hypersensitivity can be found. Perhaps as a corollary to the development of these sophisticated features, it is intriguing to comment on the phylogenetic appearance of lymphoid malignancy and autoimmune disease as immunologic diversification and sophistication become evident. For example, lymphomas of frogs and chronic biliary cirrhosis of alligators are well-accepted, albeit infrequently discussed, ailments of these species. Likewise, fish, following exposure to either radiation or carcinogens, respond similarly to humans. It is an unfortunate highlight of twentieth-century technology that the development of tumors in fish can be used to monitor pollution in our ponds and streams. Study of the phylogeny of the immune response therefore indicates that the appearance of the thymus correlates with the development of both delayed-type hypersensitivity and the bursa (or its equivalent) with antibody formation.

Ontogenetic considerations of immunity likewise illustrate the two-component nature of immunity. From studies using the chicken as a model, it is clear that the central lymphoid organs, the thymus and bursa, act as sites for the differentiation of immunocompetent cells. The products of the bursa of Fabricius are small lymphocytes known as *bursacytes* or *B cells.* In contrast, the products of the thymus gland are small lymphocytes known as *thymocytes* or *T cells.* These central lymphoid organs have a similar critical feature, namely, organization around a reticular epithelial framework. It is now known that the factors required for adequate differentiation of these bursacytes and thymocytes into mature, immunocompetent cells are derived from and are present in these reticuloepithelial frameworks (Rosen, 1968).

EXPERIMENTS OF NATURE

It has long been characteristic of clinical medicine that our knowledge and learning experience are derived largely from observations of rare congenital states and diseases that affect only a small minority of patients. This is well illustrated in clinical immunology by the overwhelming contributions of pediatric immunology and the study of patients with myeloma to our present state of the art. In particular, the association of hypergammaglobulinemia and plasmacytosis has been noted in several patients, leading to the suggestion that plasma cells are the source of immunoglobulins (Rosen, 1968; Waldmann, 1969). This hypothesis has been supported by other observations, including the association in a patient with subacute bacterial endocarditis of elevated γ globulins and extreme plasmacytosis. Earlier investigators had proposed that lymphocytes are the sole producers of antibody, but it was necessary to alter this concept as it became evident that the major source of antibody production is the plasma cell. Nonetheless, several more years were required before the relationship between differentiation of B cells into plasma cells and their subsequent production of antibody was appreciated.

The relationship between plasma cells and immunoglobulin production, however, was better illustrated and studied in multiple myeloma (Waldmann, 1969). It was well known that patients with this disease had an extensive plasma cell infiltration of bone marrow and parenchymal organs. Because myeloma is also characterized by an elevation of γ globulins, the association between plasma cells and antibodies thus became firmly established. Subsequent demonstrations revealed that the immunoglobulin elevation noted in multiple myeloma was extremely homogeneous, and that these immunoglobulins were immunochemically related to all of the others and to normal γ globulins, but were at the same time unique immunochemically. This observation laid the foundation for the developing field of molecular immunology (Edelman and Gally, 1962).

The experiments in chickens and mice noted above proved that the thymus gland was essential for the development of cell-mediated immunity as well as for the production of antibody to thymic-dependent antigens. Nevertheless, the role of the human thymus gland remained controversial. Many groups, for example, considered it little more than a vestige. Although there had been associations between human thymomas and immunodeficiency, it was the intensive study of select congenital human deficiencies that led directly to an appreciation of the significance of the thymus. The DiGeorge syndrome, in which patients are born without a thymus gland, is one such immunodeficiency syndrome (DiGeorge, 1968). Clinically, the partial or complete absence of T cells is manifested by a failure to develop either delayed or contact allergic reactions and an inability to reject skin grafts. Because the B-cell pathway of lymphocyte development is normal, immunoglobulin levels and the development of antibodies to thymic-independent antigens are normal. For example, in one patient studied, 85% of the circulating lymphocytes were B cells, as compared to only 20–30% in normals. The identification of this syndrome as secondary to a failure of T-cell development, itself due to thymic agenesis, suggested that thymic transplants may effectively replace the deficiency. This has occurred on several occasions, and DiGeorge syndrome patients have developed T-cell function following thymic transplants much more rapidly than expected.

In contrast to the selective T-cell deficiency of the DiGeorge syndrome is a selective B-cell deficiency characterized by the absence of plasma cells and agammaglobulinemia. Patients with this deficiency have a normal thymus gland and are thus capable of delayed and contact hypersensitivity as well as rejection of skin allografts. Nonetheless, they are unable to make significant antibody responses to either thymic-dependent or thymic-independent antigens (Fudenberg et al., 1971). Agammaglobulinemia therefore appears to result from a specific defect in the development of B cells. Since the equivalent of the bursa of Fabricius in mammals has not been definitely demonstrated, the site of this abnormality remains elusive. However, as will be noted below, unlike the DiGeorge syndrome, some forms of agammaglobulinemia (particularly acquired agammaglobulinemia) appear to be due not to an embryologic defect but rather to the development and appearance of a unique lymphocyte population that chronically suppresses the B-lymphocyte population.

There are a large number of other congenital immunological abnormalities in humans. These have been extensively reviewed elsewhere and will not be individually discussed here (Fudenberg et al., 1971). However, the several phenotypic variations that exist in human immunodeficiencies are critical to our understanding of the interrelationships in the development of both cell-mediated and humoral immunity and have provided investigators with fertile experimental bases for immunotherapy. Because of the selective nature of several of these congenital deficiencies, the effects of thymus, fetal liver, and bone marrow transplants can be adequately observed.

IDENTIFICATION AND PROPERTIES OF T CELLS

Lymphocytes derived from the thymus (T cells) are responsible, as noted above, for cell-mediated responses (Owen and Ritter, 1969; Schlossmann, 1972). These include the initiation of delayed allergic reactions, including solid allograft rejection, graft-versus-host disease, contact sensitivity, and recognition of immunologic responsiveness (and possibly immunosurveillance against neoplasia) (Table II). T cells also contribute a major specific component in the body's defense against a variety of pathogens, including facultative intracellular bacterial pathogens, viruses, and fungi. Morphologically, they consist of the cell population in the deep cortical areas of lymph nodes following antigenic stimulation.

Qualitative and quantitative aspects of T-cell function can be evaluated in a number of ways both *in vitro* and *in vivo*. By far the simplest clinical method involves measuring delayed hypersensitivity via skin testing. Skin testing remains the most important clinical assessment in evaluating the status of the cellular immune system. This important relationship was noted by Jenner in 1801 when he described the "disposition to sudden cuticular inflammation" following the injection of cowpox into the skin of patients previously infected with cowpox or smallpox. This concept of delayed hypersensitivity was further expanded by the astute observations of Koch following injection of extracts of tubercle bacilli into the skin of guinea pigs. These injections, when performed in tubercular guinea pigs, caused the

Table II

Characteristics of T Cells

Initiated delayed hypersensitivity
Responsible for the graft-versus-host reaction
Development of contact allergy
Form spontaneous rosettes with sheep erythrocytes
Transformed with phytohemagglutinin, concanavalin A
Respond *in vitro* to mitomycin-treated or irradiated allogeneic cells
Responsible for rejection of allografts
Function as both helper and suppressor cells

appearance of gross inflammation within 1–2 days. In contrast, injection of tubercle bacilli extracts into normal guinea pigs did not produce a reaction for 10–16 days. This relationship between previous exposure and latency periods for responsiveness initiated the concept of delayed hypersensitivity in the tuberculin test. Hypersensitivity to tuberculin could be readily separated from an Arthus or immediate reaction based on the contrasting ability of lymphocytes and sera to transfer the response. For example, Arthus reactions are mediated by IgG and can be passively transferred from an allergic to a control animal by sera, not cells. In contrast, the transfer of tuberculin sensitivity depends on the passage of lymphocytes.

Presently there are more than 20 antigens that may be used for skin testing in humans (Table III). These include, most commonly, *Candida,* mumps, purified protein derivative (PPD), streptokinase-streptodornase (SK-SD), and trichophytin. Other antigens may be used for specific diagnostic purposes. If anergy is suspected in a patient and if it is of clinical importance, a better evaluation than that gained by applying a battery of tests or by attempting sensitization with dinitrochlorobenzene (DNCB). DNCB in acetone is applied to the upper arm of the patient, and the area is allowed to dry. Approximately 2 weeks thereafter, DNCB in varying concentrations is reapplied and the development of induration is serially observed and quantitated.

There are multiple factors and clinical situations in which diminished, delayed hypersensitivity is manifested (Table IV). The common de-

Table III

Commonly Used Skin Tests for Delayed Hypersensitivity in Humans

Disease	Test extract
Tuberculosis	PPD
Leprosy	Lepromin (suspension of leprosy bacteria)
Brucellosis	Brucellin (filtrate of *Brucella abortus* or melitensis); Brucellergen (bacterial nucleoprotein)
Glanders	Mallium (filtrate of glanders bacillus culture)
Tularermia	Protein extract of *Pasteurella tularensis*
Mumps	Killed virus
Psittacosis	Killed virus
Cat scratch fever	Extract from affected lymph nodes
Candidiasis	*Candida albicans*
Coccidioidomycosis	Coccidioidin
Histoplasmosis	Histoplasmin
Dermatomycosis	Trichophyton
Lymphogranuloma venereum	Extract of the yolk sac of an infected egg
Leishmaniasis	Culture extract
Hydatid disease	Casoni antigen (hydatid cyst fluid)

Table IV

Description and Assessment of Immune Function Tests

Assessment category	Assay	Assessed function	Sensitivity	Specificity
Phagocyte activation	Monocyte polarization to FMLP	Chemoattractant receptor binding Postreceptor function	40–60% positive in normal blood	FMLP receptor mediated
Locomotion	Chemotaxis Chemokinesis	Composite assess CF receptor function Postreceptor transmission of information Orientation response Reversible adherence Directed locomotion	Very sensitive to inhibitors	Nonspecific with regard to exact nature of any inhibition
Respiratory burst	Nitroblue tetrazolium dye reduction test (NBT)	Production of reactive O_2 species in individual cells	High	Does not identify specific O_2 species being produced
	Superoxide (O_2)	Quantitative and kinetic measure of a single O_2 species produced in response to populations; individual cells not assessed	High	Very, but represents an average of all cells
Bactericidal	Killing	Ability to kill opsonized targets as a function of time	High	Defects in opsonization, phagocytosis, postphagocytic granule fusion, or respiratory burst activity are not differentiated

Test	Method	Measures	Sensitivity	Results/Comments
T-cell quantitation Monoclonal AB binding	E rosettes	Total T cells	—	95% peripheral T cells, 20% thymocytes, 30 spleen cells
	OK T3	Total T cells	—	65% peripheral T cells, 75% thymocytes, 15% spleen cells
	OK T4	Inducer/helper T-cell subset	—	70% thymocytes, normally not seen in circulating T cells
	OK T6	Thymocyte marker	—	35% peripheral T cells, 80% thymocytes, 15% spleen cells
	OK T8	Suppressor/cytotoxic T-cell subset		
Mitogen responses (PWM, concanavalin A, phytohemagglutinin)	$[^3H]$thymidine uptake	Measures mononuclear nuclear cell response to polyclonal stimulators	Very sensitive to inhibiting factors or intrinsically abnormal responses	Nonspecific in abnormalities; may indicate the presence of humoral inhibitors or imbalances of helper/suppressor function, or both
B-cell quantitation	Ig-bearing lymphocytes $[F(AB)]_2$ rabbit anti-human IgG, IgM, IgA] RID	Enumeration of lymphocytes bearing IgM, IgG, IgA on their surfaces	High	High
Humoral factors: Plasma levels of Immunoglobulins	RID	Quantitation of immunoglobulin levels	High	High
CH_{50}	Hemolytic titer	Overall functional assessment of complement	High	Nonspecific; does not differentiate low component levels from inhibitors
Natural killer cell activity measure	^{51}Cr-labeled K562 cell cytotoxicity	Ability of PBL or cells to induce release of ^{51}Cr from target cells	Moderate	Nonspecific; ability of PBL to kill standard targets

nominator of these pathophysiologic states is a defect in thymic-derived (or cell-mediated) immunity. There are nevertheless major differences, even among normal volunteers, in the ability to induce and elicit delayed hypersensitivity. These factors include genetic influence, sex, and age. Furthermore, cell-mediated immunity is present very early in life, but the ability to respond to selected antigens (e.g., PPD) may not be present in the newborn period. Moreover, viral infections, including that resulting from vaccination with attenuated measles virus, may transiently suppress delayed hypersensitivity.

CHARACTERISTICS OF B CELLS

As described above, B cells in chickens originate from the bursa of Fabricius. Mammals, however, do not have this organ, and a bursa equivalent has not yet been discovered (Cooper *et al.,* 1966). Moreover, unlike chickens, mammals may not have an exclusive source of B cells. Several groups have nonetheless proposed, on the basis of comparative considerations, that the bursa equivalent exists in mammalian gut-associated lymphoid tissues (the GALT hypothesis). However, removal of the gut in fetal lambs does not interfere with B-cell maturation. Alternatively, bone marrow, also a candidate, does not appear to be a bursa equivalent because its obliteration with 90Sr does not significantly alter B-cell ontogeny. There are also other candidates for the bursa, including fetal liver and spleen, all of which may be bursa-like contributors. On balance, however, it appears that multiple factors/organs may be involved. It is noteworthy in this regard that transplantation of fetal liver into humans with severe combined immunodeficiency (i.e., without T or B lymphocytes) may result in the appearance of both mature B cells and immunoglobulins (Buckley *et al.,* 1976).

The major functions of B cells are the secretion of immunoglobulins and the differentiation into plasma cells (Strober, 1975). Indeed, individual B cells have a receptor-specific immunoglobulin class on their cell surface that correlates with the antibody class produced. Specifically, B cells provide a primary defense against high-grade encapsulated bacterial pathogens. It is therefore not surprising that patients with multiple myeloma or agammaglobulinemia suffer from recurrent pneumococcal infections. Additionally, B cells are critical for the detoxification of protein polysaccharides and toxins (Table V).

B-cell function in humans can be rapidly evaluated by quantifying the serum level of three major immunoglobulin classes, IgM, IgG, and IgA. Moreover, the titer of antibody to several ubiquitous antigens as well as the isoagglutinins, antistreptolysin O (ASLO), and antiviral antibodies provides significant information on previous antibody formation.

Table V

Characteristics of B Cells

Contain surface immunoglobulins
Possess Fc and C′3 receptors
Secrete antibodies
Provide primary defense against high-grade encapsulated pathogens
Detoxify proteins, polypeptides, and polysaccharides
Possess receptor for Epstein-Barr virus
Can be removed with anti-immunoglobulin column
Respond with blast transformation to the mitogens LPS, PPD, and pokeweed

B cells, in a manner similar to that of T cells, can be stimulated to blast transformation with specific mitogenic agents, particularly lipopolysaccharide (LPS) and PPD. In contrast to T cells, however, B cells do not form spontaneous E rosettes with sheep red blood cells (SRBC). They do, however, form rosettes with erythrocytes coated with antibody and complement (EAC, erythrocyte antibody complement rosettes). Such EAC rosettes depend on the presence of receptors of C′3 on the surface of B cells. It should be emphasized, however, that monocytes also have a receptor for C′3 and thus form EAC rosettes. In contrast, however, B cells form rosettes with either mouse or monkey red blood cells and have surface receptors for Epstein-Barr virus.

Of particular importance to the identification of B cells is the presence of surface immunoglobulin (Table VI). Unfortunately, accurate identification of intrinsic surface membrane immunoglobulin is subject to a number of serious experimental artifacts. In particular, both B cells and monocytes have Fc receptors on their surface, and Fc receptors will bind protein aggregates present in the antisera. Ironically, commercial antisera are often packaged in lyophilized form, and the final product may therefore have a considerable amount of aggregation. This will cause fluorescence of Fc receptors and will be optically indistinguishable from the staining of surface immunoglobulin; thus, artificially high values may be obtained. This prob-

Table VI

Detection of Membrane-Bound Immunoglobulin

Fluorescent microscopy using FITC antisera or FITC F(AB)$_2$ antisera
Rhodamine conjugation
Enzyme conjugation of antisera (peroxidase)
Ferritin conjugation of antisera
Autoradiography
Radioimmunoassay

lem has been under intense investigation because it appears that the majority of studies reporting the number of peripheral blood B cells may have overestimated them. Fortunately, this experimental error can be reduced by ultracentrifugation of antisera prior to use in order to sediment and thereby remove aggregates. Similarly, one may use $F(AB)_2$ antisera or monoclonal reagents.

The relative and absolute numbers of B cells in peripheral blood have not yet been standardized. Moreover, a significant percentage of B cells have shed their immunoglobulin and will be undetected by simple direct immunofluorescence. Nonetheless, it is believed that the relative number of peripheral blood surface immunoglobulin-positive cells is 1–15%. The majority of these cells bear both IgM and IgD. The total number of IgG- and IgA-bearing cells is less than 2–5%. The number of complement receptor–bearing lymphocytes is similarly in doubt because of a heterogeneous population. It is known, however, that the two major complement receptors include C4 or the C3c region of C3b, i.e., the immune adherence receptor. Alternatively, the C3d receptor is specific for the C′3d region of C′3b. Both receptors are generally present in individual cells but may be independently expressed, particularly in lymphoproliferative disease.

CHARACTERISTICS OF NULL CELLS

In both mice and humans, subpopulations of lymphocytes lacking surface marker characteristics of both T and B cells have been demonstrated. Briefly, such cells form neither E nor EAC rosettes and lack surface immunoglobulin. They can be further distinguished from monocytes by their inability to phagocytize latex. However, *null cells,* as they are referred to, possess Fc receptors and function as efficient effector cells for antibody-dependent, lymphocyte-mediated cytotoxicity (ADLMC). In ADLMC they have been referred to as *K cells.* Specific monoclonal antibodies against such cells have been reported. However, it appears highly likely that null cells represent a heterogeneous population. It is intriguing that the percentage of null cells in human peripheral blood is often elevated in patients with autoimmune disease, e.g., systemic lupus erythematosis (Table VII) (Bentwich and Kunkel, 1973).

REGULATION OF THE IMMUNE RESPONSE

In 1966, during studies of the functions of T and B cells in the production *in vivo* of antibody to SRBC, it became clear that a profound synergism

Table VII

Characteristics of Human Null Cells

Fail to form spontaneous rosettes with sheep erythrocytes
Lack surface immunoglobulin
Effective *in vitro* as effector component in antibody-dependent
    cell-mediate cytotoxicity
Possess Fc receptors
Nonadherent
Nonphagocytic
Morphologically indistinguishable from T or B cells
Probably a heterogeneous population

---

existed between thymocytes and bone marrow cells. Insignificant titers of antibody were produced in either T or B cell—deprived animals. This critical observation introduced the concept of positive interactions in immunity and led to the proposal that antibody production to thymic-dependent antigens depends on the interaction between antigens, monocytes, T helper cells, and B cells. Moreover, similar studies have demonstrated that two different subpopulations of T cells cooperate in the induction of graft-versus-host disease and skin allograft rejection.

Until recently, the vast majority of efforts to explain the events leading to the production of the immune response against SRBC, autoantigens, and even infectious organisms were directed solely at the positive factors involved in regulation, namely, those responsible for augmentation. It has been postulated that T cells, under the influence of antigen, become activated and release a special immunoglobulin molecule known as *IgT*. The structure and function of IgT remain speculative but may be analogous to those of the immune response gene. Furthermore, the function of IgT may depend heavily on the genetic relationship between T cells and antigen recognition/responsiveness.

It is also well known that immunity is a double-edged sword. There are numerous examples of the detrimental influence of the immune system. In many of these situations, the influence on the host is due to an immunologic hyperresponsiveness in the form of either allergy or autoimmune phenomena. Therefore, attempts to understand the development and expression of the immune response are critical if immunity is to be manipulated and adjusted to prevent harmful effects. It is through our study of autoimmunity and responsiveness to both self- and foreign antigens that the field of immune regulation can be introduced.

Immune regulation is inherent in the concept of the dual-component pathway of the immune system responsible for the differentiation of antigen reactor precursor cells and the subsequent development of either cell-mediated or humoral immunity. As noted earlier, the thymus gland and the bursa equivalent produce stem cells that differentiate to form immunocompetent, antigen-reactive cells. Production of antibody is directly related to the development of precursors of antibody-producing cells (B cells), which recognize antigen by surface immunoglobulins specific for that antigen. Under this influence, B cells differentiate into plasma cells, proliferate, and secrete a specific antibody. Similarly, a select population of B cells does not produce antibody but nevertheless differentiates and survives for long periods of time as memory cells. These latter cells are capable of responding after secondary challenge or exposure to antigen and therefore produce the anamnestic response.

In contrast to humoral immunity, cell-mediated immunity is directly under the influence of thymic-derived T cells. The mechanism by which T cells recognize antigens and produce positive signals, in contrast to the above information on B cells, is unclear. It is apparent, however, that under the influence of antigens, T cells undergo repeated mitosis and differentiation into cells responsible for cell-mediated immunity. Such stimulated T cells also produce several active soluble mediators, including lymphotoxins, skin reaction factors, interferon, and macrophage inhibition factor; each plays a significant role in delayed hypersensitivity, response to infectious disease, and activation of macrophages. Similarly, a subpopulation of T cells may likewise develop into long-lived memory cells and may be responsible for the development of anamnestic responses. Additionally, under appropriate circumstances, both stimulator T and B cells are capable of becoming tolerant to select antigens. Under this influence, tolerance or immune paralysis to either cell-mediated or humoral immunity is possible.

It is also important to discuss the existence of a third cell population involved in positive regulation, the macrophage. Indeed, the macrophage appears to be important for the presentation of antigen. As such, development of the primary immune response and initiation of both cell-mediated and humoral immunity depend on the activity of monocytes. The precise role of monocytes in both positive and negative immune manipulation is under intense investigation; however, it is apparent that they function in a large variety of ways and that subpopulations of these cells may exist.

The positive mechanism by which T cells result in the development of the humoral response by B cells to complex antigens has been demonstrated for hundreds of antigens. For example, B cells both *in vivo* and *in vitro* are able to make significant antibody responses to the thymic-dependent antigen SRBC only under the influence of T cells. This positive cooperative interaction appears to be regulated by surface receptors coded by genes of the major histocompatibility complex. Additionally, certain soluble mediators, perhaps products of the *I* region of the *H-2* complex in mice, are critical in mediating this cooperative interaction between T and B cells. Similarly, although precise surface receptors on T cells have not been identified, an immunoglobulin-like material known as IgT (see above), produced by T cells after interaction with antigen, may be important for the presentation of B cells under the influence of monocytes.

There have also been several demonstrations that subpopulations of T cells exist; they are distinguishable on the basis of different surface characteristics and physical properties. These have been best studied by comparing properties of murine T cells derived from thymus, spleen, and thoracic duct. In particular, murine T cells can be further subdivided on the basis of unique mouse surface receptors, including theta, TL, and Ly antigens. Cells can be further characterized on the basis of cortisone and radiation sensitivity. These characteristics reveal that murine T cells are an extremely heterogeneous population and can be readily isolated to characterize selected discrete subpopulations. The biologic relevance of this heterogeneity is critical. It is further apparent that many of these differences are due to distinct stages in T-cell development. On the basis of surface receptors and the use of monoclonal reagents, these distinct populations may have specific immunologic properties, including, for example, positive (helper) or negative (suppressive) actions.

Thus, data are now accumulating suggesting that the functions of T cells may be carried by different sublines of T cells. These different subpopulations may be specifically detected and isolated within the thymus as well as within peripheral lymph node tissues. From a functional point of view, it is accurate to state that the study of graft-versus-host disease, development of cytotoxic lymphocytes, and immunoglobulin production have all demonstrated that T cells can function both in a positive and a negative regulatory capacity to alter the immune response.

In contrast to the development of positive immune responses, the influence of negative regulatory mechanisms (those that turn off or prevent the development of immune responses) have been investigated only relatively recently. Nonetheless, over the past several years, a number of interesting experiments have led to the concept of active suppression of immunocompetent cell populations by thymic-derived cells. Such active regulation by suppressor T cells can be readily distinguished from the influence of specific antibody or antigen-antibody complexes in regulating immune responses. Several studies of negative feedback suggest that this suppression may play a critical role in autoimmune disease.

In humoral immunity, suppression has been most easily demonstrated for antigens that do not require thymic helper cells. The antibody response to pneumococcal polysaccharide (SSS III) is enhanced by the administration of antithymocyte serum; this enhancement is reduced by the subsequent administration of thymocytes. Ironically, this observation seemed to contradict previous concepts on the use of antilymphocyte serum as an immunosuppressive agent. However, the results of these experiments were confirmed using another antigen, polyinosinic-polycytidylic acid (poly I·poly C). These studies taken together strongly suggested the existence of thymic regulation by suppression of the antibody response to several antigens requiring little thymic helper function. In addition, suppression has been demonstrated for antigens requiring thymic helper cells for a maximum antibody response. Similarly, the homocytotrophic (IgE) antibody response to dinitrophenyl-ascaris may be regulated by antigen-specific suppression. In cell-mediated systems, suppression of the induction of graft-versus-host disease by thymocytes and spleen cells has been demonstrated. The limited information to date suggests that more than one kind of thymic suppression may exist, including nonspecific and specific suppression of antibody responses and suppression of cellular immunologic phenomena. Further study may disclose more subdivisions.

The mechanism of suppression is poorly understood. Preliminary results suggest that in the antibody systems thymic suppression may act by inhibiting B-cell proliferation. A similar suppression of T-cell proliferation would be plausible for the cellular system, including graft-versus-host disease. In the normal host, however, there is probably a balance between suppressor and proliferative functions. Chronic allogeneic disease may be an example of relative reduction in suppressor function secondary to a pronounced enhancement of proliferative function. This negative influence of T-cell populations on the immune response may be either antigen specific or nonspecific.

An example of nonspecific suppression of immunity is antigenic competition mediated by thymic-derived cells previously stimulated by the antigen, inducing competition. This can be illustrated in the acute production of anergy in guinea pigs. For example, guinea pigs allergic to a variety of antigens can be rendered anergic to all of these antigens by the injection of a large quantity of one antigen in soluble form. Although this anergy is short-lived, it can be prolonged by repeated injections of the antigen but not overcome by injecting sensitized lymphocyte cells into anergic test animals. Nevertheless, lymphoid cells from anergic guinea pigs are capable of transferring delayed hypersensitivity to normal guinea pigs. The etiology of this form of antigenic competition appears to be secondary to a number of local factors, including soluble mediators produced by suppressor T cells. Other mechanisms, including the influence of the reticuloendothelial system, competition among determinants on complex antigens, and local competition with lymphoid tissues, are also critical.

A number of experiments to explain antigenic competition have heavily incriminated soluble mediator(s). A variety of protein substances released by antigen-specific stimulated T cells have been described, all of which appear to reduce the immune response to other related antigens. Although the precise chemical nature of the mediator(s) has not been determined, it is distinguishable from that of soluble materials produced by helper T cells in the development of positive immune responses.

The identification of specific populations capable of negative regulation of the immune response led to attempts to isolate and characterize this population selectively. In particular, suppression has now been demonstrated in a large number of systems both *in vitro* and *in vivo*. For example, thymocytes can suppress both cell-mediated and humoral immune responses when injected into intact syngeneic recipients. Moreover, the antibody responses to thymic-independent antigens can be enhanced either by previous injection of antithymocyte sera or by thymectomy. Similarly, it has been demonstrated that the spleen is a rich source of suppressor cells, and this splenic enrichment is particularly high in very young mice. Hence, the lack of significant maturation, i.e., the failure to produce significant humoral immune responses in young mice, may be due to the enrichment of suppressor cells in these animals.

IN VITRO METHODS FOR EVALUATION OF CELL-MEDIATED IMMUNITY

Because cutaneous anergy may result from abnormalities in lymphocytes, macrophages, neutrophils, or combinations thereof, *in vitro* tests are valuable in defining the level of the defect (Table VIII) (Dionigi, 1982). Tests that assess lymphocyte function measure surface markers and their ability to proliferate, produce mediators, and mount cytotoxic responses. The enumeration of lymphocyte subpopulations (T and B cells) utilizes the observation that unique receptors are present on each cell type. Immunofluorescence techniques are used to identify immunoglobulin receptors on B cells, and rosetting techniques are used to identify T and B cells.

Whenever possible, the clinician should use more than one *in vitro* test of lymphocyte function, since each assay may measure a distinct subpopulation of cells. Furthermore, present evidence indicates that lymphocytes are compartmentalized; that is, cells in the blood may be functionally different from those in lymph nodes or spleen. Therefore, sampling blood lymphocytes alone may not yield representative results. A thorough evaluation includes quantitation of the number of T and B cells, proliferative responses

Table VIII
Causes of Diminished Delayed Hypersensitivity in Humans

State	Cause
Congenital	
DiGeorge syndrome	T-cell agenesis
Wiscott-Aldrich syndrome	? Impaired T-cell maturation
Severe combined immunodeficiency	Stem cell defect
Ataxia Telangiectasia	Thymic hypogenesis
Immunodeficiency with thymoma	? Suppressor T cells
IgA deficiency	Relationship between thymus and IgA
Acquired infectious (viral)	
Measles	Lymphocytotoxic antibodies to T cells
Influenza	Suppressor cells
Infectious mononucleosis	Antigenic competition
Mumps	Viral infestation of T cells and/or monocytes
Hepatitis	Other
Other	
Bacterial	
Tuberculosis	Nutritional
Leprosy	Effects of suppressor cells
	Effects of lymphocyte recirculation patterns
Fungal	
Coccidioidomycosis	Nutritional
Cryptococcosis	Effects of suppressor cells
	Effects of lymphocyte recirculation patterns
	Other
Iatrogenic	
Corticosteroids	Redistribution of circulating T-lymphocyte pool
Immunosuppression	Cytotoxicity
Radiation	Other
Malignant	
Hodgkin's disease	Replacement by unregulated proliferation of B cells
Leukemia	Development of suppressor cells
Other	Other
Metabolic	
Hypothyroidism	Nutritional
Vitamin C deficiency	Other
Iron deficiency	
Protein deficiency	
Autoimmune disease	
Primary biliary cirrhosis	Lymphocytotoxic antibodies for T cells
Rheumatoid arthritis	Development of suppressor lymphocytes
Systemic lupus erythematosis	Effects on lymphocyte recirculation patterns
Sjögren syndrome	? Influence of mediators
Other	
Idiopathic diseases	
Sarcoidosis	? Influence of mediators
	? Suppressor cells
	Other

to mitogens and specific antigens, measurement of at least one lymphocyte mediator, and a cytotoxic response.

Assessment of macrophage and polymorphonuclear leukocyte function is performed by measuring the ability of these cells to ingest particles, to kill microorganisms, and to respond to certain stimuli by increased directed movement (chemotaxis), by identifying certain surface receptors, and by determining their response to lymphocyte mediators.

Because of their complexity, some of these *in vitro* assays are not routinely carried out in clinical laboratories and would be difficult in field studies in Third World nations. Moreover, because these assays measure biologic phenomena and are subject to considerable variation, the results should be interpreted with appropriate caution. These tests have a fairly high incidence (10–20%) of false-negative results. Therefore, in an individual patient, a test producing a negative result should be repeated to confirm abnormal cellular function. Although not usually diagnostic, these tests are of value clinically for identifying certain pathogenetic factors and for monitoring the results of therapy and the clinical course of patients with depressed cellular immune function.

Lymphocyte function can be assessed quantitatively *in vitro* by several methods. In particular, the selective stimulation and blast transformation of T and B cells by mitogenic agents has proved to be a major tool for the study and recognition of antigenic activation, separation of lymphoid subpopulations, and biochemical signals. It has been demonstrated, for example, that the lectins extracted from the plants *Phaseolus vulgaris* (phytohemagglutinin) and *Concanavalia ensiformis* (concanavalin A) specifically stimulate T cells. Although the degree of transformation can be quantified by morphologic counting of blast cells, the more reliable and objective means is to measure tritiated thymidine incorporation, a direct parameter of DNA synthesis.

Similarly, T cells have been found to be the principal responding population in mixed lymphocyte reactions and are the major populations recognizing histocompatibility differences. Stimulation by foreign cells therefore can be used both as a measure of T-cell function and as a means of distinguishing major genetic differences between individuals. Finally, mixed lymphocyte reactions also generate cytotoxic lymphocytes.

Several soluble mediators are produced by T cells, B cells, and monocytes that reflect in large measure the status of cellular immunity. These include mediators affecting macrophages, such as migration inhibition factor (MIF) and macrophage-activating factor (MAF); mediators affecting basophils and eosinophils; and miscellaneous others, including interferon, skin reaction factors, chemotactic factor, and the family of lymphotoxins. Although the elaboration of these factors can be shown to correlate with *in vivo* delayed hypersensitivity in humans, they do not necessariy measure the function of a particular cell type (T or B cells).

In addition to these functional parameters of T-cell function, there are a number of unique surface marker properties distinctive for T cells. One of the most important arose from the discovery that human T cells bind to SRBC. Approximately 60–70% of human peripheral blood lymphocytes bind to SRBC; such lymphocytes are T cells. Nonetheless, the E rosette assay is of minimal value compared to the sensitivity and specificity obtained using monoclonal antibodies directed at human T-cell subpopulations (Table IV). The clinical use of monoclonal reagents for diagnosis is best illustrated by the low helper/suppressor ratio in AIDS (acquired immune deficiency syndrome) (Haverkos, 1983).

Assays of lymphocyte transformation, using mitogens, provide the simplest, most reproducible, rapid, semiquantitative, and widely used *in vitro* correlate of cell-mediated immunity. Although *in vitro* assays of mediator production correlate closely with skin tests, they are in general more difficult to perform. Dissociation of cutaneous delayed hypersensitivity, *in vitro* mediator production, and lymphocyte transformation have also been observed. Sometimes only lymphocyte transformation detects defects in cell-mediated immunity, because some antigenic components induce only lymphocyte transformation, whereas others induce only mediator production. Lymphocyte transformation can be defective, even in the absence of lymphopenia, and therefore provides a sensitive indicator of defective lymphocyte function. The two most widely utilized micromethods for assessing lymphocyte transformation involve assaying protein synthesis by transforming lymphocytes, which has the advantage of rapidity, or assaying DNA synthesis, which provides greater sensitivity. These methods enable lymphocyte transformation to be used both as a routine clinical test and as a widely applicable investigative tool for experimental studies.

The battery of stimulants that can be used to evaluate lymphocyte reactivity are divided into two groups. Those classified as *nonspecific mitogens* transform 60–90% lymphocytes from all normal adults, as well as newborns, independent of immunization. The other group of stimulants is classified as *antigens* because they stimulate lymphocytes only from previously sensitized donors. Antigens initially activate only a small clone of the previously sensitized lymphocyte population to transform, but after repeated divisions during the 5–7 days of incubation, 5–35% of the lymphocytes appear to be transformed. Therefore, antigen-induced lymphoproliferation represents a secondary response *in vitro* and fails to stimulate unsensitized adults and the majority of cultures of newborn lymphocytes. Stimulants can be further characterized by whether they are thymus dependent or stimulate purified T but not B cells, or, conversely, are thymus independent and stimulate purified B but not T cells. It must be emphasized that using peripheral blood lymphocytes, the so-called T-cell stimulants activate both lymphocyte populations, presumably because they stimulate T cells to make factors that in turn enhance the reactions of B cells. Commonly used T-cell mitogens include phytohemagglutinin and concanavalin A. Pokeweed mitogen stimulates both T and B cells. In humans, pokeweed is a thymus-dependent stimulant that can stimulate B cells only in the presence of some T cells. In contrast, B-cell mitogens activate only B cells even in mixtures of B and T lymphocytes. Unfortunately, the best-known B-cell mitogens, such as thymus-independent LPS endotoxins and anti-immunoglobulin antibodies, are too limited in potency to permit evaluation of B-cell lymphoproliferative reactivity in humans using peripheral blood lymphocytes. In the case of humans, LPS stimulates only B cells of sensitized subjects and does so only in the presence of some T cells; it therefore behaves like a T-dependent B-cell antigen.

In assessing the immunocompetence of lymphocytes, it is very important to test the lymphocyte reactivity to suboptimal doses of a mitogen, such as PHA. For example, in a number of immunodeficiency states, including the Wiskott-Aldrich syndrome, the proliferative response to optimal doses of PHA will be normal, whereas subnormal reactivity will be detected only in response to suboptimal doses of PHA. Antigens that are also commonly used to evaluate the efficacy of human lymphocyte transformation are all thymus dependent and activate T- as well as B-cell proliferation. They include purified PPD (20 µg/ml), streptolysin 0 (1 : 20 final dilution), *Candida albicans* (1 : 100 final dilution of a glycerol saline extract), and tetanus toxoid (6 µg/ml).

Sensitized lymphocytes, when activated *in vitro* by a specific antigen, produce a soluble factor, termed *migration inhibition factor (MIF),* that retards the migration of macrophages or monocytes from capillary tubes. The MIF system of migration inhibition, utilizing macrophages or monocytes as indicator cells, is distinct from the system of migration inhibition that uses polymorphonuclear (PMN) leukocytes as indicator cells. The inhibition of migration of PMN leukocytes is mediated by a separate factor, termed *leukocyte inhibition factor.* Human MIF is a protein with a molecular weight of 23,000. The production of antigen-induced MIF *in vitro* correlates with the *in vivo* state of cellular hypersensitivity of the lymphocyte donor. Lymphocytes from normal subjects who manifest cutaneous delayed hypersensitivity to various antigens produce MIF *in vitro* to the same antigens, whereas lymphocytes from normal subjects who lack delayed hypersensitivity to these antigens fail to elaborate MIF when challenged *in vitro.*

Currently, two methods are available for the assay of human MIF. The direct assay (one-step procedure) involves the use of sensitized human lymphocytes mixed with guinea pig macrophages or human monocytes in capillary tubes. Specific antigen is added to the system, MIF is made locally by the lymphocytes, and the latter then acts on the macrophages or monocytes within the 24-hr period to inhibit their migration. In the indirect system (two-step procedure), sensitized lymphocytes are first cultured separately with antigen to produce MIF over a 1- to 2-day period. The cell-free supernatant is then assayed for MIF activity on nonimmune guinea pig macrophages or human monocytes in capillary tubes.

The indications for the use of the migration inhibition test fall into two main categories: (1) evaluation of lymphocyte function in general and (2) detection of sensitized lymphocytes to tissue antigens or drugs. In the former, the production of MIF in response to environmental antigens, such as PPD, *Candida,* or SK-SD gives an estimation of lymphocyte function related to cellular hypersensitivity in the skin. Skin testing to tissue antigens or drugs is not recommended because of possible reactions or sensitization of the patient, and thus MIF has the advantage of an *in vitro* test.

The *in vitro* production of MIF in normal subjects correlates with the *in vivo* state of cellular hypersensitivity of the lymphocyte donor. Recent evidence indicates that MIF production is not solely the function of human T-cell subpopulations. Human B-cell subpopulations also elaborate MIF in response to a specific antigen that is similar in size to the T-cell mediator. Furthermore, B cells make more of this material. Therefore, the MIF test may be used to assess cellular hypersensitivity generally, but it does not measure the *in vitro* response of a particular cell type (T versus B). If MIF production is absent in patients with cutaneous anergy, this presumably indicates a defect in both T- and B-cell function. It is not clear at present exactly how the B cell functions in delayed hypersensitivity or what is the role of B-cell MIF.

IN VIVO METHODS FOR EVALUATION OF CELL-MEDIATED IMMUNITY

Evaluation of cell-mediated immunity involves measurement of delayed hypersensitivity via skin testing. The development of an erythematous wheal at the site of antigen injection implies an intact afferent, central, and efferent limb of the cellular immune response, as well as confirming the patient's ability to mount a nonspecific inflammatory response.

There are many clinical situations in which diminished delayed hypersensitivity is manifested, and several factors are involved. In patients with severe or recurrent infections or in those who develop infections with unusual organisms, an underlying congenital or acquired defect in delayed hypersensitivity is frequently considered. These tests may also be used to evaluate a patient who has a disease with a known association with defects in delayed hypersensitivity, such as Hodgkin's disease or sarcoidosis. In addition, an assessment of delayed hypersensitivity may be prognostically significant in patients with certain kinds of malignancy, since diminished reactivity may be associated with poor prognosis. Nevertheless, even normal volunteers show major differences in the ability to induce and elicit delayed hypersensitivity. The factors involved include genetic influence, sex and age. Furthermore, cell-mediated immunity is present very early in life, but the ability to respond to select antigens, e.g., PPD, may not be present in the newborn period. Moreover, viral infections, including those resulting from vaccination with attenuated measles virus, may transiently suppress delayed hypersensitivity.

In each of the above cases, the standard procedure is to apply a panel of skin test antigens in an intermediate test strength. If the results with the intermediate strength are negative, then the next higher strength of antigen is utilized. Antigens selected for this purpose are those to which individuals are commonly exposed; therefore, most normal subjects will respond to at least some of them. Absence of reactivity could occur in patients who in fact have normal delayed hypersensitivity in the following circumstances: (1) There may be improper administration of antigen, degradation of the antigen by exposure to heat or light, absorption of the antigen on container walls, improper dilution, or faulty interpretation of the skin test results. (2) The patient may not have been previously exposed to the test antigens (this occurs rarely, especially in adults, when common antigens such as *Candida,* coccidioidin, mumps, tuberculin PPD, SK-SD, and trichophyton are used, but may occasionally occur in children). (3) The patient may have a skin condition that precludes the demonstration of a positive result (e.g., atopic dermatitis). (4) There may be a corresponding defect in the nonspecific inflammatory response (this differentiation may be made by using a stimulator of the nonspecific inflammatory response, such as sodium lauryl sulfate, which produces a positive result in over 90% of normal subjects; when there is a strong suspicion that the lack of reactivity may be due to local conditions or lack of inflammatory response, it may be necessary to perform *in vitro* tests to gain additional information on the status of the patient's cellular immune system). (5) A strong immediate reaction at the test antigen injection site may result in a false-negative delayed reaction; this should be suspected if there is a strong immediate reaction and no delayed reaction. Local or systemic administration of antihistamines may suppress the immediate reaction and allow visualization of the delayed reaction. When there is a question regarding previous antigenic exposure of a patient, or when the initial skin tests are negative, it is possible to gain further information by sensitizing the patient actively to an agent known to

induce delayed hypersensitivity, such as DNCB or keyhole-limpet hemocyanin, and subsequently testing for reactivity by applying a test dose of the
same antigen at a later time.

IN VITRO EVALUATION OF B CELLS

B-cell function in humans can be rapidly evaluated by quantitating the
serum levels of the three major immunoglobulin classes, IgM, IgG, and IgA
(Tables IX and X). The absolute levels must be correlated with the wide
variations seen in normal persons. IgG serum levels during the first 3 or 4
months of life depend on the amount and catabolic rate of maternally transferred immunoglobulin, with the nadir at approximately 3 months. The
values usually do not drop below 200 mg/dl. In patients older than 6
months, levels below 200 mg/dl, plus IgA and IgM levels less than 10 mg/dl,
are indicative of panhypogammaglobulinemia. When these values are accompanied by low levels of albumin or transferrin, excess loss should be
suspected and urinary or gastrointestinal sources should be evaluated. Isolated IgG subunit deficiency has been documented with normal total IgG
but appears to be rare. If conflicting or borderline quantities are obtained,
functional assessment of antibody production is needed. Titration of antibody specific for ubiquitous antigens or childhood immunizations, such as
ASLO, mumps, or rubella, gives information regarding responses to previous
antigenic challenge. Likewise, measurement of antibody titer after immunization with tetanus or pertussis provides dynamic information about current response capacity. However, live or attenuated virus should never be
used in a patient suspected of having an immune deficiency, due to the
occasionally disastrous consequences of disseminated viral infection.

During differentiation of B cells, μ, γ and α constant-region genes are
sequentially transcribed during clonal expansion, which in sequence appears to be in the order IgM to IgG to IgA. Recently, however, considerable
attention has been given to the appearance of IgD and IgM concurrently on
the surface of fetal and cord lymphocytes. This has suggested that expression of the IgD gene is an early event and that it may be critical in the
ontogeny of B lymphocytes. The method commonly employed has been
direct immunofluorescence with a fluorescein-conjugated heavy chain–
specific anti-immunoglobulin.

EVALUATION OF IMMUNOGLOBULIN STATUS

Immunoglobulin assessment in body fluids routinely involves three laboratory techniques: serum (zone) electrophoresis, immunoelectrophoresis,

Table IX
Properties of Immunoglobulins[a]

Immunoglobulin	IgG (γG)	IgA (γA)	IgM (γM)	IgD D (γD)	IgE (γE)
Serum concentration mg/100 ml (±1 SD)	1240 (±200)	390 (±90)	120 (±35)	3 (±3)	0.05
Total serum immunoglobulin (%)	70–80	10–15	5–10	0.2–1	0.002
Heavy chain designation	γ	α	μ	δ	ε
Number base units	1	1 or 2	5	1	1
Sedimentation coefficient	7 S	7 S (85%) serum 11 S secretions	19 S	7 S	8 S
Molecular weight	160,000	170,000–385,000	900,000	180,000	200,000
Biologic function	Principal serum antibody	Secretory antibodies	First antibody formed in response to antigen	Unknown	Anaphylactic reactions (reaginic antibody)
Primary distribution	Extracellular fluid	External secretion (tears, saliva, intestinal juices, colostrum)	Intravascular	Intravascular	Mast cells
Total circulating pool (mg/kg)	494	95	37	1.1	0.02
Biologic half-life (days)	23	5.8	5.1	2.8	2.3
Fractional catabolic rate (% of intravascular pool catabolized per day)	6.7	25	18	37	89
Synthetic rate (mg/kg/day)	33	24	6.7	0.4	0.02
Association with secretory component	0	+	±	0	0
Complement fixation	+	0	+	0	0

[a] Reproduced with permission from Halsted and Halsted (1981).

Table X

Levels of Serum Immunoglobulins IgG, IgM, IgA, and IgD of Normal Subjects at Different Ages[a,b,d]

Age	Number of subjects	IgG (mg/100 ml)	IgM (mg/100 ml)	IgA (mg/100 ml)	Number of subjects	IgD (mg/100 ml)
Newborn	22	1031 ± 200 (645–1244)[c]	11 ± 5 (5–30)	2 ± 3 (0–11)	90	0.12 ± 0.58 (0–3.6)
1–3 months	29	430 ± 119 (272–762)	30 ± 11 (16–67)	21 ± 13 (6–56)	26	0.22 ± 0.64 (0–2.9)
4–6 months	33	427 ± 186 (206–1155)	43 ± 17 (10–83)	28 ± 18 (8–93)		0.22 ± 0.64 (0–2.9)
7–12 months	56	661 ± 219 (279–1533)	54 ± 23 (22–147)	37 ± 18 (16–98)	22	0.56 ± 0.91 (0–3.0)
13–24 months	59	762 ± 209 (258–1393)	58 ± 23 (14–114)	50 ± 24 (19–119)	23	1.38 ± 1.39 (0–5.10)
25–36 months	33	892 ± 183 (419–1274)	61 ± 19 (28–113)	71 ± 37 (19–235)		
3–5 years	28	929 ± 228 (569–1597)	56 ± 18 (22–100)	93 ± 27 (55–152)	50	1.84 ± 2.31 (0–11.0)
6–8 years	18	923 ± 256	65 ± 25	124 ± 45	25	4.92 ± 3.80

Age	n	IgG (mg/dl)	IgM (mg/dl)	IgA (mg/dl)	n	IgD (mg/dl)
9–11 years	9	(559–1492) 1124 ± 235	(27–118) 79 ± 33	(54–221) 131 ± 60		(0–14.0) 4.87 ± 3.19
12–16 years	9	(779–1456) 946 ± 124	(35–132) 59 ± 20	(12–208) 148 ± 63	21	(0.72–12.5)
17–49 years	12	(726–1085) 950 ± 0.090	(35–72) 103 ± 0.239	(70–229) 79 ± 0.161	62	5.84 ± 3.16 (0–17)
50–59 years	60	890 ± 0.045	82 ± 0.107	81 ± 0.722		
60–69 years	46	880 ± 0.046	80 ± 0.122	78 ± 0.875		
> 70 years	25	940 ± 0.062	85 ± 0.166	97 ± 0.112		

[a]Reproduced with permission from Halsted and Halsted (1981).

[b]IgG, IgM, and IgA levels of newborns through 16 years are given as mean ± standard deviation from E. R. Stiehm and H. H. Fudenberg. Serum levels of immune globulins in health and disease: survey. *Pediatrics* **37**, 15 (1966). IgG, IgM, and IgA levels of adults given as mean ± standard error of the estimate are from C. E. Buckley, E. G. Buckley, and F. C. Dorsey. Longitudinal changes in serum immunoglobulin levels in older humans, *Fed. Proc., Fed. Am. Soc. Exp. Biol.* **33**, 2036 (1974). IgD levels given as means ± 1 standard deviation are from G. A. Leslie, R. H. Lopez Correa, and J. N. Holmes. Structural and biological functions of human IgD. IV. Ontogeny of human serum immunoglobulins D (IgD) as related to IgG, IgA, and IgM. *Int. Arch. Allergy Appl. Immunol* **45**; 350 (1973).

[c]Ranges are in parentheses.

[d]Serum levels of immunoglobulins IgG, IgM, IgA and IgD of normal subjects with age. From E. R. Stiehm and G. S. Rachelefsky. Control of antibody synthesis. In "Allergy: Principles and Practice" (E. Middleton, Jr., C. E. Reed, and E. F. Ellis, eds.). p. 000. Mosby, St. Louis, Missouri, 1978.

and quantitation of major immunoglobulin classes. Serum electrophoresis provides an overview of the five major electrophoretic groups of serum proteins (Fig. 2). Zone electrophoresis also provides ready qualitative assessment of serum or urine abnormalities. This is particularly valuable for the detection of myeloma proteins and Waldenstrom macroglobulins (and Bence Jones proteins) as discrete bands discernible in addition to the usual serum or urine protein peaks. Immunoelectrophoresis permits identification of the major classes of normal immunoglobulin and of myeloma proteins and other anomalous proteins, e.g., Bence Jones protein, heavy chain disease that cannot be done by zone electrophoresis. It is not, however, a good quantitative technique. Quantitation of specific immunoglobulins by radial diffusion or other methods allows precise definition of the amounts of each immunoglobulin class.

These three measurements are sufficient in most cases for the evaluation of immunoglobulins in body fluids. In some situations, however, such as heavy chain disease, additional physicochemical techniques such as exclusion (Sephadex) chromatography, ion-exchange chromatography, or special electrophoretic procedures may be needed. Furthermore, monoclonal antisera to immunoglobulin subclasses, e.g., IgG_1, IgG_2, IgG_3, IgG_4, or to Gm groups may be of assistance.

Results of analytic tests may differ between laboratories as a consequence of variations in technique and in the antisera employed as reagents. Reference samples of human serum with agreed-on immunoglobulin content (provided by the World Health Organization) help to standardize data. Reference kits containing known myeloma protein, Waldenstrom macroglobulins, Bence Jones proteins, and hypogammaglobulinemia sera permit laboratories to check their controls regularly.

Clinical laboratories now include total serum protein (TSP) determinations and serum electrophoresis (SE) as screening procedures for patient sera. Whenever the gamma globulin region is increased or decreased on the SE scan, further examination by immunoelectrophoretic analysis (IEP) and/or quantitation of immunoglobulins G, A, and M (IgG, IgA, and IgM) is indicated. Excluded from routine testing are IgD, which has unknown clinical significance, and IgE, which requires different methodology. Quantitation of the first three serum immunoglobulins should be performed in all patients with suspected immunoglobulin abnormalities.

Radial immunodiffusion (RID) with limited or timed diffusion is the most widely used of several methods available for quantitation of the serum immunoglobulins (and other serum proteins) and is the accepted method for standardization of reference sera. Despite the greater incubation time and antibody requirement, limited diffusion is probably the better choice to

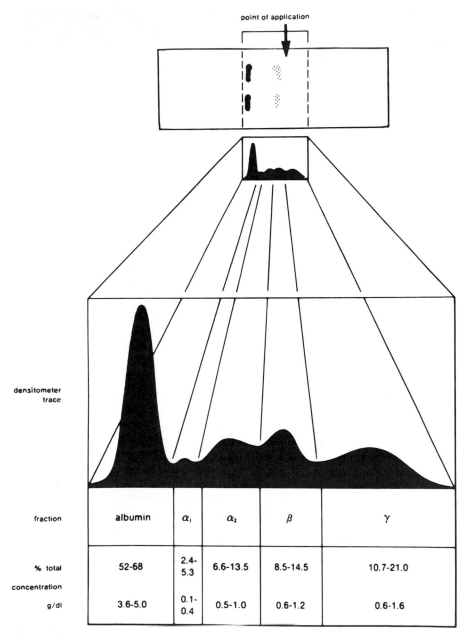

Fig. 2. Serum protein electrophoresis. Reproduced with permission from Halsted and Halsted (1981).

obviate variables (time, temperature, etc.) affecting timed diffusion and to obtain the highest accuracy. RID was the earliest of the modern methods and is simple, not requiring sophisticated laboratory equipment. It is often employed in field studies of malnourished individuals. However, in a survey to assess its accuracy as performed in a number of laboratories, the results varied widely, although many of the discrepancies could be attributed to differences in the reference sera employed. The clinical interpretation of quantitative immunoglobulin levels should not be undertaken unless the total serum protein value and either SE or IEP patterns are also available. Quantitation alone, for example, may not reveal the early stages of myeloma in a patient, whereas properly applied IEP will.

EVALUATION OF PHAGOCYTOSIS

Phagocytes can be tested in four broad categories of cell function: activation, directed locomotion, respiratory burst capabilities, and microbicidal activity. Due to the limited quantity of cells available (especially monocytes) from subjects, the tests discussed are not meant to be comprehensive but rather to reflect functional categories that are felt to be important in the phagocytes' role in host defense.

First, monocytes can be readily identified as esterase-positive cells, and their polarization can be quantified in a purified mononuclear cell fraction by a cytoprep technique employing a nonspecific esterase stain. *Polarization* refers to the change in shape that follows the exposure of monocytes and neutrophils to a chemoattractant, and is felt to represent an early activation response as well as being a necessary but not sufficient prerequisite for directed locomotion. Morphologically, unstimulated cells, which are generally round in suspension, assume a more triangular shape with a broadened, ruffled pseudopod in front and a narrowed uropod in back.

Neutrophils can be evaluated for nitroblue tetrazolium (NBT) reduction (spontaneous and stimulated), chemotactic response, superoxide production, and bactericidal capacity.

The NBT test is a relatively nonspecific measure of the cells' respiratory burst activity, since the tetrazolium dye can be reduced by any number of reactive oxygen species that are produced upon PMN stimulation. Its usefulness and uniqueness from a more specific assay (e.g., superoxide production) lie in its ability to identify and enumerate in a semiquantitative way the metabolic responsiveness of individual cells. PMN functional heterogeneity is being appreciated by many investigators using many different assay systems, and its role in relation to PMN host defense capabilities is an area of active investigation.

PMN chemotaxis involves multiple functional activities that are normally coordinated in order to allow appropriate directed locomotion. Thus, it measures the composite abilities of chemotactic receptor function, receptor-mediated shape changes (polarization), and reversible changes in adherence, as well as continued gradient sensing and locomotor activity.

The chemotaxis assay is very sensitive to any abnormalities in the described component functions. For the same reason, it is nonspecific in that a demonstrated defect in chemotactic ability may be the consequence of abnormalities in any and/or all of the above functions.

The specific evaluation of superoxide production using two soluble stimuli yields information on both the quantity and rate of O_2 production. From the literature, it seems clear that there is more than one mechanism for activation and/or expression of the respiratory burst. The use of two different classes of stimuli, N-formylmethionyl-leucylphenylalanine (FMLP), which results in a discrete quantum of O_2 production, and phorbol myristate acetate (PMA), which results in a more prolonged and continuous production of O_2, will yield increased information on the qualitative as well as quantitative nature of any abnormalities seen in this aspect of oxygen metabolism by stimulated PMN.

The killing assay is sensitive to abnormalities in phagocytic capability, respiratory burst, and/or secretory function, with a normal killing curve indicating the functional integrity and coordination of these various systems. Again, the nature of the endpoint (i.e., bacterial killing) makes the assay relatively nonspecific in that a measured abnormality in killing does not indicate where the defect may actually arise.

COMPLEMENT

The complement system comprises a group of interacting serum proteins, many of which are enzymes, which together function as initiators, regulators, and effectors of cell lysis and inflammation. The major serum antibody components, IgM and IgG, utilize complement activation via the classic pathway, with resulting induction of the inflammatory response for elimination of antigens. It has become increasingly apparent that the system may also become significantly activated by another or "alternate" pathway, initiated by such factors as IgA, endotoxin, and certain drugs. As in the clotting system, the two pathways intersect at a common reaction point sharing the final reaction sequence.

At least 11 complement proteins are involved in mediating antibody-initiated hemolysis. These make up the classic complement pathway and are termed *complement* (abbreviated *C*) *components* or *subcomponents*. They are designated with numerals in order of their activation sequence, with two exceptions: (1) after its discovery, C1 was found to be a macromolecule consisting of three proteins linked by calcium, and these are designated *C1q, C1r,* and *C1s,* respectively; (2) the fourth component discovered was found to be the second to react in the hemolytic sequence, but its original designation as *C4* was retained. The classic C pathway has been divided into recognition (C1q, C1r, C1s), activation (C4, C2, C3), and attack (C5, C6, C7, C8, C9) portions with respect to their function in cytolysis.

The alternate or properdin pathway consists of at least four additional proteins, which have been termed *initiation factor* (*IF*), *factor D, factor B,* and *properdin,* along with C3 and C3b. Other pathways to activation of the terminal C components have been shown, but their physiologic importance is unknown.

Several proteins that act as inhibitors of C components have been identified. The most important clinically is the C1-esterase inhibitor (C1-INH), which, as one of its many functions, inhibits the ability of C1s to act on C4 and C2. Inborn deficiency of this inhibitor is responsible for hereditary angioneurotic edema (HAE). An inactivator of C3b, termed *C3b-INA,* has been defined, and its deficiency has been associated with hypercatabolism and, therefore, depletion of C3. Other inhibitors and inactivators have been reported but have not yet been associated with clinical symptomatology.

All the proteins of the primary C pathway are required to obtain hemolysis in assays for hemolytic C activity. However, multiple functions that do not require the activation of the complete C component result from activation of individual or groups of C components. These include agglutination, adherence, opsonization, and generation of anaphylatoxins (which initiate the release of histamine from mast cells). These may involve single proteins (C1q), cleavage products (C4b, C3b, C5b), activation peptides (C3a, C5a), or multimolecular assembly units (C567). Since hemolysis of sensitized erythrocytes requires all the classic pathway factors, is convenient, quantitative, and has been the most widely used, it remains the functional C assay of choice. Functional assays selective for the properdin pathway have not become generally useful.

In recent years, immunochemical assays for specific C and properdin proteins have received wider use. This is because of their simplicity, accuracy, less rigid requirement of serum volume, collection, and storage, and adaptability to laboratory routines that involve similar immunochemical assays. Of these, RID assays for C3, C4, and perhaps C1q in the classic pathway, and for factor B and properdin in the alternate pathway, have been of the greatest clinical value. Technology directed to the identification and quantification of cleaved components has also been developed but remains more useful in the specialty laboratory.

3

Nutritional Assessment

INTRODUCTION

It has long been recognized that an inappropriate diet, including the intake of either too much or too little food, is a major factor in predisposition to disease. This has best been shown using dietary manipulation of experimental animals.

Gathering information to prove this point, as well as to monitor the nutritional status of humans, is considerably more difficult. There are, for example, major differences in specific populations (e.g., young versus old, hospitalized patients and pregnant women). Nutritional status is related to metabolism, and thus some specific laboratory indices are available. In addition, the use of anthropometrics in nutritional assessment, as well as specific quantitation, is essential to an adequate evaluation.

A detailed physical examination is the first step in evaluating nutritional status. The traditional methodology of clinical science can be applied, including the determination of vital signs, temperature, pulse, blood pressure, height, and weight (Table I). Tables and statistics are valuable in correlating these data with age and sex. Virtually anyone, even with almost no medical training, can be taught to do a general physical examination, at least one based on the evaluation of chronic rather than acute changes.

The use of anthropometry in nutritional evaluation was first applied in the diagnosis and evaluation of protein-energy malnutrition (PEM). It has many disadvantages, including observer subjectivity, difficulty in adequate quantitation, and the fact that it is a relatively gross measurement. In virtually all such studies, the height, weight, mid-arm circumference, and triceps muscle skinfold are measured. In some studies, both head and chest circumference are also included. These measurements provide some assessment of muscle mass and fat reserves. In addition, by doing correlations between these

Table I

Anthropometric Evaluation

Weight
Height
Mid-arm circumference
Skinfold thickness
Head circumference

various measurements, it is possible to estimate the acuteness and chronicity as well as possibly the severity of malnutrition.

Laboratory evaluations are dependent, to a large extent, on the facilities available. Although, ideally, one would like to quantify all of the major groups of nutrients, this is generally impossible. Nonetheless, there are some standard measurements, as well as some specific nutrient deficiencies, that should be considered (Table II). First, a general measurement of nutritional status should include a complete blood count, with hemoglobin and hematocrit determinations as well as red cell counts and red cell indices. The last measure provides information on the iron, vitamin B_{12}, and folic acid status. Concurrently, and where indicated, measurements of serum iron and total iron-binding capacity provide important supplemental information. Other laboratory tests include the measurement of serum or plasma zinc, vitamins A, C, D, B_6, and B_{12}, thiamin, riboflavin, and folic acid. All of these are readily determined either by atomic absorption spectrophotometry, by radioimmunoassays, or by specific assays.

Measurements of food intake, including specific estimates of individual dietary components, are receiving considerable attention because of their value in the field. One technique, known as *replicate plate analysis,* is often used. While dietary records can be used for the determination of macronutrient and energy intake, the calculation of intake based on dietary records and published nutrient composition tables can lead to erroneous results due to regional differences in the trace mineral content of foods. To overcome this problem, replicate plate analysis is used. This method, also known as the *duplicate portion technique,* requires that a copy of what is served and eaten be used for chemical analysis.

APPLICATION OF TECHNIQUES

One of the most important factors in using this information concerning the effects of host nutrition on immunocompetence in a clinical setting is

Table II

Clinical Assessment of Nutritional Status[a]

Organ	Sign[b]	Deficiency to be considered
General appearance	Emaciated, edematous	PEM, (marasmus, kwashiorkor)
	Obese	Obesity
Skin (face and neck)	Nasolabial dyssebacia	Riboflavin, niacin
Mucous membranes	Pale	Anemia
Skin (general)	Petechiae, purpura	Vitamin C
	Scrotal and vulval dermatitis	Riboflavin
	Symmetrical dermatitis, exposed skin, thickened pressure points	Niacin
	Follicular hyperkeratosis	Vitamin A
	"Crazy-pavement" dermatitis	Vitamin A, protein
	Dependent edema	Protein, thiamin
Subcutaneous tissue	Decreased	PEM
	Increased	Obesity
Hair	Altered color, texture, easily plucked	Protein-calorie malnutrition
Eyes	Xerophthalmia, keratomalcia	Vitamin A
	Bitot spots	Vitamin A
	Circumcorneal injection	Riboflavin
	Conjunctival pallor	Anemia
Lips	Bilateral angular lesions, scars, cheilosis	Niacin, riboflavin
Gums and teeth	Acute periodontal gingivitis, dental caries	Vitamin C
Tongue	Smooth, pale atropic	Anemia, riboflavin
	Red, painful, denuded, edema	Niacin
Glands	Goiter	Iodine
	Parotid enlargement	? Protein
Skeletal	Costochondral beading	Vitamins C and D
	Cranial bossing, craniotabes	Vitamin D
	Epiphysial enlargement (especially the wrists)	Vitamin D
Neurological	Loss of vibratory sense, deep tendon reflexes; calf tenderness	Thiamin
Extremities	Painful on movement	Vitamin C
	Frog-leg position	

[a]Reproduced with permission from McLaren and Burman (1976).

[b]The clinical signs, interpreted in the light of dietary intake and subsequent biochemical change, are useful in assessment of an individual patient.

the ability to assess the patient's nutritional status. Without accurate data on a wide variety of nutritional parameters, it would be difficult to ascertain the relevance of the experimental information and impossible to apply any of it in a clinical context. Fortunately, considerable effort has been expended in the past 3 decades to develop meaningful measurements of such nutritional parameters. Early studies focused on obtaining data regarding the nutritional status of entire communities in Third World nations (Jelliffe, 1966). Malnutrition in such settings was overt, was frequently the cause of or a major contributor to the exceptionally high infant mortality rates, and was widespread in many sectors of these communities. More recent studies have attempted to develop means to assess less severe forms of malnutrition that may accompany a variety of pathological, often subclinical, processes. Surveys of hospitalized patients in Western nations have shown that well over half of them may be suffering from significant malnutrition (Bistrian *et al.,* 1976). In addition, large surveys in the United States have indicated that a broad segment of the population may be suffering from one or more nutrient deficiencies. While many of the earlier studies and methodologies emphasized the nutritional status of children, more recent ones have focused on procedures for adults.

The nutritional status of any patient, whether an elderly adult in an institution or a protein-energy malnourished infant in a Third World country, is assessed by obtaining information in the following general areas: (1) medical history (e.g., chief complaint, past medical history, treatment regimens), (2) dietary assessment, (3) clinical examination, (4) anthropometric measurements, (5) biochemical measurements, and finally, (6) hematological and immunological measurements (Tables II, III). It is very important to realize that such nutritional assessment is not based on any single measurement, but rather on the integrated and corroborative picture of all of the measurements obtained (Table IV). For instance, data obtained from biochemical measurements should confirm those abnormalities observed on clinical examination or should corroborate any dietary deficiencies that were suspected on the basis of dietary surveys. Of course, the accuracy and clinical significance will vary with the parameter considered, since some are more reliable, more easily obtained, and more clinically relevant than others. We will focus on the methodology that has been developed for the nutritional assessment of children. We will also consider some of the more recent developments that apply particularly to adults living in institutions.

A large body of information obtained while eliciting the medical history may be useful in establishing the patient's nutritional status. While the chief complaint and the past medical history may provide obvious clues to possi-

Table III

Useful Tests for Biochemical Nutritional Assessment

Nutrient	Approximate value (ml)	Normal values	Comments
Albumin	0.1	$\geq$3.0 g/100 ml	Simple radial immunodiffusion
Transferrin	0.1	>100 ml/100ml	
Prealbumin	0.1	$\geq$20 mg/100 ml	
Iron	1–2	$\geq$40 mg/100 ml	
Transferrin saturation	1–2	$\geq$16%	All serum
Ferritin	1–2	$\geq$10 ng/ml	
Vitamin A	1	$\geq$20 μg/100 ml	Serum or plasma
Carotene	1	$\geq$100 mg/100 ml	Serum or plasma
Vitamin D (alkaline phosphatase	1	<40 King-Armstrong units <15 Bodansky units	
Vitamin E	3	$\geq$0.7 mg/100 ml	Serum
Vitamin K (prothrombin time)	5	11–18 sec	Prothrombin time
Folic acid-serum	0.5	$\geq$3 ng/ml	
RBC	0.5	$\geq$140 ng/ml	Whole blood serum
Thiamin	0.1	<15%	Erythrocytes used
Riboflavin	0.1	<1.2	Erythrocytes used
Pyridoxine	0.1	<1.25	Erythrocytes used
Vitamin B_{12}	1	$\geq$150 pg/ml	Serum
Vitamin C	0.4	>.02 mg/100 mg	Whole blood
Zinc	7	>10 μg/100 ml	Serum

[a]Reproduced with permission from Neumann et al. (1982).

ble nutritional deficiencies, the clues may be far more subtle. Indeed, specific questions regarding parameters not normally scrutinized may be necessary to establish a hypothesized nutritional deficiency. Many of these questions may be asked when the sociocultural history is taken, for instance, those regarding food choices, allergies, intolerances, eating behavior, feeding skills, and the developmental level in children. In addition, specific disorders such as cancer frequently result in nutritional problems and raise many questions relevant to the nutritional status of the child or adult, e.g., those regarding the site of the lesion and treatment regimens such as chemotherapy (see below), radiation, or surgery (Fig. 1). In addition, infections

Table IV

Common Errors of Measurement[a]

All measurements	Inadequate instrument
	Restless, anxious child
	Reading part of instrument not fixed when value taken
	Reading and recording errors
Length	Incorrect age for instrument
	Footwear or headwear not removed
	Head not in correct plane
	Head not firmly against fixed end of board
	Child not straight along board
	Body arched
	Knees bent
	Feet not vertical to movable board
	Board not firmly against heels
Height	Incorrect age for instrument
	Footwear or headwear not removed
	Feet not straight nor flat on vertical platform or wall
	Knees bent
	Body arched or buttocks forward (body not straight)
	Shoulders not straight on board
	Head not in correct plane
	Headboard not firmly on crown of child's head
Weight	Room cold, no privacy
	Scale not calibrated to zero
	Child wearing unreasonable amount of clothing
	Child moving or anxious
Head circumference	Occipital protuberance; supraorbital landmarks poorly defined
	Hair crushed inadequately, ears under tape
	Tape tension and position poorly maintained by time of reading
Triceps fatfold	Wrong arm (should be left arm)
	Midarm point or posterior plane incorrectly measured or marked
	Arm not loose by side during measurement
	Examiner not comfortable or level with child
	Finger-thumb pinch or caliper placement too deep (muscle) or too superficial (skin)
	Caliper jaws not at marked site
	Reading done too early or too late (should be 3 sec)
	At time of reading, pinch not maintained, caliper handle not fully released
Arm circumference	Tape too thick, stretched, or creased
	Wrong arm (should be left arm)
	Mid-arm point incorrectly measured or marked
	Arm not loosely hanging by side during measurement
	Examiner not comfortable or level with child
	Tape around arm, not at midpoint; too tight (causing skin contour indentation), too loose (inadequately opposed)

[a]Reproduced with permission from Neumann *et al.* (1982).

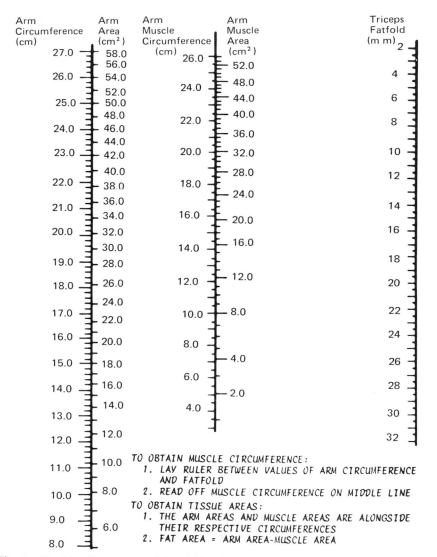

Arm Circumference (cm)	Arm Area (cm²)	Arm Muscle Circumference (cm)	Arm Muscle Area (cm²)	Triceps Fatfold (m m)

TO OBTAIN MUSCLE CIRCUMFERENCE:
1. LAY RULER BETWEEN VALUES OF ARM CIRCUMFERENCE AND FATFOLD
2. READ OFF MUSCLE CIRCUMFERENCE ON MIDDLE LINE
TO OBTAIN TISSUE AREAS:
1. THE ARM AREAS AND MUSCLE AREAS ARE ALONGSIDE THEIR RESPECTIVE CIRCUMFERENCES
2. FAT AREA = ARM AREA-MUSCLE AREA

Fig. 1. Nutritional assessment of the child with cancer. Reproduced with permission from Neumann *et al.* (1982).

may further complicate the picture, and the resultant sequelae (e.g., diarrhea, sepsis) may markedly alter the nutritional parameters (e.g., serum protein and serum iron levels).

The second major category of information involves calculating the nutritional intake of the patient after determining the foods that comprise the diet. The most widely utilized methodology is the 24-hr recall (in which the patient is asked to recall all of the foods consumed within the past 24 hr), which must be repeated on several occasions. When done on 3–4 successive days, this method has been found to be surprisingly accurate. Indeed, there was little improvement when such recall procedures were expanded to 3 days (72 hr). Such information must be obtained utilizing common household measures; many nutrient composition tables have been compiled with such measures in mind. Other methods involve keeping a dietary inventory for a week or describing how frequently an extensive list of foods is consumed. A variety of tables is available for calculating the nutrient value of such diets. The point of this assessment is to reveal diets that are grossly imbalanced in terms of any of the nutrients. In Third World countries, this may be the result of excessive consumption of one or two staple crops. In the more developed nations, it may also be the result of limited diets, fad diets, or eccentric diets. Such dietary inventories provide important clues on what to look for in the physical examination. Correlations between the findings of dietary assessment and the clinical examination (particularly if confirmed by biochemical findings) provide strong evidence of nutritional deficiency.

The clinical examination itself will most likely be performed as part of the physical examination. Those portions of the body that most readily give evidence of nutritional deficiency are the skin, eyes, mouth, teeth, tongue, mucous membranes, hair, skeleton, and nervous system (Neumann *et al.,* 1982). The most useful indicators are listed in Table II. It should be re-emphasized that such clinical signs are only clues and cannot be used diagnostically; they must always be confirmed with dietary data, biochemical measurements, and, in some cases, therapeutic trials (Table III). Subjectivity is one of the major drawbacks of such clinical findings. It has been noted that agreement among even expert practitioners seldom approaches 50% in the detection of a given clinical sign of nutritional deficiency (Brook, 1971). It is also important to realize that clinical signs of nutritional deficiency are generally pathognomonic for more than a single nutrient. It should be noted that many of these symptoms may also be due to non-nutritional causes. For instance, while edema may be due to a low-protein diet and resultant hypoproteinemia, it may also be due to obstruction of the lymphatic system, nephrosis, or heart failure. Finally, it should be pointed out that clinical signs are useful in identifying only advanced cases of nutritional deficiency; they are seldom useful in early or mild cases.

Growth monitors have proven to be the most useful tool in assessing the nutritional status of children. The critical sign to monitor is a decrease in the slope of the growth curve, which in severe cases may be flattened. It is frequently difficult to obtain accurate data on children, particularly in Third

World countries. However, well-trained ancillary health care personnel can make such measurements. The most useful measurements are weight, length or height, arm circumference, head circumference, and sub-cutaneous tissue fatfold measurements (Tables I, V, VI, Fig. 1, 2). In addition, a number of parameters can be extrapolated from these initial measurements, including the circumference of the upper arm muscle and fat, as well as the percentage of body weight composed of fat and muscle mass. Various combinations of these measurements (e.g., weight for height, weight for age, height for age) can be used to judge whether the malnutrition is acute or chronic. The most important drawbacks are a lack of accuracy in the individual measurements, the need to find the appropriate reference data, and the clinical relevance of any data obtained (Table IV) (Figs. 3–7).

Measurements of the patient's weight are particularly helpful in determining acute nutritional disturbances. It should be recalled at all times, however, that nonnutritional factors such as abdominal ascites or excessive intestinal contents (e.g., heavy parasitism) can obscure such changes in body weight and therefore may overshadow changes in nutritional status. Length or height (length measured in children under 2 years of age, height measured after that age) are better indicators of long-term nutritional status; however, these parameters are not sensitive to any short-term alterations in nutritional status. It has been noted that these measurements, more than any others, must be obtained with great care (Neumann et al., 1982). A variety of reference standards are available, largely dependent upon the age group observed (Jelliffe and Jelliffe, 1982; Waterlow, 1976). In general, children are categorized according to their standing relative to those children having values near the 50th percentile (Fig. 8). For instance, the Wellcome Trust Working Group has set up four basic categories: (1) normal, (2) wasting, but no permanent stunting (acute malnutrition), (3) wasting with stunting (concomitant acute/chronic malnutrition), and (4) stunting with no apparent wasting (children recovered from previous episodes of malnutrition as well as nutritional dwarfs). Head circumference has also been frequently measured in nutritional surveys. It is considered to correlate closely with the number of brain cells and to be an indicator of brain growth (Winick and Rosso, 1969). Reference data also exist for these measurements.

The measurement of mid-upper arm circumference (MUAC) has recently gained increasing acceptance as an objective means of measuring nutritional status, particularly the degree of protein-energy malnutrition (PEM) present in a given child (Jelliffe and Jelliffe, 1979). A high correlation between MUAC and body weight has also been noted. In combination with the triceps fatfold measurement (see below), it is possible to quantify the compartments attributed to muscle and fat. A further advantage is that there is very little change in MUAC between the ages of 1 and 4 years (Jelliffe and

Table V

Arm Muscle Area: Reference Data[a]

Arm muscle area percentiles (cm)

Age	Male					Female				
	5th	15th	50th	85th	95th	5th	15th	50th	85th	95th
0–5 months	52.2	70.3	89.2	124.4	141.4	59.1	67.0	86.6	105.8	127.2
6–17 months	79.1	92.8	120.1	150.0	169.0	75.6	82.1	108.4	130.4	146.0
1.5–2.5 years	97.8	108.2	128.4	152.5	168.6	88.5	99.1	124.1	155.1	169.3
2.5–3.5 years	102.7	116.3	138.4	167.0	184.2	92.8	106.8	129.8	151.6	162.8
3.5–4.5 years	110.6	122.4	145.1	180.5	197.3	104.0	114.3	139.0	169.3	182.8
4.5–5.5 years	117.1	134.2	157.9	193.0	219.3	111.9	122.7	151.6	182.5	204.5
5.5–6.5 years	127.5	143.5	170.0	201.9	222.0	116.3	133.3	156.3	190.2	217.4
6.5–7.5 years	134.2	148.5	181.5	215.2	238.6	121.3	138.4	170.0	209.6	243.3
7.5–8.5 years	150.6	164.7	198.7	239.8	272.9	132.2	151.3	181.8	223.9	275.8
8.5–9.5 years	152.2	163.7	207.4	264.5	318.8	147.3	162.5	195.5	247.7	297.8
9.5–10.5 years	160.8	183.2	223.9	275.3	323.9	152.8	172.7	211.5	263.7	306.6
10.5–11.5 years	180.1	198.7	240.6	300.0	354.4	155.1	184.2	233.5	301.8	348.6
11.5–12.5 years	187.4	212.6	260.3	340.1	390.2	178.1	205.2	255.8	318.3	358.2
12.5–13.5 years	201.2	227.3	301.3	399.8	466.1	190.5	217.8	271.1	338.2	401.4
13.5–14.5 years	223.1	264.5	354.4	435.8	560.1	218.6	243.0	295.2	388.3	435.8
14.5–15.5 years	237.5	272.9	386.7	506.0	582.6	212.6	238.7	303.1	383.8	427.9
15.5–16.5 years	274.1	333.1	418.4	536.3	626.6	231.6	251.0	319.8	409.6	538.6
16.5–17.5 years	337.3	374.3	477.1	582.6	671.3	231.6	250.2	305.8	396.8	461.2

[a]Reproduced with permission from Frisancho (1974).

Table VI

Arm Muscle Circumference: Reference Data[a]

Arm muscle area percentiles (cm)

Age	Male					Female				
	5th	15th	50th	85th	95th	5th	15th	50th	85th	95th
0–5 months	8.1	9.4	10.6	12.5	13.3	8.6	9.2	10.4	11.5	12.6
6–17 months	10.0	10.8	12.3	13.7	14.6	9.7	10.2	11.7	12.8	13.5
1.5–2.5 years	11.1	11.7	12.7	13.8	14.6	10.5	11.2	12.5	14.0	14.6
2.5–3.5 years	11.4	12.1	13.2	14.5	15.2	10.8	11.6	12.8	13.8	14.3
3.5–4.5 years	11.8	12.4	13.5	15.1	15.7	11.4	12.0	13.2	14.6	15.2
4.5–5.5 years	12.1	13.0	14.1	15.6	16.6	11.9	12.4	13.8	15.1	16.0
5.5–6.5 years	12.7	13.4	14.6	15.9	16.7	12.1	12.9	14.0	15.5	16.5
6.5–7.5 years	13.0	13.7	15.1	16.4	17.3	12.3	13.2	14.6	16.2	17.5
7.5–8.5 years	13.8	14.4	15.8	17.4	18.5	12.9	13.8	15.1	16.8	18.6
8.5–9.5 years	13.8	14.3	16.1	18.2	20.0	13.6	14.3	15.7	17.6	19.3
9.5–10.5 years	14.2	15.2	16.8	18.6	20.2	13.9	14.7	16.3	18.2	19.6
10.5–11.5 years	15.0	15.8	17.4	19.4	21.1	14.0	15.2	17.1	19.5	20.9
11.5–12.5 years	15.3	16.3	18.1	20.7	22.1	15.0	16.1	17.9	20.0	21.2
12.5–13.5 years	15.9	16.9	19.5	22.4	24.2	15.5	16.5	18.5	20.6	22.5
13.5–14.5 years	16.7	18.2	21.1	23.4	26.5	16.6	17.5	19.3	22.1	23.4
14.5–15.5 years	17.3	18.5	22.0	25.2	27.1	16.3	17.3	19.5	22.0	23.2
15.5–16.5 years	18.6	20.5	22.9	26.0	28.1	17.1	17.8	20.0	22.7	26.0
16.5–17.5 years	20.6	21.7	24.5	27.1	29.0	17.1	17.7	19.6	22.3	24.1

[a]Reproduced with permission from Frisancho (1974).

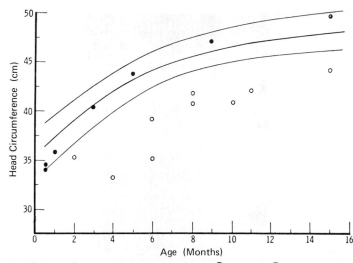

Fig. 2. Head circumference versus postnatal age. ●, normal; ○, marasmus; lines indicate United States normal values. Reproduced with permission from Winick and Rosso (1969).

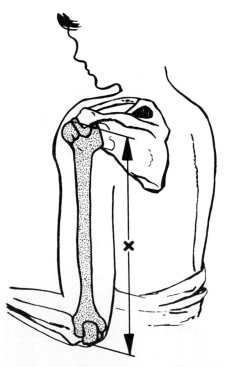

Fig. 3. Landmarks for the midpoint of the upper arm. Reproduced with permission from Neumann *et al.* (1982).

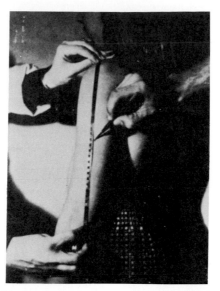

Fig. 4. Locating the midpoint of the upper arm. Reproduced with permission from Fomon (1978).

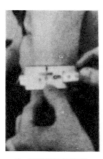 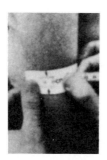 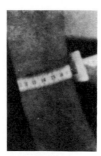 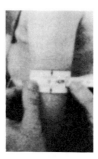

1. THREADING
THE TAPE

2. STABILIZING
AT SLOT

3. INSPECTION
AROUND ARM

4. READY FOR
READING

5. RECORDING THE RESULT

STEPS IN MEASURING THE MID-UPPER ARM CIRCUMFERENCE USING THE INSERTION TAPE

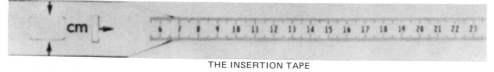

THE INSERTION TAPE

Fig. 5. Use of Zerfas insertion tape to obtain arm circumference. Reproduced with permission from Zerfas (1975).

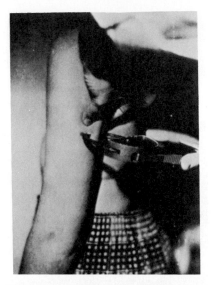

Fig. 6. Measuring the triceps fatfold with a Lange caliper. Reproduced with permission from Fomon (1978).

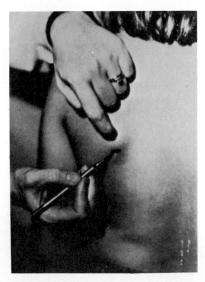

Fig. 7. Location for subscapular fatfold-measuring site. Reproduced with permission from Fomon (1978).

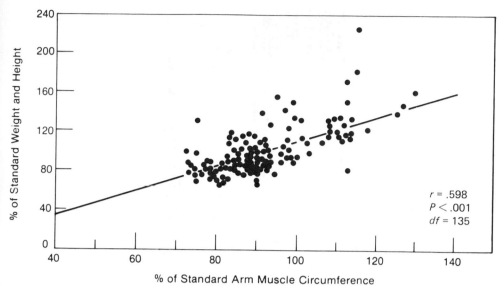

Fig. 8. Relation of weight/height to arm muscle circumference in a composite medical survey. Reproduced with permission from Bistrian *et al.* (1976).

Jelliffe, 1979). It should once again be pointed out that adequately trained personnel are most important in obtaining accurate data. In the case of MUAC, it may prove particularly difficult to get good data on young infants. However, in older children, when such measurements are accurate, they provide a particularly helpful means of differentiating lack of weight gain due to nutritional causes from that due to nonnutritional causes (e.g., severe constipation, ascites).

The final widely employed objective anthropometric measurement is fatfold measurement. It is highly useful in both children and adults, and is only minimally invasive in patients who are quite ill. Indeed, it is the only convenient clinical method that allows objective, direct assessment of body fat content (it can be useful as an estimate of "energy reserve") (Neumann, 1979). Indeed, such measurements, utilizing accurate calipers (plastic calipers produced by drug companies are *not* recommended due to inadequate springs and resultant inconsistent pressure), correlate closely with both electrical conductivity and ultrasound investigations (Neumann, 1979). While the triceps fatfold is the easiest to measure and is the most frequent measurement obtained, it is recognized that fatfolds taken at multiple sites provide a more accurate estimate of total body fat (Fig. 9). Such measurements are particularly useful in children, in whom nearly all body fat is found subcutaneously, whereas in adults significant amounts of fat

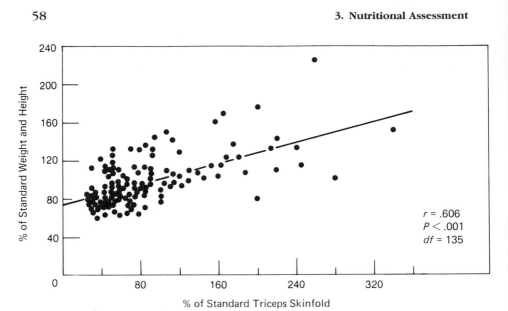

Fig. 9.   Relation of weight/height to triceps skinfold in a composite medical survey.   Reproduced with permission from Bistrian *et al.* (1976).

surround the organs and viscera. Subscapular fatfolds are also frequently measured. It should be noted that significant sexual differences exist in these measurements, particularly after puberty. There are also racial differences as well, with black children exhibiting notably smaller fatfolds than white children.

It should be pointed out that all of these measurements are subject to substantial error. Further, they should ideally be correlated with biochemical markers. The Center for Disease Control (1975) monitored such measurements in a variety of settings and found that a substantial proportion were seriously errant due to poor techniques and instruments. It has been suggested that revision and refinement of these techniques is of utmost importance.

Perhaps the most reliable means of assessing nutritional status involves monitoring biochemical parameters. Such measurements are particularly useful in establishing deficiencies of a less overt nature, enabling clinicians to intervene early in the course of a nutritional deficency. Such biochemical measurements should only be obtained for a limited number of nutrients, because a complete panel of measurements would prove costly and time consuming and would generally involve the drawing of large amounts of blood from patients who are in a precarious state of health. Emphasis should be placed on those nutrients that appear to be deficient on clinical examination and dietary assessment of those nutrients likely to be deficient given the patients' condition and/or treatment regimen. It is most important to comply meticulously with the most appropriate protocol (volumes of serum needed for the test, type of container necessary to avoid contamination, etc.) in order to minimize the need to draw large volumes of blood. Moreover, the results of such biochemical testing will also depend on the presence of superimposed infectious disease, timing of the last meal, circadium rhythms, and the administration of any pharmacological agents. A listing of the most commonly employed tests, the most useful means of obtaining the data, and the normal values is shown in Table III.

Standard procedure is to classify the range of values obtained into four general categories: (1) normal, (2) borderline or marginal, (3) low, and (4) deficient. As a general rule, such values are considered abnormal when they fall outside of the 95% confidence limits. A full discussion of the measurement of each nutritional parameter would require an entire chapter itself. Such information has been reviewed by others (Jelliffe, 1966; Sauberlich *et al.,* 1973; Neumann *et al.,* 1982).

Hematological and immunological status are also used in the establishment of a diagnosis of nutritional abnormalities. A number of specific nutritional deficiencies result in precisely characterized syndromes of anemia. The most common causes of nutritional anemia are a lack of iron and folic acid; lack of vitamin B_{12} is also seen on occasion. PEM is also associated with an anemia which has been attributed to an insufficient level of hemoglobin production. Measurements generally obtained include hematocrit, hemoglobin, and total peripheral red cell number. From these values further indices can be extrapolated (e.g., mean corpuscular hemoglobin, mean corpuscular hemoglobin concentration, etc.). In addition, the presence of either hyperchromicity or hypochromicity and cell size is valuable in establishing a diagnosis. The parameters to watch are shown in Table IV. It must be emphasized that a large number of nonnutritional factors may also result in such anemias. In addition to hematological parameters, immunological parameters are also being used at present to diagnosis malnutrition; this is the general subject of this volume.

4

Malnutrition and Infectious Disease: Studies from the Field

INTRODUCTION

In developing overall concepts regarding the impact of nutritional factors on host susceptibility to infectious disease, field studies have provided a wealth of important information. However, they have also led to premature conclusions. It is certain that continued deprivation of adequate nutrition throughout life, as observed in many parts of the world, comprises a large *in vivo* experiment. Sufficient evidence has been accumulated to indicate that malnourished individuals are far more susceptible than well-nourished ones to a wide variety of infectious maladies. Such heightened susceptibility to disease has often been correlated with defective immune function, as measured in a variety of ways. However, when one attempts to gain an overall perspective, perhaps one of the most striking features of the data is the variability and the frequency of contradiction. There are, in actuality, good reasons why the evidence is not consistent and is not easily interpreted. These reasons are best exemplified in considering research on protein-energy malnutrition (PEM). While PEM is frequently regarded as a single syndrome, it is not. It has proven quite difficult to assess the nutritional status of human populations quantitatively with regard to PEM. The methods currently employed under field conditions have not proven to be very reliable; the more reliable biochemical and anthropometric assessments frequently require equipment too cumbersome and analytical methodologies too technically complicated for most field conditions. Recent evidence seems to indicate that nutritional assessment based on multiple anthropometric and biochemical parameters is the best alternative at present. The search continues for reliable indicators of nutritional status; quantitative assessment of immune dysfunction remains a promising technique.

Much of the variation in the results of field studies may be the direct result of variability in the degree of nutritional deprivation. Only recently have many investigators begun to differentiate between marginal or mild, moderate, and severe forms of PEM. In fact, many earlier works failed to characterize the magnitude of the nutritional deficit under investigation. These studies tended to focus on the severely malnourished child with overt clinical symptoms. Most investigations of immunological function in malnutrition have focused on such markedly affected subjects, particularly undernourished Third World children brought to hospitals and nutritional rehabilitation centers for treatment of long-term, severe nutrient deficits. The majority of these children also had a long history of complicating infectious diseases. While such forms of severe PEM do affect massive numbers of individuals, smaller nutritional deficiencies no doubt constitute a much greater public health problem. Recent studies, as described below, have begun to investigate the influence of milder forms of undernutrition; some of them are focusing on appropriate measures to detect marginal forms of malnutrition and their impact on immunological function. Such marginal malnutrition represents a much more significant problem in developed nations and may be far more prevalent than was previously surmised. As the methodology to assess marginal nutritional status is developed, it will become possible to determine the influence of such deficits on immune function.

In addition to the variable severity of nutritional deficiencies, another factor that is seldom given appropriate attention is their timing. The influence of PEM during critical periods of development may be much more pronounced than its effect during a later stage. In general, if PEM is experienced during the fetal period, when the foundations of immunological responsiveness are established, a variety of immune defects may persist throughout life and immunodeficiency may even be observed in subsequent generations. Therefore, when immunological surveys are conducted among protein-energy malnourished children, it is critical to attempt to determine if the child being studied has been undernourished since birth, if similar nutritional insults were suffered *in utero,* and if the mother suffered from nutritional deprivation throughout her life. Without such longitudinal analysis of nutrient intake and nutritional status, the results of field studies, no matter how comprehensive, are of only limited value. Part of the considerable variation in field studies throughout the world is, no doubt, the result of significant differences in the timing and duration of the nutrient deficiencies investigated. Nonetheless, we can utilize the results of some of these studies; when interpreted with caution, they can provide some information.

NUTRITIONAL SURVEYS

A serious complication in many field studies of immunocompetence in malnourished children is that of single or multiple nutrient deficiencies. Nutritional surveys of malnourished children often indicate deficiencies of many vitamins and minerals, thereby complicating the interpretation of data (Neumann *et al.,* 1975) (Table I). In some studies, the clinical symptoms of vitamin or mineral deficiencies are monitored, but with many nutrients the deficiency must be quite severe before clinical symptoms develop. There-

Table I

Age, Sex Distribution, and Selected Clinical Features Among Severely Malnourished, Moderately Malnourished, and Control Children Studied[a]

Groups	Group I, severely malnourished $n = 34$	Group II, moderately malnourished $n = 42$	Group III, controls $n = 41$
Age[b]			
6–12 months	6	9	5
1–3 years	22	28	20
3–6 years	6	5	16
Sex			
Male	21	21	18
Female	13	21	23
Clinical infections by total children having a given infection (%)			
Pyoderma	30	7	19
Skin fungus	18	5	0
Pneumonia	15	2	0
Urinary tract infection[c]	7	5	0
Stomatitis	3	5	0
Tuberculosis	3	0	0
Intestinal parasites by total children having a given parasite (%)			
Strongyloides stercoralis	20	2	2
Ascaris lumbricales	12	19	15
Giardia lamblia	12	10	17
Ancylostoma duodenale	3	2	0
Other (nonpathogenic)	3	5	7

[a]Reproduced with permission from Neumann *et al.* (1975).

[b]Age is approximate in about one-third of study children, particularly among the 3- to 6-year-old group due to lack of birth records.

[c]Diagnosed by urine culture.

Table II

Cellular Immune Responses in Group I Children with Kwashiorkor
versus Children with Marasmus[a,b]

	Kwashiorkor ($n = 22$)	Marasmus ($n = 11$)
Peripheral lymphocyte counts	2781 ± 320	3054 ± 595
Percent lymphopenic (<1000 cells/mm^3)	2/20 (10%)	1/11 (9%)
Lymphocyte response (*in vitro*) to PHA		
Ratio: unstimulated/stimulated cells ± 1 SEM[c]	65.4 ± 7.4	60.3 ± 10.3
Percent with reduced response	4/18 (22%)	1/7 (14%)
Delayed cutaneous hypersensitivity		
PHA—size, mm[d]	5.3 ± 0.9	6.2 ± 1.7
Percent nonreactors	9/22 (41%)	5/11 (46%)
Monilia—size, mm	4.6 ± 1.2	6.4 ± 1.6
Percent nonreactors	14/22 (64%)	4/11 (36%)
SK-SD—size, mm	2.6 ± 0.9	5.6 ± 2.4
Percent nonreactors	17/22 (77%)	8/11 (73%)
Tonsil size: none or trace seen grade 0 (10)	7/23 (30%)	5/11 (46%)

[a]Reproduced with permission from Neumann *et al.* (1975).
[b]Differences between means of the kawashiorkor and marasmus group are not statistically different by Student's *t* test except for monilia skin tests.
[c]SEM: standard error of the mean.
[d]Size measured in millimeters of diameter of indurated area.

fore, the presence of complicating single nutrient deficiencies cannot be easily ruled out. Moreover, single nutrient deficiencies often have a major impact on immune function and have often been shown to be correlated with the immune dysfunction seen in PEM (Neumann *et al.,* 1975; Golden *et al.,* 1978;) (Table II). Even when a single nutrient deficiency does not directly affect immune responsiveness, it may, through nutrient interactions, have an indirect effect on immune function by altering the metabolism of a nutrient that directly alters immunological responsiveness. As knowledge grows of the influence of specific nutrient deficiencies on immunocompetence, nutrient interactions, and methodology to detect nutrient deficits, especially under field conditions, it should prove more feasible to determine the impact of such nutrient deficiencies in field studies of nutritional immunological interactions. At present, they must be interpreted with these limitations in mind.

Many field studies, particularly early ones, focused on hospitalized patients, generally infants and young children. Frequently, by the time the studies were completed, the children had been subjected to weeks of nutritional repletion. In addition, such children were seldom brought to the hospital until death was imminent. These studies are most useful as indicators of the status of children when they enter the hospital and how they respond to the early stages of therapeutic intervention. The type of diet that such children are fed has been shown to affect their overall metabolic state and to influence significantly the type of tissue that is laid down during the repletion stage (B. E. Golden and Golden, 1981; M. H. N. Golden and Golden. 1981) (Fig. 1, 2). Substantial influences on immunological function are, no doubt, manifested as well. Future studies of this type should specify, as carefully as possible, the timing of nutritional repletion with regard to the tests of immune function that are to be performed, as well as the precise composition of the formula utilized in the nutritional rehabilitation.

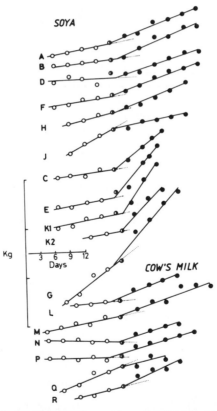

Fig. 1. The effect of zinc supplementation on the rates of weight gain of children receiving a soya–based formula diet (upper lines) or a cow's milk–based diet (lower lines). Plotted are the median weights for 3-day periods. $\bigcirc$, before supplementation; $\bullet$, after supplementation; $\pmb{\bigcirc}$, median for the day before, the day of, and the day after supplementation. This point was used in both regression equations. Initials refer to the individual patients.   Reproduced with permission from B. E. Golden and Golden (1981).

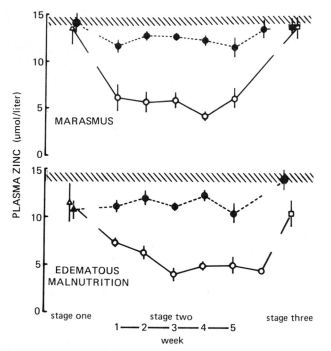

Fig. 2. Plasma zinc concentration during recovery from severe malnutrition. The upper graphs are for children with an admission diagnosis of marasmus and the lower graphs for children with edematous malnutrition. △ and ▲, maintenance diet; ●, cows milk–based formula; ○, soya protein–based formula; □ and ■, mixed diet. The open symbols are for children given the soya diet and the closed symbols for those given the cow's milk diet. the shaded bar represents the mean ± SEM for the control children. Errors shown are SEM. Reproduced with permission from B. E. Golden and Golden (1981).

The other major type of study is the survey of immunological function conducted among children in rural communities. While such studies reflect a sample representative of the population as a whole, they also present inherent difficulties. First, the determination of nutritional status is much more difficult, since the diagnostic capabilities of the large urban hospital are not available. It may prove impossible to determine the presence of complicating single nutrient deficiencies, since the methodology for assessing the status of vitamins and trace elements is not readily adapted to field conditions. Second, most of the assays of immunological function, e.g., the response of peripheral blood lymphocytes to mitogens, are highly susceptible to environmental influences and have a substantial range of variation even under the best laboratory conditions in developed countries. Seldom are such assays easily adapted to the conditions prevalent in rural areas of the tropical, arid, and high-altitude regions where so many malnourished children are found. Moreover, it has not been established what degree of malnutrition revealed by immunological tests represents a biologically significant alteration in immunocompetence and thus indicates an increased susceptibility to infection. Clearly, a substantial amount of work still needs to be done to refine the tools necessary to investigate interactions between nutritional status, the immune response, and resistance to infectious disease in human populations.

BRIEF CHARACTERIZATION OF PEM

An abbreviated description of the pathophysiology and biochemistry of protein-energy malnutrition (PEM) is in order here to understand the pervasive changes that take place in the undernourished organism. Only those aspects considered to be of possible importance to the interaction between malnutrition, the immune response, and infectious disease will be covered here (Deo, 1978).

Traditionally, PEM has been divided into two major categories: kwashiorkor, predominantly a protein deficiency, with sufficient intake of total calories; and marasmus, basically undernutrition or starvation, with a diet deficient in most nutrients, most notably total calories. However, in practice, PEM generally presents as a combination of these two classic disorders. Additionally, the variable stages of the disease, complicating single nutrient deficiencies, and the presence of infection or other forms of stress further complicate the picture. PEM has been considered a range of pathological conditions arising from a coincident lack of varying proportions of protein and calories, occurring most frequently in infants and young children, and commonly associated with infections. Consequently, *marasmus* frequently refers primarily to a deficit of total dietary calories and *kwashiorkor* refers primarily to a protein deficiency, although many other nutrients may also be present in the diet in quantities inadequate to support optimal growth and health. The term *protein-energy malnutrition* refers to a continuum of disease entities that generally involve a deficiency of both protein and calories, and possibly other nutrient deficits as well.

Consideration of the factors underlying the development of PEM lends further credence to the concept that PEM is actually a group of closely related disorders. In some areas of the world, it was proposed that the nutrient density of the major dietary staples is a critical factor in determining whether kwashiorkor or marasmus developed. In contrast, other studies began to demonstrate that the development of kwashiorkor or marasmus did not seem to depend on the protein/energy ratio of the diet (Gopalan,

1968). Currently, the most prevalent hypothesis is the one first proposed by Waterlow (1968): that the marasmic form of PEM is mainly the result of a long-term chronic adaptation to a deficiency of several essential nutrients, most notably total calories, whereas kwashiorkor is an inefficient and ineffective adaptation to a severe, acute nutritional insult. The time course of disease development seems to confirm this possibility, being quite rapid in kwashiorkor and much more gradual in marasmus (Viteri *et al.,* 1964). Additional stresses such as infection and weaning tend to predispose to kwashiorkor (Morley, 1962; Poskitt, 1971). As our knowledge of both nutrient requirements and interactions and the ramifications of their insufficiency grows, our understanding of the pathophysiology of these deficiency disorders should increase.

Perhaps the most prominent feature of PEM is a reduction or failure of growth. When nutrient availability becomes limiting, the rate of growth is decelerated, and deprivation of sufficient severity and duration can halt the growth process. Reversibility depends on providing adequate levels of dietary essentials while growth is still possible. If nutritional repletion does not occur, lack of adequate nutrition can lead to permanent stunting. Different organ systems are altered to varying degrees by PEM, those tissues with the highest rates of turnover being most severely affected. Two types of tissue experience especially high rates of turnover and therefore are particularly susceptible to deprivation of essential nutrients (Deo, 1978). First, there are tissues with a high rate of cell turnover, such as intestine, testis, and bone marrow. These organ systems manifest some of the primary lesions observed in PEM, and while the number of cells is affected, cytoplasmic lesions are minimal. In such cells, the DNA synthetic machinery is altered and a prolongation of the cell cycle results; the major increase is in the S phase, with G_2 being variably altered (depending on the specific organ system being considered) and G_1 generally being shortened.

The other type of tissue that is notably susceptible to an insufficiency of essential nutrients contains cell types that, while undergoing little cell renewal, are metabolically very active and experience a high rate of cytoplasmic turnover, such as liver and pancreas. These tissues tend to show cytoplasmic lesions, such as those that lead to fatty liver in PEM. Biochemical alterations in PEM in this type of tissue include decreased synthesis of protein and RNA, while DNA synthesis remains intact. In most organ systems, the delay in growth and development reflects a decrease in cell proliferation due to prolongation of the cell cycle and a decrease in the number of stem cells. In many developing organ systems, cell migration may be delayed, but differentiation may often be unaffected (Deo, 1978). This is because, in many individuals with PEM, rapid cell proliferation continues beyond the period associated with this phenomenon in normally nourished individuals, possibly due to the cumulative delay in the cell cycle. In some systems, there may also be a decline in cell loss, which may assist in balancing the decreased cellular genesis (Deo, 1978). However, the precise limits of growth and development in many tissues remain ill-defined.

PEM of sufficient severity and duration is associated with a wide variety of aberrations in homeostasis and biochemical function; nearly all organ systems are affected to some extent. Of particular importance in the resistance to infectious disease are alterations in the basal metabolic rate (BMR); thermoregulation; gastrointestinal, renal, and cardiac function; endocrine parameters; and a wide variety of abnormalities in the metabolism of proteins, amino acids, lipids, carbohydrates, and minerals. The BMR may be altered whether considered on a whole body basis or with reference to a particular organ (e.g., brain, liver) (Montgomery, 1962; Brooke and Cocks, 1974). This finding is consistent with many of the classic clinical features of PEM such as hypothermia, bradycardia, physical inactivity, and an unresponsive emotional state (Alleyne *et al.,* 1977). The BMR has been shown to return to normal with suitable dietary treatment (Ashworth *et al.,* 1968; Brooke and Ashworth, 1972). Inability to maintain normal body temperature has also been reported among malnourished children (Brenton *et al.,* 1967; Brooke, 1972); some investigators feel that hypothermia is associated with a particularly poor prognosis (Brenton *et al.,* 1967; Wharton, 1970). The ability of children with PEM to respond to both cold stimuli and heat stress has been shown to be impaired (Wayburne, 1968; Brooke *et al.,* 1973; Brooke and Salvosa, 1974). This must be of particular importance to children with PEM who live in tropical as well as high-altitude areas.

The physiological functions of the gastrointestinal tract and the cardiac and renal systems are all compromised to some extent during PEM. Perhaps most significant in the development of PEM are the changes in the gastrointestinal tract, most of which tend to decrease further the absorption of those meager nutrients that are taken in. PEM results in a substantial reduction in the intestinal mass (Passmore, 1947), the size of enterocytes, the mitotic index of intestinal cells (Brunser *et al.,* 1968), and secretion of dipeptidases, disaccharidases, and pancreatic enzymes (Barbezat and Hansen, 1968; James, 1971; Hazuria *et al.,* 1974) (Tables III, IV). Deficiencies of sucrase, maltase, and lactase have been demonstrated, and lactose intolerance is frequently observed in malnutrition (Bowie *et al.,* 1963; Chandra *et al.,* 1968; Wharton *et al.,* 1968; Dahlquist, 1971). Tests for malabsorption utilizing D-xylose have also shown an impaired absorptive capacity (Viteri *et al.,* 1973), but this method has been questioned. Malabsorption has been shown for a large number of nutrients, including fats, fat-soluble vitamins, carbohydrates, and nitrogen (Gomez *et al.,* 1956; Arroyave *et al.,* 1959). Gastroenteritis, frequently observed in association with PEM, results in a further reduction in the absorption of a wide variety of nutrients. In the

Table III
Total Thickness of the Mucosa of Normal Infants and of Infants with Kwashiorkor
and Marasmic-Type Malnutrition[a]

Mucosa	Normal (8)[b]	Kwashiorkor (10)	Marasmus, all cases (18)	Marasmus before recovery (8)	Marasmus during recovery (10)
Total thickness (μm)[c]	506 ± 72	473 ± 71	413 ± 100	387 ± 104	434 ± 107
P <		0.10	0.01	0.02	0.10

[a]Reproduced with permission from Brunser et al. (1968).
[b]Numbers in parentheses are numbers of infants.
[c]The total thickness is the mean of 10 measurements for each specimen studied.

small intestine, bile salt metabolism is altered with an increased turnover of bile salts, a decrease in the size of the bile salt pool, and an increase in the deoxycholate/cholate ratio, the overall result being an impaired ability to form micelles and therefore absorb fat (Viteri and Schneider, 1974). Thus, the function of the gastrointestinal tract is significantly impaired and the capacity to absorb nutrients is severely limited, thereby further accelerating the state of malnutrition.

The heart and circulatory system, as well as the kidneys, are also markedly affected by PEM. There is a decrease in cardiac output, a prolongation of the systemic circulation time, and a decreased peripheral blood flow (Alleyne, 1966; Brooke, 1973). Postmortem examinations often reveal a reduction in heart size, and congestive heart failure may be the cause of death in some

Table IV
Mitotic Index and Number of Epithelial Cells Per Mitosis in the Crypts of Lieberkühn
of Jejunal Biopsies of Normal Infants and of Infants with Kwashiorkor and Marasmus[a]

	Normal (8)[b]	Kwashiorkor (10)	Marasmus, all cases (18)	Marasmus before recovery (8)	Marasmus during recovery (10)
Mitotic index	3.9 ± 0.2	3.0 ± 0.6	1.9 ± 0.8	1.3 ± 0.5	2.4 ± 0.8
Range	2.6–4.5	1.8–3.7	0.7–3.6	0.7–2.1	1.4–3.6
Number of crypt cells per mitosis[c]	26 ± 5	35 ± 9	65 ± 32	87 ± 34	46 ± 16
P<		0.02	0.01	0.001	0.01

[a]Reproduced with permission from Brunser et al. (1968).
[b]Numbers in parentheses are numbers of infants.
[c]The number of crypt epithelial cells per mitosis is the reciprocal value of the mitotic index.

cases (Viteri *et al.* 1964). Various forms of concomitant anemia may further complicate the picture. A decrease in renal function is also frequently observed, with a decline in the rates of glomerular filtration and renal plasma flow; gastroenteritis further depresses the efficiency of both of these functions. The presence of aminoaciduria, phosphaturia, and inefficient excretion of the acid load confirm the impairment of tubular function (Alleyne, 1967). Many of the derangements in renal function are related to alterations in endocrine parameters (e.g., the level of antidiuretic hormone, aldosterone). Altered renal function takes on increased importance in light of the widespread prevalence of dehydration in cases of PEM complicated with gastroenteritis.

Metabolic and biochemical abnormalities affect nearly all aspects of homeostasis in the malnourished organism. Altered metabolism of protein and amino acids has been studied perhaps most extensively, and a number of widely used diagnostic criteria (e.g., levels of serum proteins and plasma amino acids, ratios of amino acids) are based on these aberrations. Much of this information was generated in the 1960s and early 1970s, when it was felt that protein deficiency was possibly the most serious nutrient deficiency. Since that time, due to revisions in the estimates of protein requirements and a better understanding of the world food situation, it has been recognized that a deficiency of total food intake is probably the most widespread and serious nutritional problem. Nonetheless, our understanding of the alterations in protein and amino acid metabolism that take place in PEM was greatly increased by this major emphasis on protein.

Perhaps the best indicator of altered protein metabolism in PEM is depression in the level of circulating plasma proteins, the albumin fraction being particularly affected (Waterlow and Alleyne, 1971; Whitehead and Alleyne, 1972). There is a 50% reduction in the total albumin pool, which is especially apparent in the extravascular fraction of the pool, even though there is a marked reduction in the catabolic rate (Cohen and Hansen, 1962; Picou and Waterlow, 1962; James and Hay, 1968). Other plasma proteins such as transferrin and retinol-binding protein (RBP) are also significantly reduced (Antia *et al.,* 1968). In notable contrast, the globulin fraction of plasma proteins is less affected by the nutritional state (Cohen and Hansen, 1962). It has been shown in experimental animals that in protein deficiency, turnover of total body protein is significantly decreased (Waterlow and Stephen, 1968); however, in humans, definitive studies are limited (Picou and Taylor-Roberts, 1969). It is known that the polysomal profile is markedly affected by nutritional conditions, which would certainly have a major impact on the rates of protein synthesis and degradation (Deo, 1978). It is well established that protein synthesis and degradation in specific organs are affected to a different extent by PEM; muscle experiences a substantial decline in total protein turnover, while such turnover is maintained at nearly normal levels in liver (Millward *et al.,* 1975). It is hypothesized that in general, rates of protein turnover in various organs are adjusted to allow for a redistribution of endogenous amino acids from muscle tissues to metabolically active visceral organs such as liver.

The total plasma levels of amino acids are reduced to approximately 50% of the normal levels in severe PEM (Whitehead and Alleyne, 1972). Amino acid metabolism is especially deranged in patients with kwashiorkor, with a marked decrease in the plasma concentration of most essential amino acids, particularly the branched chain amino acids and threonine; far less alteration in plasma levels of phenylalanine and lysine is observed (Arroyave *et al.,* 1962; Holt *et al.,* 1963). The nonessential amino acids are generally maintained at a normal level or may possibly be increased (Arroyave *et al.,* 1962). The concentration of alanine has been suggested to reflect the balance between the relative effects of the dietary deficit of protein or energy that occur in most cases of PEM (Waterlow and Alleyne, 1971). These alterations in amino acid metabolism have been used as a means of assessing nutritional status.

Both plasma and urinary urea have been demonstrated to be low in severe PEM (Picou and Phillips, 1972). In general, total urinary nitrogen closely parallels dietary nitrogen, and as the latter falls to a minimum, urinary excretion of urea decreases. The low-protein diet in PEM leads eventually to considerable nitrogen conservation, due largely to a decrease in the output of urinary urea (Picou and Taylor-Roberts, 1969) (Fig. 3). In contrast, ammonia excretion is not decreased to the same extent (Waterlow, 1963); in fact, it can exceed the excretion of urea in some cases of PEM. Continued excretion of ammonia is essential because of the increased

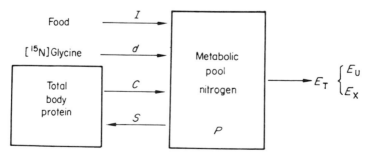

Fig. 3. Model of protein metabolism. *I,* rate of intake of protein (N mg/hr); *d,* rate of infusion of ^{15}N-labeled amino acid (^{15}N mg/hr); *C,* rate of catabolism of protein (N mg/hr); *S,* rate of synthesis of protein (N mg/hr); E_T, rate of excretion of total urinary N (mg/hr); E_u, rate of excretion of urinary urea N (mg/hr); E_x, rate of excretion of urinary nonurea N (mg/hr). Reproduced with permission from Picou and Taylor-Roberts (1969).

uric acid excretion due to the accelerated breakdown of protein to supply energy and amino acids, to increases in fatty acid metabolism, and to the potassium deficiency that frequently develops in PEM.

Alterations in lipid metabolism are also observed in PEM, one of the cardinal signs of kwashiorkor being fatty liver. On postmortem examination, it has been found that liver lipids comprised up to 30–40% of the total body fat in children with kwashiorkor (Garrow *et al.,* 1965) (Table V). Indeed, the development of fatty infiltration of the liver is associated with a very high risk of death. While fatty liver is found in marasmus, most observers believe that it is uncommon (Truswell, 1975). Currently, it is felt that fatty liver develops as a result of the impaired ability of hepatic tissue to dispose of triglycerides, probably due to decreased synthesis of the protein portion of very low density lipoproteins (Flores *et al.,* 1973). Children who develop marasmus tend to have normal or increased concentrations of plasma triglycerides, cholesterol, and β-lipoprotein; however, subnormal levels have occasionally been reported (Pretorius and Weymeyer, 1966; McLaren *et al.,* 1967). Plasma levels of free fatty acids are quite variable (Lewis *et al.,* 1966; Truswell, 1975). In children with kwashiorkor, low levels of fasting serum triglycerides, as well as low levels of cholesterol and phospholipids, have been observed (Truswell, 1975). Serum levels of β-lipoprotein are reported to be variable (Coward and Whitehead, 1972).

Carbohydrate metabolism is also markedly altered in PEM; many of these changes may be related to reciprocal alterations in the levels of insulin and the corticosteroids (Whitehead and Harland, 1966; Kerpel-Fronius and Kaiser, 1967). Most investigators now concur that PEM is generally associated with a depressed fasting blood glucose level, although wide variations have been reported. Liver glycogen stores are significantly reduced, but metabolic adaptation (e.g., elevated activity of hepatic glucose-6-phosphatase) allows for reasonable preservation of blood glucose levels (Alleyne and Scullard, 1969). The efficient use of gluconeogenesis, as well as effective recycling of glycolytic intermediates and products, helps to maintain glucose homeostasis to a degree compatible with survival.

While very little is known regarding vitamin metabolism in PEM, some data have been accumulated on mineral metabolism. Decreases in total body and exchangeable potassium have been reported (Garrow *et al.,* 1965; Nichols *et al.,* 1974). Indeed, hypokalemia is a frequently reported symptom, especially in severe PEM (Halliday, 1967). Potassium levels in brain, muscle, red blood cells, and leukocytes have all been demonstrated to be low (Garrow, 1967; Alleyne *et al.,* 1969; Khalil *et al.,* 1974). Any complicating infectious disorder that involves vomiting and/or diarrhea would be expected to increase the possibility of potassium deficiency. During treat-

Table V

Nutritional Status of Subjects[a]

| Clinical class | A[b] | | B | | C | | D | | E |
Child	L.S.	C.W.W.	R.H.	E.W.	C.W.	S.D.	C.B.	A.C.	C.A.
Sex	M	F	F	F	F	F	F	M	M
Age, months	10	14	9	13	6	16	14	12	11
Weight before postmortem, kg	4.69	4.17	7.50	7.70	4.10	6.70	5.67	6.30	7.60
Height, cm	57	58	65	71	55	65	67	70	70
Severity of edema	—		—	—	++	++	+	+	++
Birth weight, kg	3.1	1.6	4.3	(3.4)[b]	3.4	(3.4)†	(3.4)†	3.4	2.9
Expected weight for age,[c] kg	9.75	8.85	9.61	10.30	7.26	10.66	10.25	9.75	10.25
Expected weight for height, kg	4.65	5.25	7.15	9.05	4.42	7.15	7.75	8.70	8.70
Weight as percentage expected for age	48	47	78	75	57	63	55	65	74
Weight as percentage expected for height	101	79	105	85	93	94	73	73	87
Body fat as percentage of body weight	22.5	19.2	25.5	18.4	4.6	3.9	16.0	15.4	20.0
Liver fat as percentage of liver weight	2.4	3.7	17.9	7.6	27.0	6.0	50.1	43.7	39.0
Liver fat as percentage of body fat	0.4	0.8	2.7	1.9	36.5	6.5	30.2	39.6	9.1

[a]Reproduced with permission from Garrow et al. (1965).

[b]Class A: clinically well nourished and with normal liver fat; class B: clinically well nourished but with increased liver fat; class C: marasmic kwashiorkor with gross edema, dyspigmentation, and loss of subcutaneous fat; class D: kwashiorkor with gross fatty liver, dyspigmentation, and edema; class E: malnutrition plus proteinuria.

[c]Assumed birth weight.

[d]Corrected for birth weight.

ment, normal potassium levels are very slowly repleted (Garrow, 1965; Alleyne, 1968). Most studies of sodium levels indicate a general elevation in most organs in PEM, e.g., brain, muscle, and red cells (Halliday, 1967; Nichols *et al.,* 1973; Khalil *et al.,* 1974). This intracellular accumulation of sodium may be related to the impaired activity of the ATP-requiring sodium-potassium pump, which may also explain the relative potassium deficiency (Patrick *et al.,* 1980). In some children with PEM, low levels of plasma sodium have been observed; this is considered an ominous prognostic sign (Garrow *et al.,* 1968).

In both biopsy and postmortem examinations, magnesium levels are frequently found to be low in a variety of organs (Alleyne *et al.,* 1969; Caddell and Olson, 1973). Further indications of deficient magnesium levels in PEM include low urinary excretion of magnesium and greater than expected retention of magnesium upon repletion (Montgomery, 1960; Caddell *et al.,* 1973). Initial reports indicate that the metabolism of iron, zinc, and copper may also be altered in PEM (Golden and Golden, 1979). With these elements, as with many nutrients, it is particularly difficult to distinguish between altered nutrient metabolism due to PEM and a deficient dietary intake of the nutrient itself. No doubt, alterations in gastrointestinal tract function and absorptive capacity, renal function, endocrine factors, and the presence of complicating infections, as well as nutritional interactions between the minerals themselves, may all contribute to the altered mineral metabolism in PEM.

Changes in body water balance are also seen in PEM. Total body water, as measured by both *in vivo* isotopic and postmortem techniques, indicates overhydration in a variety of tissues in both marasmus and kwashiorkor (Garrow *et al.,* 1968). This has generally been attributed to an expansion of the space occupied by the extracellular fluid. The magnitude of this expansion closely parallels the degree of edema. When individual tissues were analyzed for water content, children with PEM were found to have consistently higher levels of water, particularly those with edema (Frenk *et al.,* 1957; Smith, 1960). Extracellular water has been reported to be increased by all investigators (Brinkman *et al.,* 1965), while results regarding the percentage of total body water in the intracellular fraction have been quite variable (Hansen *et al.,* 1965; Alleyne, 1968). The pathogenetic mechanism of edema in kwashiorkor and marasmus remains unclear. Retention of water and sodium is, of course, critical and is closely related to the degree of hypoproteinemia. Serum albumin is the fraction of plasma protein that is most apparently affected by PEM, and it is known that albumin is the single most important factor contributing to serum colloidal osmotic pressure, especially with very low concentrations of serum albumin (Coward, 1975). Increases in the globulin fraction can partially balance the decline in serum albumin. In addition, total body levels of potassium and other related minerals, as well as multiple hormonal changes, no doubt figure prominently in the development of edema.

Numerous alterations in endocrine parameters are also seen in PEM. Many of them have a potential impact on immunological function and responsiveness to infectious challenge. Both kwashiorkor and marasmus are frequently associated with increased levels of human growth hormone, and there is a significant negative correlation between levels of plasma growth hormone and serum levels of albumin in PEM (Pimstone *et al.,* 1968; Lunn *et al.,* 1973). In PEM, particularly the marasmic form, low fasting levels of plasma insulin have been observed (Lunn *et al.,* 1973). After stimulation with an intravenous infusion of glucose or glucagon, the insulin response is reduced or absent (Hadden, 1967; Alleyne *et al.,* 1972). Marked structural changes in the pancreas have been noted on postmortem examination; these alterations may be the basis of the impairment. The deranged insulin response may also be related to an abnormal intake and/or metabolism of other nutrients, e.g., potassium or chromium (Hopkins *et al.,* 1968; Gurson and Saner, 1973). Elevated levels of plasma 17-hydroxycorticosteroids and plasma cortisol have been seen in both kwashiorkor and marasmus (Leonard and MacWilliam, 1964; Schonland *et al.,* 1972; Lunn *et al.,* 1973). The levels of plasma cortisol and insulin may be important in determining whether marasmus or kwashiorkor ensues in an individual child with deficient nutrition. The initial stages of marasmus are generally associated with elevated levels of plasma corticosteroids, emphasizing the reduced synthesis of muscle protein, allowing for relatively intact synthesis of plasma proteins such as albumin (Lunn *et al.,* 1976a). High levels of cortisol are not found in the earliest stages of kwashiorkor; instead, elevated levels of plasma insulin are observed as a result of the consumption of starchy foods. This favors protein synthesis in muscle at the expense of hepatic protein synthesis, resulting in a rapid drop in plasma albumin, resultant hypoproteinemia, and edematous PEM (Lunn *et al.,* 1976b). Superimposed stress, such as infection or hypoglycemia, can further contribute to elevated levels of corticosteroids (Alleyne and Young, 1967; Lunn *et al.,* 1973). Diurnal rhythms are altered, and an impaired clearance of exogenous cortisol has been demonstrated (Alleyne and Young, 1967). In the advanced stages of kwashiorkor, the percentage of free cortisol is greatly elevated, especially in children with severe hypoalbuminemia (Schonland *et al,* 1972). There seems to be a reciprocal relationship between serum levels of insulin and cortisol (Lunn *et al.,* 1973). While some reports of hypothyroidism do exist, the precise status of the thyroid in PEM has not been established (Beas *et al.,* 1966; Ingenbleek and Malvaux, 1980).

In general, the biochemical picture in children with PEM is one of multiple aberrations, many of which have a notable impact on immunocompetence and the ability to respond effectively to challenge by pathogenic organisms. The digestion, absorption, and metabolism of nearly all types of nutrients are substantially altered to facilitate the continued survival of the total organism. The efficiency and effectiveness of these adaptive mechanisms may well determine whether a given child develops kwashiorkor or marasmus. Whichever syndrome does develop, the child with PEM is in a metabolically precarious state, a fragile creature. Such a child is ill-equipped to handle the dual requirements of rapid growth and challenge by a continual barrage of infectious microorganisms. Thus, common communicable diseases that only rarely present a serious health hazard in the Western world frequently prove fatal, and the result is the high child mortality rate observed in less developed countries.

PEM AND INFECTIOUS DISEASE: SYNERGISTIC INTERACTIONS

While an interaction between nutritional intake and resistance to infectious disease has long been postulated, only recently have data begun to accumulate to support this hypothesis. Much of the early information was derived from wartime experiences, when severe food shortages resulted in a sharp increase in incidence and mortality from a variety of infectious diseases. It should be noted, however, that such populations were under extreme duress, and stress has been shown to alter immunological function markedly. During these early stages of study, tuberculosis was the disease that attracted the greatest attention. Mortality attributed to tuberculosis increased substantially in various European countries during both World Wars I and II (Faber, 1938; Grafe, 1950; Palmer *et al.,* 1957). Moreover, studies of primitive tribes indicated that differences in dietary staples were associated with a sixfold difference in the incidence of tuberculosis. In general, malnutrition attributed to a variety of causes was associated with an increased incidence and greater severity of tuberculosis.

Other observations of the interaction between nutritional factors and disease suceptibility included an increased incidence and severity of typhus, infectious hepatitis, infection with *Entamoeba histolytica,* and acute respiratory and diarrheal diseases (Gordon *et al.,* 1964). In addition, it has long been known that children who developed measles, chronic tuberculosis, severe chickenpox, whooping cough, meningitis, or infantile diarrhea, or especially a number of these infectious maladies concurrently, had a greater tendency to develop symptoms of overt vitamin A deficiency, xerophthalmia, or keratomalacia (Table VI). Infectious episodes, particularly if repeated, were correlated with the development of scurvy, pellagra, beriberi

Table VI

Clinical Characteristics of Inpatients with Severe Protein-Calorie Malnutrition, Outpatients, and Village Comparison Subjects[a]

	(n)	Age (months)[b]	Sex M	Sex F	Weight (kg)	Length (cm)	% expected wt/age[b]	% expected length/age[b]	% expected wt/length[b]	Plasma-protein (g/dl)	HCT (%)	Xerophthalmia No.	Xerophthalmia (%)	Night blindness No.	Night blindness (%)	Angular Stomatitis No.	Angular Stomatitis (%)
Inpatients																	
Marasmus	56	13[c] (12–18)	50	50	4.43[d] ±2.12	65.0[d] ±11.8	40.5[d] ±8.6	80.5[d] ±7.2	63.1[d] ±7.0	6.6[d] ±1.0	30.5[d] ±6.1	9	(16)	1	(2)	2	(4)
Marasmic Kwashiorkor	28	40 (30–60)	46	54	7.43 ±3.00	80.0 ±14.0	46.7 ±10.7	81.0 ±7.5	67.4 ±10.0	5.0 ±0.8	24.4 ±6.8	9	(32)	2	(7)	8	(28)
Kwashiorkor	14	25 (14–42)	57	43	7.25 ±3.16	74.4 ±14.4	53.0 ±9.1	82.2 ±4.7	76.4 ±8.8	4.0 ±0.6	25.2 ±6.4	5	(36)	1	(7)	5	(36)
All inpatients	98	20 (18–30)	50	50	5.70 ±2.92	70.7 ±14.4	43.8 ±10.0	80.9 ±7.0	66.3 ±9.4	5.8 ±1.4	28.0 ±6.9	23	(23)	4	(4)	15	(15)
Outpatients	146	24 (22–32)	60	40	8.8 ±3.4	79.8 ±16.4	68.5 ±11.8	89.0 ±8.0	84.3 ±10.3	7.3 ±0.8	34.1 ±4.1	NA	—	NA	—	NA	—
Village comparison subjects	94	32 (29–44)	65	35	10.06 ±2.54	82.3 ±10.0	67.2 ±10.5	85.6 ±5.6	86.1 ±8.1	7.8 ±0.6	35.6 ±3.4	0	(0)	3	(3)	2	(2)

[a] Reproduced with permission from Brown et al. (1981).

[b] Age is not known with certainty in Bangladesh. These data must be interpreted as best approximations based on family histories and "local events" calendars. Anthropometrics were compared to CDC/NCHS reference data.

[c] Median (95% confidence limits)

[d] Mean ± 1 S.D.

(Scrimshaw *et al.,* 1968), and megaloblastic anemia (Luhby, 1959). Some observers believe that the most readily apparent sign of the nutritional consequences of infection is the widespread retardation of growth and development observed throughout the world (Mata *et al.,* 1972b; Whitehead, 1977b).

More recent studies have tended to focus on the increased incidence of infectious disease and high infant mortality rates observed in less developed countries (Table VII). An Inter-American study on the causes of infant and child mortality provided considerable data regarding the influence of nutritional status on the susceptibility to infection and the consequently high rates of mortality. Among children who died before reaching their fifth birthday (50% of all children in most locations studied), nutritional deficiency or immaturity was a primary or associated cause of death in 57% of the cases. Nutritional deficiencies were found to be associated with 61% of all deaths due to infectious disease; for example, 59% of the deaths were attributed to measles, as opposed to only 33% to noninfectious causes. Moreover, in kwashiorkor the outstanding epidemiological feature was the large number of cases caused by an immediately antecedent episode of measles, diarrheal disease, or another common communicable disease of childhood (Scrimshaw *et al.,* 1968).

The greatest health hazard facing the child growing up in poverty-stricken rural and periurban areas of the Third World is the vicious cycle of interaction between PEM and diarrheal disease. Because of the high mortality rates attributed to gastroenteritis during the weaning stage of infancy/childhood, a disease entity called *weanling diarrhea* has been defined (Gordon *et al.,* 1963). The weaning period, rather than the period immediately postpartum, is associated with the greatest threat to survival. In addition, during the first 2 years of life, episodes of gastroenteritis are likely to cause kwashiorkor or marasmus (Jelliffe, 1953). This is especially true if breast feeding is discontinued early. The incidence of all infectious disease in India, most notably diarrheal diseases, was approximately threefold higher in babies who were fed infant formulas than in those who continued to breast-feed (Chandra, 1981c). A similar influence on mortality rates due to a variety of infectious disorders has been observed throughout the developing world (Jelliffe and Jelliffe, 1978). Indeed, prolongation of breast feeding or administration of banked human milk with a high titer of IgA to rotavirus resulted in decreased rotavirus excretion, and significant weight gains were finally observed. The immunological aspects of breast feeding will be covered in detail elsewhere in this volume.

Many children in less developed countries are subjected to a continued barrage of diarrheal disease episodes, and the true pathogenic agent is often difficult to identify. The rate of growth and development in such children

Table VII

Nutritional Status of 122 Children Who Died in 12 Matlab Villages, August 1975–July 1976[a]

Cause of death	Number	Median age (months)	Percentage of standard weight for height[b] (mean ± SE)	Percentage of standard weight for age (mean ± SE)	Days between rash onset and death (mean ± SE)	Days of diarrhea prior to death (mean ± SE)
Measles deaths	33	37	85.7 ± 3.0	62.6 ± 2.1	14.5 ± 1.7	7.9 ± 1.3
With diarrhea	15	36	82.1 ± 3.4	60.5 ± 2.3	17.5 ± 3.1	12.9 ± 1.8
With pneumonia	10	37	91.8 ± 3.0[c]	66.0 ± 2.7	9.7 ± 1.3	2.3 ± 1.0
With other[d]	8	43	84.9 ± 3.3	62.7 ± 3.4	13.9 ± 1.9	6.2 ± 2.3
Nonmeasles deaths	89	38	82.5 ± 2.8	59.9 ± 4.9	—	—
diarrhea alone	29	38	73.5 ± 4.0[e]	52.0 ± 6.4	—	24.7 ± 3.9
Living controls[f]	33	38	88.2 ± 0.9	—	—	—

[a]Reproduced with permission from Koster et al. (1981).

[b]Weight and height recorded prior to onset of illness leading to death.

[c]Nutritional status of children dying of measles with pneumonia is significantly better than that of children dying of measles with diarrhea or other; $p = $ <.05, Wilcoxon rank sum test.

[d]Deaths associated with a combination of diarrhea and respiratory symptoms or with seizures, anasarca, oral ulceration, and anorexia.

[e]Nutritional status of children dying of diarrhea alone is significantly lower than that of controls or all measles-associated deaths, $p <.01$, Wilcoxon rank sum test.

[f]Survivors without history of measles during 12-month study period, age- and sex-matched to measles-associated deaths.

can be shown to be strongly correlated with the rate of infection due to enteropathogens (Mata *et al.,* 1972a). The major pathogenic culprits in the etiology of gastroenteritis are enterotoxic and enteropathogenic *Escherichia coli, Shigella,* and the rotoviruses; by far the most important pathogen in the etiology of PEM is toxigenic *E. coli* (Brown *et al.,* 1981). Infection with these pathogens is particularly critical in younger children (below 2 years of age) and in children who concurrently have measles (Koster *et al.,* 1981) (Table VII). Diarrheal disease is particularly severe when it occurs in conjunction with measles, and the mortality rate is markedly elevated when these conditions occur simultaneously (Koster *et al.,* 1981).

The growth rate of children in Bangladesh has been shown to be highly seasonal, with up to a fourfold difference in various months (Brown and Black, 1981). This seasonal difference has been attributed to the increased burden of infectious disease during specific seasons; during warm, wet months, bacterial disease is the major cause of gastroenteritis, and during colder, dry months, viral pathogens are the principal cause of diarrheal disease. In countries such as Bangladesh, the presence of monsoons and seasonal food shortages may also contribute to the increased incidence of diarrheal disease. During months when enterotoxigenic *E. coli* predominates, a direct correlation between growth failure and the incidence of diarrheal disease has been established (Brown and Black, 1981). In contrast, no such correlation could be established between rotovirus titers and growth velocity. Therefore, growth (and growth failure) tends to be seasonal. Neumann *et al.* (1975) have shown that children in such an environment are frequently anergic in response to skin test antigens, and the depression of this response has been related to their impaired nutritional status. Indeed, the degree of anergy is particularly useful in predicting morbidity due to diarrheal disease. T-lymphocyte numbers in children with mild and moderate PEM are a valuable prognostic index of morbidity during the following 6 months and are especially useful in predicting the duration of a diarrheal episode (Keusch, 1981) (Table VIII). Indeed, in this and other instances, it was found that certain immunological parameters were better predictive indicators of growth and diarrheal morbidity in mild/moderate malnutrition then were traditional anthropometric measurements.

There are a number of mechanisms whereby diarrheal disease can profoundly influence nutritional status. Gastroenteritis is characterized by a decrease in intestinal transit time, with less time allowed for nutrient absorption. Bacterial toxins have a direct effect on intestinal structure and function, producing flattening of villi and microvilli. Protein-energy malnourished children with gastroenteritis have an abnormal gut flora and aberrant bile salt metabolism; these features were present in 75% of the children who did not even have diarrhea on the day of the examination

Table VIII
Stages in T-Cell Differentiation and Observed Effects of Protein-Energy Malnutrition[a]

Cell type	Role in T-cell differentiation	Changes in malnutrition
Stem cell	Uncommitted, pluripotential precursor cell	? Normal
Prothymocyte	Early cell in committed T-cell lineage Responsible for NK (natural killer) cell activity in peripheral blood null cells	May be increased
Thymocyte	Intrathymic lymphocyte population that bears specific detectable antigens during differentiation process	Decreased by morphologic assessment of thymus tissue
T cell	Postthymic peripheral blood mature T cell	Decreased by study of surface markers and functions

[a]Reproduced with permission from Keusch (1981).

(Whitehead, 1981). Moreover, there can be bacterial overgrowth extending into the small intestine (Scrimshaw, 1981). The overall result is a malabsorption syndrome that encompasses inefficient absorption of a wide variety of essential nutrients. For instance, Rosenberg et al. (1977) have estimated that young Guatemalan children with only a moderate form of diarrheal disease lose more than 500–600 calories/day. Caloric intake is not the only nutritional component that is reduced; malabsorption of nitrogen (Cook, 1974), carbohydrates (Dossetor and Whittle, 1975), and fat also occurs. In addition, gastroenteritis is associated with malabsorption of vitamins, including vitamin A, folate (Matoth et al., 1964), and vitamin B_{12}. Absorption of minerals under similar circumstances has been studied far less thoroughly but is most likely affected to a similar extent.

In addition to gastroenteritis, a number of systemic infections including tuberculosis, measles, streptococcal infections, and systemic bacterial sepsis have been shown to alter the efficient absorption of a wide range of nutrients (Cook, 1974; Dossetor and Whittle, 1975). A variety of intestinal parasites can also cause malabsorption. Thus, a child who is malnourished prior to the onset of diarrhea faces a serious problem. Moreover, recovery of normal absorptive function after an acute diarrheal episode requires much more time than would be expected; absorptive losses can continue for more than 2 weeks (along with the continued alteration of metabolism, such as negative nitrogen balance, during convalescence).

Measles is another disease that has a profound impact on a host with a compromised nutritional status. Mortality rates for measles in less developed countries are far higher than those in the developed world; for instance, mortality rates in 1968 were 268 times as high in Guatemala and 214 times as high in Ecuador (Scrimshaw *et al.,* 1968). In some African countries, infection with measles culminates in a mortality rate of 25–50% in young children with the edematous form of PEM. Such marked differences in the mortality rates for measles between developed and developing countries have resulted in investigations of the virus itself. However, no study has ever shown that there are any significant differences in the virulence of the measles virus found in the Latin American countries compared to the United States. In addition, the mortality rate for measles in well-nourished upper-class Guatemalan children are not unlike those of the developed areas. The difference must therefore be in the susceptibility of the host to the measles virus; while measles is generally a harmless childhood malady in developed countries, it is one of the most feared child killers in less developed nations (Morley, 1962; Ristori *et al.,* 1962; Taneja *et al.,* 1962).

The incidence of serious complications from measles such as pneumonia, diarrhea, corneal ulceration, and blindness is far higher in the malnourished child than in the well-nourished one (Dekkers, 1981). The widespread confluent epidermal rash, severe inflammation, and widespread cytotoxic mucosal pathology, in combination with anergy attributed both to the viral infection and to nutritional insufficiency, make the skin and mucosal membranes of such children ideal targets for life-threatening infections. Such children often fall victim to a variety of secondary bacterial, protozoal, and/or fungal infections; at times there may be a reactivation of latent infections such as malaria or tuberculosis. This relationship between nutritional deficiency and measles infection is further underscored by the fact that nutritional supplementation has been demonstrated to reduce fatalities and serious complications attributed to measles. (Scrimshaw *et al.,* 1966).

With the onset of infection in children in Third World countries, there is a notable drop in serum albumin levels; for instance, both gastroenteritis and measles are associated with such a decrease, and the simultaneous combination of these infectious diseases is particularly critical (Lunn *et al.,* 1979b). Indeed, the survival rate is often directly correlated with the level of serum albumin. A marked drop in serum albumin is also seen in many children with PEM, especially those who develop kwashiorkor (Alleyne *et al.,* 1977). These children develop a syndrome known as *protein-losing enteropathy,* which leads to a marked loss of albumin into the intestinal lumen during infection (Dossetor and Whittle, 1975). The intestinal wall is generally abnormally thin in a child with chronic PEM; infection with measles and/or gastroenteritis has an additional influence on all epithelial tissues, including the intestinal mucosa (Passmore, 1947; Creamer, 1964). Thus, the functional and structural integrity of the intestinal wall is further compromised, allowing for leakage of albumin and other plasma proteins into the gut lumen. It is most likely that the same changes in the integrity of the gut wall, and thus in intestinal permeability, permit macromolecular substances obtained from the digesta to pass from the intestine into the bloodstream and lymph; this is why one sees elevated titers of serum antibodies to antigens from common foods (Chandra, 1974). Intestinal helminths, such as hookworm, and systemic parasites, such as malaria, also seem to have such an impact on plasma albumin, with both young children and experimental animals showing sharp drops in plasma albumin concentration on infection with the intestinal parasite (Blackman *et al.* 1965; Nielsen, 1976; Crompton *et al.,* 1978).

In the case of diarrheal disease, there is also a clear correlation between the onset of acute disease and the sharp decline in serum albumin levels. In Gambia, of 19 children from a rural village who experienced a rapid and precipitous decline in serum albumin, a concurrent episode of diarrhea was observed in 17 (Lunn *et al.,* 1979b). Longitudinal studies have also shown that infection with measles is often followed by a sudden, precipitous drop in serum albumin, and kwashiorkor often appears shortly thereafter (Frood *et al.,* 1971; Mathews *et al.,* 1972; Poskitt, 1972). The magnitude of this drop in serum albumin can also be correlated with growth faltering and failure, and ultimately with mortality from diseases such as gastroenteritis and measles (Whitehead, 1981).

It is conceivable that the syndrome of protein-losing enteropathy is one of the mechanisms by which infection contributes to the development of kwashiorkor in children with chronic PEM (Whitehead, 1981). In the child who develops an acute infectious episode, there is a sudden drop in plasma albumin levels, with subsequent development of hypoproteinemia and edema. Such children show an increased leakage of plasma proteins into the lumen of the gastrointestinal tract (Lunn *et al.,* 1979b). Therefore, infection may not only contribute to the ultimate development of malnutrition but may also alter its course, thereby determining the form of PEM that ensues.

All in all, the picture is one of an intensive interaction between deficient nutritional status and impaired resistance and response to infectious challenge. The end result is the high rate of mortality seen in less developed countries, especially among infants and young children. In addition, many of those who do survive bouts of these common communicable diseases of childhood such as measles suffer permanent disabling handicaps.

It is now over 20 years since Scrimshaw *et al.* (1959, 1968) first proposed the idea of synergism between malnutrition and infection (see Chapter 1). Scrimshaw and co-workers (1968) used the term *synergism* to describe this interaction because the simultaneous presence of malnutrition and infection resulted in more serious clinical consequences than would be expected from the additive effects of the two. The overall result is a strain on the viability of the host that is so great that mortality frequently occurs. Unfortunately, in many instances, we still have no clear idea of the biological basis of the mechanisms leading to the severe outcome of these interacting influences. The framework proposed by these investigators is still the most influential one in the study of nutritional immunological interactions.

IMMUNOLOGICAL DEFENSES IN PEM: CELL-MEDIATED IMMUNITY

Taken together, studies conducted in children with PEM in the Third World indicate that the aspect of the immune response most profoundly altered is cell-mediated immunity. Perhaps the first substantial evidence that PEM resulted in defective cell-mediated immunity was the severe thymic atrophy observed by Jackson (1925) at autopsy in children dying of kwashiorkor in Central Africa. However, because the central role of the thymus in immunobiology was yet to be established (Miller, 1964), little attention was paid to these findings. More recent studies assessing thymic size by radiographic shadow have confirmed decreased thymic weights in PEM children (Golden *et al.,* 1977; Chandra, 1981d). Further studies have indicated that the weights of both the thymus and the spleen were low at autopsy in children with PEM; chronic thymic atrophy was marked (Smythe *et al.,* 1971) (Table IX). On histological examination, the thymus was found to be depleted of small lymphocytes, with significant degeneration of the Hassel's corpuscles (Chandra, 1981a). Peripheral lymphoid tissues were also notably affected; lymph nodes showed paracortical depletion, and germinal centers were largely absent (Smythe *et al.,* 1971). Tonsil size was also shown to be significantly affected by PEM, paralleling the influence on the thymus and other lymphoid tissues. This has been suggested as a useful bedside indicator for the diagnosis of immunodeficiency secondary to malnutrition (Chandra, 1981a). In general, the lesions found in children with kwashiorkor were more serious than those in children with marasmus, this being consistent with the framework developed above (Smythe *et al.,* 1971).

The numbers of various cell types in peripheral blood have been considered indicative of the degree of impairment in the immune response in children with PEM (Table X). A substantial percentage of such children have absolute lymphocyte counts of less than $2500/mm^3$ (Smythe *et al.,* 1971). More importantly, the absolute lymphocyte count was demonstrated to be an important predictive indicator of impending mortality in children with PEM (Smythe *et al.,* 1971; Alleyne *et al.,* 1977; Keusch, 1981). For

Table IX

Postmortem Findings in Groups A and B (without features of PCM), Group C (Marasmus), and Group D (Kwashiorkor)[a]

	Group			
	A	B	C	D
Number	27	21	23	47
Mean body weight (%)	102	82	59	69
Thymus (%)				
Thymic weight (%)	96	69	37	30
Normal histology (%)	48	29	8	0
Acute involution (%)	45	33	22	15
Chronic atrophy (%)	7	38	70	85
Mean thickness thymic lobule (μm)	1172	911	538	476
Spleen				
Splenic weight (%)	69	68	70	54
Lymphoid tissue				
Mean tonsillar area (mm^2)	44	43	23	22
Mean thickness Peyer's patch (μm)	765	720	575	405
Mean lymphoid tissue of appendix (μm)	675	540	405	360
Paracortical depletion (%)				
None	74	65	59	30
Partial	22	15	36	40
Marked	4	20	5	30
Germinal centers				
Present all sites (%)	56	33	22	10
Mixed (%)	29	48	48	45
Absent (%)	15	19	30	45

[a]Reproduced with permission from Smythe et al. (1971).

instance, in one study, a total peripheral lymphocyte count of less than $2500/mm^3$ was found in only 1/63 children who survived, as opposed to 13/49 who subsequently died (Smythe et al., 1971). More recent studies have shown that the percentage of rosette-forming cells, an indicator of the number of T lymphocytes, seemed to be consistently decreased in PEM (Chandra, 1977; Neumann et al., 1977; Salimonu and Osunkoya, 1980; Keusch, 1981; Salimonu et al., 1982a,b). In addition, the mean percentage of null cells, i.e., lymphocytes that do not bear surface markers of either T or B lymphocytes and that may represent incompletely differentiated pre-T lymphocytes, was significantly increased (Chandra, 1977, 1979a)

The increase in the number of null cells may be directly related to the impaired production of thymic hormones, as reflected by reduced levels of thymic hormone activity found in serum obtained from children with PEM (Chandra, 1979b). Most recently, this finding has been further supported by

Table X

Lymphocyte Subpopulations in Ten Malnourished Children and Matched Controls[a]

Subject	Age (months)/sex	Weight (% of standard)	Total leukocytes/ mm³	Absolute lymphocytes/ mm³	E-rosetting lymphocytes (%)	sIg-bearing lymphocytes (%)	EAC-rosetting lymphocytes (%)	F-receptor-bearing lymphocytes (%)	Null cells (%)
				Malnourished ($n = 10$)					
1	6/M	55	8,600	2838	35	20	16	18	45
2	10/M	50	5,200	1560	18	17	15	14	65
3	12/M	64	8,100	3564	30	20	19	15	50
4	12/F	60	10,500	2205	41	25	20	15	34
5	15/M	58	7,600	1520	35	22	20	19	43
6	18/M	68	7,200	2376	25	18	15	16	57
7	18/M	75	12,500	5000	44	16	12	14	40
8	20/F	70	9,800	3038	32	22	21	21	46
9	24/M	60	8,400	2940	15	20	15	15	65
10	30/M	62	5,600	2240	18	21	16	18	61
Mean ± SEM	16.3 ± 2.2	62.2 ± 2.3[b]	8250 ± 1124	2726 ± 686	20.9 ± 3.1[c]	20.9 ± 0.9	16.9 ± 0.9	16.5 ± 0.7	50.6 ± 3.1[c]
				Healthy ($n = 10$)					
Mean ± SEM	16.5 ± 2.2	87.8 ± 1.9[b]	7650 ± 1098	3243 ± 415	68.0 ± 1.4[c]	23.0 ± 1.7	18.3 ± 1.1	17.8 ± 0.9	9.0 ± 1.1[c]

[a]Reproduced with permission from Chandra (1981a).
[b]Statistically significant difference ($p < .01$).
[c]Statistically significant difference ($p < .001$).

evidence that the percentage of cells able to form rosettes that were obtained from children with PEM could be enhanced *in vitro* by supplying biological factors obtained from thymus (Jackson and Zaman, 1980; Olusi *et al.,* 1980). Indeed, it has been suggested that such biologically active products obtained from the thymus might be employed as a means of therapeutic intervention, at least to ameliorate partially cell-mediated immunity defects in individuals with PEM (Chandra, 1981b). The mechanism probably involves an alteration in stem cell development; in addition, elevated levels of plasma corticosteroids, such as those observed in PEM, are known to affect immune cell populations and probably contribute to the phenomenon as well.

Functional parameters of cell-mediated immunity have also been studied in protein-energy malnourished subjects, and defective cellular immunity has often been seen. The *in vitro* test perhaps most widely utilized is peripheral blood lymphocyte transformation in response to stimulation with mitogens, which results in nonspecific activation of lymphocyte proliferation. The response to mitogens known to activate T cells specifically, e.g., concanavalin A and phytohemagglutinin, has frequently been demonstrated to be depressed (Smythe *et al.,* 1971; Chandra, 1972; Sellmeyer *et al.,* 1972; Work *et al.,* 1973; Kulapongs *et al.,* 1977a,b). Nutritional supplementation of such individuals has been shown to be associated with recovery of normal or even elevated mitogen responsiveness (Kulapongs *et al.,* 1977a,b). However, the results have proven quite variable, with some investigators finding normal responses to mitogens (Schlesinger and Stekel, 1974). The mitogenic response varies substantially depending on the source and especially the dose of mitogen, the culture conditions including the duration of incubation in the presence of the mitogen, and the type of serum utilized to sustain the cells. Moreover, Chandra (1980a,b,) found that while the total response to mitogens was depressed, when considered on the basis of stimulation per rosetting T lymphocyte, much of the decrease in mitogen responsiveness could be accounted for by a fewer number of cells.

Intensive investigation has revealed that serum obtained from malnourished children contains factors capable of inhibiting immunological responses such as *in vitro* lymphocyte transformation (Chandra, 1974; Moore *et al.,* 1974; Heyworth and Brown, 1975). Other investigators have shown that autologous plasma obtained from PEM patients fails to promote optimal responsiveness of T cells to mitogens (Beatty and Dowdle, 1979). Such factor(s) may be related to those responsible for decreased rosetting of T cells in PEM (Salimonu and Osunkoya, 1980; Salimonu *et al.,* 1982a,b). It is possible that prolonged or abnormal synthesis or impaired degradation of immunosuppressive embryonal proteins such as α-fetoprotein may be involved (Chandra and Bhujwala, 1977). The precise nature of this defect in lymphocyte responsiveness remains to be elucidated and deserves attention.

Another means of assessing cell-mediated immunity *in vitro* involves the study of those factors elaborated by lymphocytes that have been sensitized to mitogens or antigens. The production of macrophage MIF was found to be depressed in children with PEM (Chandra, 1980a,b). Reports concerning leukocyte MIF have been mixed, with some investigators reporting low levels of activity (Lomnitzer *et al.,* 1976) and others reporting levels within normal ranges. All have been unable to demonstrate a correlation between the production of these factors and the degree of PEM or the incidence and/or severity of infection. The production of interferon by lymphocytes obtained from marasmic children and activated *in vitro* by Newcastle disease virus was shown to be reduced (Schlesinger *et al.,* 1976). However, a study of *in vivo* interferon production in response to challenge with measles virus failed to show defective production of this lymphokine (Whittle *et al.,* 1980). These investigators found that rather than a defect in interferon production, there was another unexplained factor responsible for the increased virus production observed in cultured cells obtained from PEM children. These authors also found that peripheral blood cells obtained from malnourished children killed HeLa cells infected with measles virus as effectively as did cells taken from healthy, adequately nourished donors (Whittle *et al.,* 1980). This was true of both antibody-dependent and antibody-independent cytotoxicity. Of particular interest was the fact that antibody-dependent cellular cytotoxicity in children with PEM who subsequently died was significantly below that in cells obtained from children who eventually survived (Whittle *et al.,* 1980).

The principal means of assessing cell-mediated immunity *in vivo* is to examine the delayed hypersensitivity response to a variety of antigens; this procedure has been widely employed with undernourished children (Cunningham-Rundles, 1982).The depressed tuberculin reaction following vaccination with bacille Calmette Guérin (BCG) was the initial functional evidence that cell-mediated immunity and cutaneous hypersensitivity might be impaired in PEM (Harland and Brown, 1965). In rural East Africa, far less than half of the children with PEM had a positive Mantoux test after vaccination with BCG (Brown and Katz, 1965; Harland and Brown, 1965; Lloyd, 1968). Indeed, Brown and Katz (1965) found that not 1 of 31 children hospitalized with PEM had a positive skin test for tuberculosis. Of even greater significance was the fact that impaired tuberculin reactions occurred with even marginal changes in nutritional status (Harland and Brown, 1965). These alterations in host response to cutaneous administration of antigens have important implications for screening programs for diseases such as tuberculosis among malnourished populations.

A substantial depression of delayed hypersensitivity to a wide variety of antigens has been shown in children with severe PEM (Smythe *et al.,* 1971; Chandra, 1972, 1974; Abassy *et al.,* 1974a; Schlesinger and Stekel, 1974; Neumann *et al.,* 1975). PEM affects the total number of children who are able to respond at all, as well as the magnitude of the response (Chandra, 1980a,b). In addition, children described as having only moderate PEM also experienced a depression of delayed cutaneous hypersensitivity (Ziegler and Ziegler, 1975; Reddy *et al.,* 1976b). It should be kept in mind that this defect in immunological function may involve impaired recognition of the specific antigenic determinant, a defective proliferative response of specific lymphocyte subsets, a depression of the acute inflammatory response, or any combination of these phenomena. The degree of the defect remains to be established, and may vary with the type and severity of malnutrition being studied.

Thus, in general, cell-mediated immunity seems to be affected fairly substantially by PEM. However, nearly all of the attempts to establish the nature of the defect in cellular immunity have been equivocal. A substantial amount of information has also been derived from studies in experimental animals; this will be presented in subsequent chapters. While such experimental evidence no doubt helps to define the nature of the interaction between nutritional status, immunological function, and resistance to infectious disease, the implications of these findings for the situation in Third World countries are not always clear. As has been pointed out, the PEM syndrome is quite variable and thus cannot be characterized easily in precise clinical terms. However, the need at present is to find the mechanisms that lead to impaired immune function in the inadequately nourished host. This will require the utilization of the most sophisticated laboratory and diagnostic techniques being developed in both immunology and nutrition. It is quite possible that many of the inconsistencies that have plagued field studies may be attributed to variation in the degree of PEM in the individuals studied and to deficiencies of specific nutrients, many of which have now been shown to alter immunocompetence and which thereby further complicate the study of nutritional immunological interactions. With elucidation of the levels of this synergistic interaction, much more efficient consideration of potential therapeutic regimes will be possible

HUMORAL IMMUNITY IN PEM

In general, there are two ways to assess the functional competence of humoral or antibody-mediated immunity. The first is to quantify the levels of total immunoglobulin present in serum or other bodily fluids. The second is to quantify the response to a challenge with a specific antigen. Because of the relative ease of RID, the first method has been widely employed worldwide with reasonably consistent results. In nearly all instances, total levels of serum immunoglobulins were either similar to those seen in control children or, in many cases, were elevated above these norms (Brown and Katz, 1965; Keet and Thom, 1969; McFarlane *et al.* 1970; Watson and Freesemann, 1970; Alvarado and Luthringer, 1971; Purtilo *et al.,* 1976) (Tables XI, XII, Fig. 4). An informative study by Cohen and Hansen (1962) showed that while albumin synthesis was decreased to one-third the level observed in well-nourished controls, synthesis of γ globulins remained relatively stable; in response to infectious challenge, an appropriate threefold elevation in the rate of immunoglobulin synthesis was noted. While increased levels of IgM, IgG, and IgA are frequently observed, children with PEM are most likely to have elevated levels of serum IgA (Fig. 5). Such increases in all of the immunoglobulins are most likely due to continual exposure to infectious challenge, and the particularly high titers of IgA in the serum probably reflect the chronic stimulation of cells in the gut that secrete IgA in response to the bacterial pathogens in the gut and the constant diarrheal disease that ensues.

Elevated levels of serum IgE are also seen in children with PEM (Johansson *et al.,* 1968). One possible explanation for this is the frequency of helminth infections in such individuals, which are known to result in elevated titers of IgE (Purtilo *et al.,* 1976). It may also indicate an increased hypersensitivity to a variety of allergens, perhaps secondary to defective suppressor cell function. While reactions to common allergens may not be elevated in children with PEM (Abassy *et al.,* 1974a,b) this may be due to an inability to generate the inflammatory response of the cutaneous hypersensitivity reaction (Neumann *et al.,* 1975). Increased levels of serum IgE may

Table XI
Immunoglobulin Levels (Mean ± SE) in Malnourished and Normal Children[a]

Immunoglobulin class	Group I: severe malnutrition	Group II: moderate malnutrition	Group III: normal	U.S. standards
IgG, mg/100 ml	1830 ± 85	1645 ± 55	1690 ± 70	700–1100
IgM, mg/100 ml	175 ± 10	155 ± 7	145 ± 7	40–80
IgA, mg/100 ml	125 ± 10	135 ± 11	120 ± 10	40–100
IgD, mg/100 ml	9 ± 1	7 ± 1	8 ± 0.5	0.7–17
IgE, IU	1115 ± 245	805 ± 195	585 ± 120	40–210

[a]Reproduced with permission from Work *et al.* (1973).

Table XII

Serum Immunoglobulins in the Groups of Children Studied[a]

Group	Immunoglobulins		
	IgG	IgA	IgM
Malnourished	1201 ± 465	203 ± 98	126 ± 118
	(25)	(25)[b,c]	(25)
Recovered	1210 ± 456	130 ± 87	97 ± 44
	(12)	(12)[b]	(12)
Controls	977 ± 136	83 ± 40	64 ± 30
	(14)	(14)[c]	(14)

[a]Reproduced with permission from Alvarado and Luthringer (1971).

[b]$p < .05$ within groups.

[c]$p < .001$ within groups.

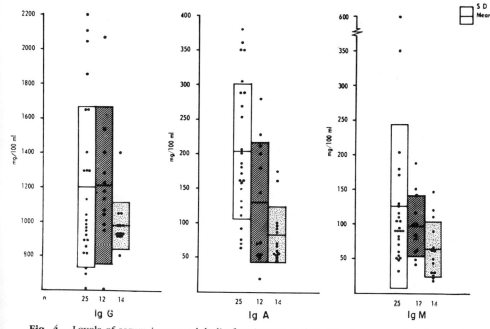

Fig. 4. Levels of serum immunoglobulin fractions in malnourished, recovered and control children. □, PCM; ▨, recovered; ▨, controls. Reproduced with permission from Alvarado and Luthringer (1971).

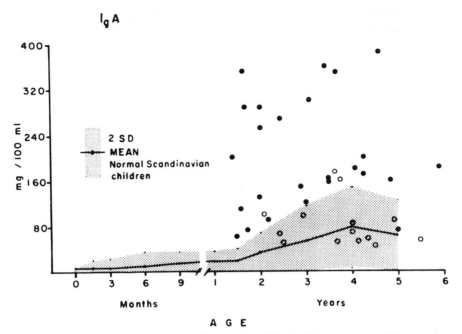

Fig. 5. Serum IgA levels in protein-calorie malnourished children and normal Guatemalan controls, compared with healthy Scandinavian children. ●, PCM children; ○, normal controls. Adapted from D. O. Johansson and T. Berg, *Acta Paediatr. Scand.* **56**; 572–579 (1967). Reproduced with permission from Alvarado and Luthringer (1971).

be related to the increased uptake of a variety of macromolecules from the intestinal lumen and the elevated levels of antibodies to common food antigens (Chandra, 1974). It is interesting to note that on nutritional supplementation, a certain percentage of PEM children develop eczema. There are exceptions to these observations of normal or elevated serum immunoglobulin levels in children with PEM. If malnutrition occurred during gestation or early in lactation, when the lymphoid system and normal intact immunocompetence develop, levels of serum immunoglobulins may be low and such children may require a protracted period in which to develop a normal serum immunoglobulin profile (Aref *et al.,* 1970). The importance of nutritional factors during the development of the immune system will be covered in Chapter 5.

The other means of evaluating the functional capability of humoral immune responses is to determine the response to challenge with a specific antigen. Often the antigens employed are vaccines that are routinely utilized throughout the developed and developing worlds to prevent disease. Thus, the response to these antigens in PEM individuals has enormous practical implications, as well as being helpful in attempting to define nutritional immunological interactions. As early as 1948, Gell found that antibody titers to antigens such as heterologous erythrocytes and to tobacco mosaic virus were significantly depressed in adult prisoners of war (Gell, 1948). Since that time, the response to a wide variety of antigenic determinants has been studied in children with PEM. In general, it seems that the response to a specific antigen is determined by the nature and dose of the antigen and the degree of malnutrition present in the subjects being evaluated. For instance, responses to diphtheria, typhoid, and yellow fever are all reduced in PEM (Reddy and Srikantia, 1964; Brown and Katz, 1965, 1966a; Chandra, 1972). In contrast, the specific antibody response to challenge with tetanus and polio virus is essentially normal (Pretorius and de Villiers, 1962; Chandra, 1972; Salimonu *et al.,* 1982a,b). The response to measles virus and measles vaccination has proven quite variable, being reported as either normal or decreased (Hafez *et al.,* 1977; Ifekwunigwe *et al.,* 1980; Salimonu *et al.,* 1982a,b) (Table XIII). These findings are of critical signifi-

Table XIII

Seroconversion Rates to Measles Vaccination by Age, Sex, and Nutritional Status—
Eastern Nigeria (Biafra),1970[a]

Variables	n	Seroconversion[b] (%)	Geometric mean titer rise at 4 weeks (± SD)	P[c]
Age (years)				
<1	14	100	8.9 ± 2.0	
1	17	94	8.4 ± 2.4	
2–4	58	90	7.6 ± 3.2	NS[d]
5+	22	96	7.8 ± 2.5	
Sex				
Male	58	95	8.2 ± 2.5	
Female	53	92	7.6 ± 3.0	NS
Nutritional status (by Gomez[e] criteria of median weight for age)				
Normal (>90%)	19	95	7.5 ± 2.2	
Malnutrition				
Mild (75–90%)	9	89	8.8 ± 3.8	
Moderate (60–75%)	71	92	7.9 ± 3.0	
Severe (<60%)	12	100	7.9 ± 1.9	NS
Total	111	94	7.9 ± 2.7	

[a]Reproduced with permission from Ifekwunigwe *et al.* (1980).
[b]Convalescent sera had a titer ≥ 1:20
[c]By one-way analysis of variance.
[d]Not significant.
[e]From Gomez, 1956.

cance in the worldwide attempt to reduce mortality from measles. Indeed, because of the importance of responsiveness to such specific antigens for vaccination programs throughout the world, it is critical to define the conditions under which vaccination programs will be reasonably successful. Under some conditions, nutritional supplementation has resulted in enhanced antibody production to specific antigens; some such preliminary remedial measures may be necessary before vaccination programs can be successful in some areas (Matthews *et al.,* 1972).

It is possible that one mechanism contributing to the decreased response to certain antigens is a reduction in antibody affinity (Reinhardt and Stewart, 1979). Such a reduction has been observed under certain circumstances, especially with the thymic-dependent as well as macrophage-processed antigens. This decreased antibody affinity in PEM may be related to a number of factors, including (1) inadequate availability of essential amino acids required for synthesis of the combining variable of the antibody molecule, (2) dysfunction of the T-cell subsets responsible for regulating the synthesis and assembly as well as the specificity of the combining variable region of the immunoglobulin molecule, and (3) high levels of serum corticosteroids that may interfere with antibody-binding capacity.

The final aspect of humoral immunity that may be affected by PEM and thus may contribute substantially to immunodeficiency and impaired resistance to disease is the secretory antibody response. In general, in PEM, levels of secretory IgA and lysozyme are low in a variety of bodily secretions, tears, mucus, saliva, etc. (Chandra, 1975a; McMurray *et al.,* 1977; Watson *et al.,* 1978). However, not all investigators have found such changes; Bell *et al.* (1976) found normal or even increased levels of secretory IgA in children with PEM and concurrent infection. It is interesting to note that while serum antibody responses to polio immunization were normal in the protein-energy malnourished child, secretory antibody responses to polio virus vaccine and measles virus vaccine were markedly depressed (Chandra, 1975a). Indeed, some children showed no detectable levels of secretory IgA at all. The mechanism involved in the impairment of the secretory immune responses may involve decreased synthesis of an essential constituent of the secretory IgA molecule, e.g., secretory component, or an alteration of immune cell populations in gut-associated lymphoid tissue, and/or decreased numbers of mucosal plasma cells producing IgA (Chandra, 1980b). This impairment of the secretory antibody response may be part of the elusive explanation of the inability of the malnourished host to respond to measles virus (Whittle *et al.,* 1980). In addition, defective secretory immune responses would seem to have serious implications for other infectious disorders that involve the immune mechanisms in mucous membranes, e.g., gastroenteritis and upper respiratory tract infections. Deficient secretory immunity may also contribute to the above-mentioned inappropriate absorption of foreign macromolecules that may facilitate allergic reactions.

NONSPECIFIC IMMUNE FUNCTION IN PEM

Nonspecific host defense mechanisms include a very diverse group of body structures and serum factors that defend the host organism against pathological challenge. Such nonspecific host defense mechanisms include (1) normal microbial flora (gut flora), (2) anatomic barriers (skin, mucous membranes, endothelial surfaces, (3) secretory substances (lysozyme, hydrochloric acid, mucus), (4) febrile responses, (5) metabolic responses (e.g., endocrine alterations), and (6) an altered physicochemical environment (e.g., alterations in serum and tissue trace element levels) (Douglas, 1981).

The effects of PEM on some of these nonspecific defense mechanisms are obvious and have already been noted. The gut flora are notably altered in malnutrition, which probably contributes to the increased incidence of diarrheal disease in children with PEM. The first apparent signs of many nutritional deficiencies are alterations in the integrity of the anatomic barriers such as epidermis and mucous membranes. Such lesions are characteristic features of PEM and, no doubt, predispose the child to a variety of local and systemic infections. In sharp contrast, virtually nothing is known about the effects of nutritional factors on the development and maintenance of endothelial cell surfaces and basement membranes; this is an area that demands attention.

As noted above, levels of many secretory substances with important host defense functions are altered by PEM, e.g., gastric acid and lysozyme in lacrimal secretions (McMurray et al., 1977; Watson et al., 1978). Impaired secretion of hydrochloric acid may result in increased pH in the gastrointestinal tract, allowing the multiplication and passage into the small intestine of pathogens responsible for diarrheal disease. It may even allow the survival of sufficient numbers of the pathogen *Vibrio cholerae* to threaten the life of the patient. Faulty body temperature regulation, noted above, may preclude the development of the normal febrile response; the latter is an integral part of the intact host defense (Keusch, 1977). Moreover, overall homeostatic regulation is markedly altered in PEM, and these changes may counteract or obviate many of the normal homeostatic responses to infectious challenge.

Phagocytic cell function in PEM has been examined fairly extensively, with somewhat variable results. Populations of circulating phagocytic cells

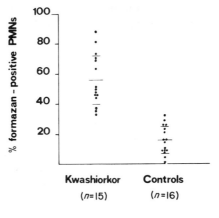

Fig. 6.   NBT test. Individual cases are plotted and mean ± SD are indicated.   Reproduced
with permission from Schopfer and Douglas (1976b).

are essentially normal or increased; very little is known regarding the
number of analogous phagocytes in tissues. Examination of neutrophils obtained from children with PEM shows cytologic abnormalities, with the
presence of Dohle bodies and frequent cytoplasmic vacuolization (Schopfer
and Douglas, 1976b). When such neutrophils were studied *in vivo* utilizing
the Rebuck skin window technique, elevated neutrophil chemotaxis and
depression of mononuclear cell chemotoxis were demonstrated (Schopfer
and Douglas, 1976b). The actual phagocytic process consists of two phases:
(1) the engulfment or uptake of foreign material, and (2) intracellular killing. Initial studies indicated that polymorphonuclear leukocytes (PMNs)
obtained from malnourished children and adults show deficient energy
production via the glycolytic pathway, as evidenced by reduced lactate
production (Balch and Spencer, 1954; Selvaraj and Bhat, 1972a,b; Seth and
Chandra, 1972). Despite these metabolic alterations, no defect in the actual
phagocytic uptake process has been demonstrated (Table XIV, Fig. 7). Engulfment of artificial substances such as IgG-coated sheep erythrocytes and
polystyrene latex, and actual organisms such as *Candida albicans* and *Staphylococcus aureus,* was normal in blood monocytes and neutrophils isolated from protein-energy malnourished children (Schopfer and Douglas,
1976b). However, once particle uptake occurred, the bactericidal capacity
of PMNs was substantially compromised. While the nitroblue tetrazolium
(NBT) test has been shown to be normal at times, it is generally abnormal in
PEM (Kendall and Nolan, 1972; Schopfer and Douglas, 1976b) (Fig. 6). As
with other immunological parameters, these studies have been complicated
by specific nutrient deficiencies and methodological inconsistencies. The

Table XIV

Enzyme Activities and Glycolysis[a]

	Controls (n = 8)	Kwashiorkor[b] (n =11)
Enzyme activities (μmol/10⁶ PMN/min)		
Hexokinase (10^{-3})	0.48 ± 0.35	0.63 ± 0.45
Fructokinase (10^{-3})	3.93 ± 1.8	4.86 ± 0.45
Glycerate kinase (10^{-1})	1.12 ± 0.17	1.36 ± 0.42
Pyruvate kinase (10^{-2})	10.29 ± 0.34	9.71 ± 1.2
Glucose-6-phosphate dehydrogenase (10^{-3})	2.49 ± 0.78	2.58 ± 1.8
Myeloperoxidase (10^{-1})	7.83 ± 2.35	8.55 ± 4.9
NADPH-oxidase (10^{-5})	3.28 ± 2.35	3.55 ± 0.74
NADH-oxidase (10^{-5})	0.38 ± 0.26	0.26 ± 0.18
Glutathione reductase (10^{-5})	0.26 ± 0.08	0.25 ± 0.11
Lactate production (nanmol/10⁶ PMN)		
Resting	28.3 ± 8.6	13.4 ± 9.5
Phagocytizing	37.6 ± 5.2	38.5 ± 7.4

[a]Reproduced with permission from Schopfer and Douglas (1976b).
[b]Mean ± SD.

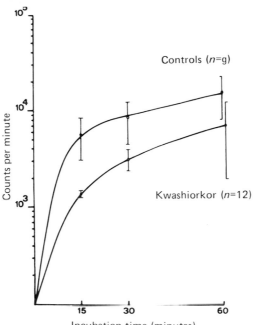

Fig. 7. Kinetics of leukocyte iodination (mean ± SD). ^{131}I incorporation into TCA proteins by phagocytizing PMNs. Count per minute per 5 × 10⁶ cells. Reproduced with permission from Schopfer and Douglas (1976b).

defective bactericidal capacity is most likely the result of a decrease in the activity of one of the enzymes central to the killing function (Selvaraj and Bhat, 1972a,b).

Investigation of the complement system in PEM has indicated decreased levels of total hemolytic activity attributed to complement as well as a decrease in the level of all complement components except C4 (Suskind *et al.,* 1976a,b). However, not all studies report such a total depletion of all complement components (Haller *et al.,* 1978). Results of some studies have suggested a possibly increased consumption of complement components, particularly C3 by the alternative pathway (Haller *et al.,* 1978). It is possible that PEM may be characterized by deficient synthesis and secretion of those factors associated with the alternative complement pathway.

Experimental animals with induced PEM have been shown to be deficient in serum opsonic activity for a number of *E. coli* strains tested, especially these opsonized by the alternative complement pathway (Keusch *et al.,* 1978a,b). In human studies, opsonization was shown to be deficient in severely protein-energy malnourished Thai children. Keusch *et al.* (1981) have found that more moderate PEM did not depress the acute inflammatory response to a variety of stimuli of the serum level of components considered responsible for the mediation of inflammation. Opsonic activity of C3, C4, and IgA, and hemolytic activity of complement, were not low for these same children with moderate to mild malnutrition. In contrast, children whose severe PEM developed acutely had low levels of these opsonics and defective complement activation.

There are a number of acute-phase proteins that seem to be important in regulating the inflammatory response; in PEM, there may be a decreased response of acute-phase reactants to infectious challenge. Metalloproteins such as ceruloplasmin, lactoferrin, and transferrin seem to be altered in PEM (Antia *et al.,* 1968). Ceruloplasmin and other copper metalloproteins such as copper-zinc superoxide dismutase may modulate various inflammatory responses, e.g., enzyme release from lysosomes (Ackerman *et al.,* 1980), neutrophil chemotactic response (Ackerman *et al.,* 1980), scavenging of superoxide anions (Goldstein *et al.,* 1979), and possible modulation of some lymphocyte responses (Lipsky and Ziff, 1980). Transferrin is an iron-containing protein that has a role as a bactericidal agent. When serum levels of transferrin decrease, unbound free iron that is absorbed from the gut may favor the multiplication of bacteria (Alleyne *et al.,* 1977). It has been shown that human T lymphocytes also synthesize and secrete iron-binding proteins, and these proteins may also mediate immunological surveillance (Dorner *et al.,* 1980). Indeed, it has been shown that levels of serum transferrin are a good prognostic index of the eventual outcome of PEM (Antia *et al.,* 1968).

5

Nutritional Factors and Immune Ontogeny

INTRODUCTION

In considering the influences of nutritional factors on immunocompetence, it is extremely important to distinguish the effects of nutrition on immunological function in adults from those on neonatal or developing organisms. Young animals undergo rapid growth and development, and are therefore subjected to heightened physiological stress; thus, insufficient availability of essential nutrients is more critical in this age group than in adults. Nutritional deficiencies that may not result in an impaired immune response in adult animals or humans may cause notable dysfunction in the developing fetus or neonate, rendering it more susceptible to a variety of infectious agents. Moreover, should the essential nutrient deficiency occur during a particularly critical period of development or embryogenesis, the capacity for normal immune ontogenesis may be permanently compromised. Consequently, even prolonged periods of subsequent nutritional rehabilitation in such animals may not result in an acceptable level of immunological function. A wide variety of nutrients have now been shown to be essential during gestation and/or lactation for the normal development and maintenance of immunocompetence in mammals.

HUMAN STUDIES

While the influence of nutritional deficiencies in adult life has been fairly well characterized, much less is known regarding the impact of very early nutrient shortages. Several types of protocols have been developed to study the immediate and long-term effects of nutritional stress during gestation or the postnatal period, i.e., while the immune system is developing. In this chapter, we have grouped studies into prenatal and postnatal categories, although in many field surveys in which postnatal malnutrition is being considered, it is quite likely that substantial prenatal nutritional deprivation may also have occurred.

Most clinical studies of the fetal period have focused on fetuses characterized as displaying intrauterine growth retardation (IUGR) (also known as *small for gestational age* or *small for date*), which means that gestation was of normal duration (38–40 weeks) but that the birth weight was low when compared with some arbitrary standard (e.g., the 3rd percentile of the Harvard growth standard, 2500 g). A number of factors may contribute to IUGR, including maternal malnutrition, environmental insults such as viral infections, or various pathological conditions such as placental insufficiency. Studies of IUGR related to nutritional factors ideally should be confined to cases in which maternal malnutrition can be adequately demonstrated; in addition, premature infants should be considered separately, since in these infants it is very difficult to distinguish between the influences of gestational age and low birth weight. Thus, the most important of these studies have confined observations to infants of normal gestational length, low birth weight, and born to mothers who experienced nutritional deprivation during pregnancy. Studies of postnatal influences are plagued by similarly variable causative factors and circumstances.

The initial indication that immunological function may be impaired for long periods came from studies showing that children who had experienced IUGR were more than normally susceptible to infection during later childhood (Chandra, 1975a). In actuality, children of inadequately nourished mothers in Third World countries are the product of both a prenatal and a postnatal environment characterized by a synergistic interaction between infection and an inadequate supply of nutrients, as was pointed out in Chapter 4. Fetuses carried by such mothers often experience early and excessive antigenic stimulation (Table I), as exemplified by high levels of cord blood IgM that cannot cross the placenta (Mata *et al.,* 1971; Urrutia *et al.,* 1975). Approximately 40% of newborns studied in rural Guatemala and more than 60% of those examined in Peru had elevated levels of cord blood IgM, demonstrating levels higher than 0.2 mg/ml (Mata and Urrutia, 1971; Urrutia *et al.,* 1975). Levels of complement component C3 were also elevated in over 50% of the Peruvian cord blood samples, confirming this premature antigenic stimulation. In addition, newborn infants also had a high frequency of elevated antibody titers to specific bacterial and viral antigens immediately after birth, indicating prior antigenic confrontation.

It has also been noted that if antigenic components of bacteria and viruses

Table I

Incidence of Elevated Serum IgM Level in Newborns[a,b]

Localities	Number of infants	Number (%) of cases[c] with IgM level >0.20 mg/ml
Santa Maria Cauque, Guatemala[d]	263	111 (42)
Santo Domingo Xenacoj, Guatemala[e]	211	80 (38)
Four ladino villages in Guatemala[f]	132	18 (14)

[a]Reproduced with permission from Urrutia et al. (1975).
[b]Umbilical cord serum IgM level measured in Guatemalan newborns from rural communities, 1964–1973.
[c]Specimens with values of IgA >0.10 mg were excluded from tabulation.
[d]Blood collected by traditional folk midwives.
[e]Blood collected by a trained midwife.
[f]Blood collected by a physician.

cross the placenta at an early age, such infants may be partially or wholly tolerized to these particular antigens, thereby impairing their ability to respond to them later in life (Koster et al., 1981). More attention is now being directed to the possibility that such interactions, though of lesser magnitude, may also affect children in developed nations (Sever, 1975). However, it is far more difficult to establish such a relationship due to the more moderate maternal malnutrition and the reduced antigenic stimulation.

The consequences of nutritional deprivation occurring during gestation can be quite pervasive and may persist for many years, possibly compromising immune function permanently. Studies of small-for-date infants at autopsy indicated a notable atrophy of lymphoid tissue, particularly spleen and thymus (Watts, 1969; Naeye et al., 1971). With regard to humoral immunity, Chandra observed a significant correlation between low birth weight and serum immunoglobulin levels (Chandra, 1976). He found that infants with IUGR have a significant correlation between infant birth weight when less than 2500 g, and particularly if below 2250 g, and cord blood levels of IgG. The placental transfer of IgG_1 is affected more than that of IgG_2, especially in infants with a demonstrated defect in placental function (Chandra, 1976). In a 1-year follow-up of the latter group, serum IgG_1 levels were shown to remain, low with a pronounced physiological hypogammaglobulinemia (Chandra, 1976). These low levels of IgG_1 also correlated with increased susceptibility to bacterial infection.

Other studies have found a significant relationship between cord blood IgA levels and birth weight in small-for-gestational-age infants when the birth weight was less than 2550 g. In addition, IgA titers following immunization were depressed (Figs. 1, 2) (Chandra, 1975a). For such a profound decrease in serum immunoglobulin levels to occur, the nutritional insult must occur prior to the seventh month *in utero.* Ghavami *et al.* (1979) confirmed some of these findings and found a correlation between severe infections, low levels of IgG, and birth weights below 3500 g; this included many infants who were only marginally malnourished. Serum levels of IgA were in the low-normal region; considering the excessive antigenic stimulation these children received, this may indicate relatively deficient serum IgA production. In many of these infants, elevated levels of IgM were found, and the authors suggested that this may represent compensatory serum immunoglobulin production in the face of decreased levels of IgG. It may also represent excessive antigenic stimulation *in utero,* leading to elevated levels of IgM synthesis. Virtually nothing is known regarding the effects of gestational nutrient deficits on titers of serum IgD or IgE. Certainly, both merit considerable attention: studies of serum IgD levels may help elucidate the role of nutritional factors in the evolution of a normal immunoglobulin profile, and studies of IgE may unlock some of the mysteries surrounding the burgeoning pediatric problem of food allergies.

Low-birth-weight infants (birth weights ranging from 1800 to 2800 g) were also demonstrated to have a sharply decreased percentage of surface immunoglobulin-positive cells (only 380 ± 195 Ig$^+$/mm^3 compared with

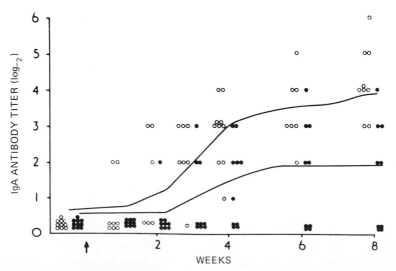

Fig. 1. Level of specific IgA antibody to poliovirus type 1 before and after a single oral dose of live attenuated trivalent poliovirus vaccine. O, healthy children; ●, malnourished children. Reproduced with permission from Chandra (1975a).

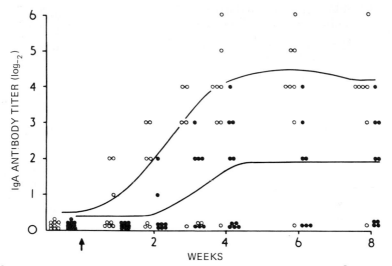

Fig. 2. Preimmunization and postimmunization measles IgA antibody titers. ○, healthy children; ●, malnourished children. Reproduced with permission from Chandra (1975a).

1485 ± 810 Ig$^+$/mm^3 in age-matched control subjects) (Moscatelli *et al.,* 1976) (Table II). In most cases, differences between IUGR infants and controls were narrowed after 3–4 weeks of nutritional supplementation, but in some children no significant improvement was observed even at 2–3 months of age.

The influence of IUGR on the antibody response to specific antigenic challenge seems to depend on the nature of the antigen in question. When typhoid and tetanus toxoid vaccines were administered, antibody responses were within normal ranges in infants who had suffered significant degrees of

Table II

Absolute Numbers (mean $\pm$ 1 SD) of B and T Lymphocytes in Peripheral Blood of Small-for-Date Infants Compared with Newborns of Normal Birth Weight[a]

	Lymphocytes/mm^3	Ig-bearing lymphocytes/mm^3	Rosette-forming cells/mm^3
Small-for-date infants ($n = 19$)	2936 ± 1312	380 ± 195	900 ± 616
Infants with appropriate birth weight ($n = 30$)	5500 ± 1800	1485 ± 810	2915 ± 1150

[a]Reproduced with permission from Moscatelli *et al.* (1976).

IUGR (Chandra, 1975a). In contrast, when live attenuated poliovirus vaccine was administered, while most IUGR infants did experience seroconversion, the mean titer of specific antibodies was significantly low at both 4 and 8 weeks postimmunization. Such findings are significant for any public health vaccination programs, including those for infants with IUGR.

One of the first studies to follow up on humoral immune parameters of infants malnourished early in postnatal life indicated that marked immunosuppression resulted from such nutritional deficiencies and that this defective immunocompetence persisted for prolonged periods. Children with kwashiorkor who experienced clinical disease prior to the age of 7 months showed deficient production of all immunoglobulins studied (IgM, IgA, and IgG). Serum levels of IgA and IgM were especially low even at 4 months of age, with most of the children studied having no detectable IgM; many children still had undetectable levels of IgM even at 7–8 months (Aref *et al.,* 1970). In children aged 1–4 years who had experienced early-onset kwashiorkor, the aberrant levels of serum immunoglobulins continued to persist. While total serum immunoglobulin levels were normal or high, IgG tended to be high, and IgM was consistently quite low, children as old as 4.5 years had no detectable IgM. IgA levels in serum were quite variable. For example, many infants subjected to early nutritional deprivation showed only a trace of IgA, while others had slightly reduced or even elevated levels. Thus, despite years of nutritional rehabilitation, the serum immunoglobulin profile remained highly aberrant if nutritional insults occurred early in life. Although not specifically stated, it is quite possible that nutritional deficiencies also occurred *in utero,* since most of these children were born to mothers from a deprived socioeconomic environment. Different degrees of coincident nutritional deficiencies during gestation, along with complicating specific nutrient deficiencies, may have contributed to the variability in some immune parameters.

More recently, the persistence of defects in serum immunoglobulin levels in children who had experienced early postnatal nutritional deprivation (e.g., during the first 6 months of life) has been confirmed. Children between 1 and 9 years of age continued to exhibit significantly decreased levels of serum IgM, while most other immune parameters were within normal ranges. The influence of protein in the diet during this early postnatal period has been studied, both retrospectively (Table III) and prospectively (Table IV). In particular, studies have been performed utilizing isocaloric diets containing either 2.5 or 4.0 g/kg body weight/day throughout the first year of life (Zoppi *et al.,* 1978). Both serum IgG and total γ globulin levels were significantly lower in children on the lower-protein diet monitored at 5, 7, or 10 months of age (Table IV). Serum IgM and IgA levels were also slightly lower, but these differences were not

Table III

Morbidity of Infants in Retrospective Study

	2.5 g/kg/day protein diet	4.0 g/kg/day protein diet
Number of infants studied	180	107
Number of infants with infections	176	93
Number of episodes of infections	510	145
Number of episodes per infant	2.89	1.56

[a]Reproduced with permission from Zoppi *et al.* (1978).

significant. As expected, reduced serum immunoglobulin levels correlated with morbidity in children fed the lower-protein diet, both in terms of the number of children experiencing infections and the number of infectious episodes per child; this was especially true of upper respiratory tract infections, bronchitis, and gastroenteritis (Zoppi *et al.,* 1978). Serum levels of IgD and IgE have been studied to a far lesser extent; titers of both have been shown to be elevated in children deprived of essential nutrients during the early postnatal period. In many malnourished children, detectable and often markedly elevated titers of IgD and especially IgE were observed, whereas in age-matched controls, titers of these two serum constituents were not detectable. Titers of IgG were particularly high in children with early-onset marasmus and marasmic kwashiorkor, and in most cases remained elevated even after extensive nutritional rehabilitation. Levels of IgE, in contrast, generally responded to nutritional treatment and may have been related to the high incidence of parasitism seen in association with all forms of PEM. Although high levels of IgE are frequently seen in PEM, allergy is seldom associated with such nutritional deficiencies. Nonetheless, antibodies to a variety of food proteins (e.g., eggs, milk, gluten) are frequently observed in children with PEM (Chandra, 1975a).

Not all studies of the development of humoral immunity following nutritional deprivation during the early postnatal period have found such depressed levels of serum immunoglobulins. Berg (1968) found a significant correlation between serum levels of IgG and gestational age, but no correlation between full-term low-birth-weight infants and serum IgG levels. Infants of lower gestational age had a tendency toward pronounced hypogammaglobulinemia during the first months of life. In addition, the early ability to synthesize IgM by premature infants was notably impaired, and this persisted for some time. Such defects could not be found in full-term infants of

Table IV

Serum Total Protein, Protein by Electrophoresis, and Immunoglobulin Levels in Infants in Prospective Study[a][b]

	2.5 g/kg/day protein diet			4.0 g/kg/day protein diet		
	Age 164 ± 8 days	Age 194 ± 18 days	Age 301 ± 31 days	Age 165 ± 9 days	Age 217 ± 26 days	Age 297 ± 32 days
Protein (g/dl)	6.32 ± 0.28	6.58 ± 0.30	6.70 ± 0.34	6.81 ± 0.35	6.55 ± 0.25	6.83 ± 0.31
Albumin (g/dl)	4.18 ± 0.28	4.34 ± 0.33	4.34 ± 0.30	4.21 ± 0.25	3.91 ± 0.31	4.24 ± 0.36
α_1-Globulin (g/dl)	0.16 ± 0.04	0.17 ± 0.05	0.14 ± 0.03	0.15 ± 0.03	0.17 ± 0.04	0.16 ± 0.04
α_2-Globulin (g/dl)	0.75 ± 0.11	0.84 ± 0.04	0.81 ± 0.24	0.83 ± 0.08	0.83 ± 0.06	0.82 ± 0.12
β-Globulin (g/dl)	0.72 ± 0.14	0.77 ± 0.09	0.77 ± 0.23	0.80 ± 0.07	0.81 ± 0.06	0.80 ± 0.08
γ-Globulin (g/dl)	0.49 ± 0.05	0.45 ± 0.10	0.50 ± 0.06	0.82 ± 0.09	0.83 ± 0.10	0.82 ± 0.10
IgA (mg/dl)	21.67 ± 5.57	23.92 ± 8.36	28.00 ± 9.42	30.71 ± 12.32	33.31 ± 18.65	25.5 ± 9.98
IgG (mg/dl)	414.17 ± 93.51	420.00 ± 83.44	466.10 ± 71.60	596.43 ± 73.81	641.25 ± 138.06	660.7 ± 85.38
IgM (mg/dl)	79.7 ± 12.99	85.15 ± 25.49	77.20 ± 26.17	100.00 ± 33.09	104.17 ± 39.06	79.0 ± 32.40

[a]Reproduced with permission from Zoppi et al. (1978).
[b]Values are means ± SD.

low birth weight. In all infants studied, the levels of serum IgA and IgD were within normal ranges. Other investigators were also unable to document an influence of prenatal nutritional deprivation on levels of serum immunoglobulins (Bhaskaram *et al.,* 1977). It should be pointed out, however, that none of the infants in these studies showed evidence of severe nutritional deprivation (nearly all birth weights were approximately 2000 g). In addition, excessive antigenic stimulation in these children may have resulted in serum immunoglobulin levels within normal ranges, but perhaps the specific immune response would have been compromised.

Studies of cell-mediated immune function have also proven somewhat variable, although there is general agreement that if nutritional insults occur during critical periods of gestation or postnatally within 6 months after parturition, such children will have impaired cell-mediated immune responses and the defective immunological function may be long-term. In infants of low birth weight, there is thymic atrophy (Naeye *et al.,* 1971) and a reduced number of rosette-forming T lymphocytes, especially in those with birth weights of less than 2550 g (Chandra, 1974; Ferguson *et al.,* 1974; Moscatelli *et al.,* 1976; Bhaskaram *et al.,* 1977) (Figs. 3, 4) In addi-

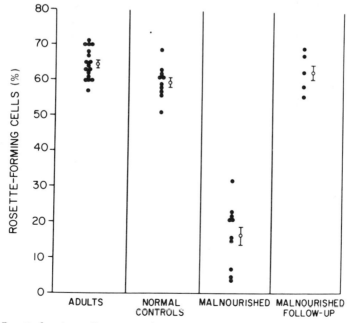

Fig. 3. Rosette-forming cells expressed as a percentage of peripheral blood lymphocytes (●) comparing Caucasian adults, normal and malnourished Ghanaian children, and malnourished children after dietary therapy. ○, mean ± SE of the mean. Reproduced with permission from Ferguson *et al.* (1974).

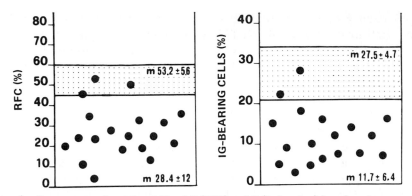

Fig. 4. Percentages of peripheral blood T (RFC) and B (Ig-bearing) lymphocytes compared with those in newborns with normal birth weight. ⊡, normal values.   Reproduced with permission from Moscatelli *et al.* (1976).

tion, those cells that formed rosettes bound significantly fewer sheep erythrocytes (Moscatelli *et al.,* 1976). Moscatelli *et al.* (1976) showed that when T lymphocytes obtained from IUGR infants were incubated with thymosin prior to the rosette assay, there was a significant increase in the proportion of lymphocytes that formed rosettes with SRBC. As has been demonstrated with older children who experienced PEM, it is possible that the serum of these IUGR infants contained some factor that inhibits rosette formation by T lymphocytes (Olusi *et al.,* 1978). Even after years of nutritional rehabilitation, the percentage of lymphocytes forming rosettes, i.e., T lymphocytes, remained significantly low in older children who had experienced IUGR, even though the difference in the absolute number of T cells, although lower in IUGR children, was not statistically significant.

As a further indication that cell-mediated immunity is impaired in IUGR, delayed cutaneous hypersensitivity responses to a battery of skin test antigens including phytohemagglutinin, SK-SD, DNCB, *Candida,* and *Trichophyton* have all been found to be consistently low (Chandra, 1974; Ferguson *et al.,* 1974; Ghavami *et al.,* 1979). Not only did IUGR children respond poorly to these skin test antigens, most small-for-gestational-age children responded to only one of these antigens and many IUGR children failed to respond to any of them. Additionally, as with the reduced ability of T lymphocytes to form rosettes, this decreased ability to demonstrate a delayed-type hypersensitivity response to skin test antigens persisted for many years (Ghavami *et al.,* 1979). Defective cell-mediated immunocompetence often coincided with low levels of serum immunoglobulins (Ghavami *et al.,* 1979). Many small-for-gestational-age infants also demonstrated a decreased level of *in vitro* blast transformation in response to mitogens such as phytohemagglutinin (Chandra, 1974; Bhaskaram *et al.,* 1977).

Decreased responsiveness to T-cell mitogens in IUGR infants has not always been a consistent finding. In one study, investigators found that when such infants were followed later in life (i.e., up to 9 years of age), many exhibited a hyperresponsiveness to phytohemagglutinin. This suggests that defects in immune regulation occurred at the level of suppressor T-cell function. The hyperresponsive reaction may also represent an inherent hyperactivity of a specific T-cell subpopulation, e.g., helper T cells. These children also expressed persistently low levels of serum IgM, although all had experienced intensive antigenic confrontation; however, other parameters of immunological function were within normal ranges. While the pathogenesis of such immune dysfunction remains unclear, the potential importance of malnutrition during either the prenatal or early postnatal period is altogether too clear. The result in such children is a high rate of infection by opportunistic pathogens, e.g., *Pneumocystis carinii,* as well as greatly accentuated sequelae of common childhood infectious disorders (Puffer and Serrano, 1973).

Nonspecific parameters of immunity, e.g., phagocytic cell function, complement component levels, and total hemolytic complement activity in children subjected to IUGR have also been investigated. While phagocytosis is normal in such children, intracellular bactericidal killing is significantly low. Nitroblue tetrazolium reduction by PMNs is markedly depressed (Chandra, 1974). In low-birth-weight infants, phagocytic cell mobility, whether directed or random, is also substantially decreased (Chandra, 1974). Keusch *et al.* (1976) confirmed many of these findings in infants who had been severely malnourished during the gestational period. However, they were able to localize the defect in these IUGR children more precisely. Cord blood phagocytic cell intracellular bactericidal killing activity with preopsonized *Staphylococcus aureus* or *Escherichia coli* was within normal ranges. However, without preopsonization, the intracellular bactericidal killing activity was defective, indicating an opsonic defect (Keusch *et al.,* 1976). The limiting humoral factor was found to be heat labile, suggesting that it was a complement component. Chandra (1974) found that such IUGR infants had significantly low serum levels of complement component C3, which correlated closely with the observed opsonic defect and the decreased level of intracellular bactericidal activity. While this opsonic defect was most serious in infants with very low birth weights, it was also present in many infants with only moderately low birth weights. Very little is known regarding the possible persistence of these nonspecific immune defense deficits in later life.

EXPERIMENTAL ANIMAL STUDIES

A number of studies have attempted to reproduce in experimental animals dietary manipulations similar to the dietary conditions of malnourished human populations. While it is difficult to duplicate such dietary deficiencies, studies in animals allow one to observe serially the effects of early nutritional deficiencies and to allow for specific antigenic challenge. The results have helped to elucidate the role of specific nutrients in the immunodeficiency observed in undernourished populations.

On the basis of field studies suggesting possible long-term impairment of immune function in humans (Jose et al., 1970) and studies in experimental animals indicating that the thymus is one of the organs most affected by nutritional deprivation during development (Dubos et al., 1969), Jose et al. (1973) investigated the influence of a defined period of nutritional deficiency during postnatal development on immunological function in mice. In addition to a carefully defined period of nutritional deprivation, some animals were subjected simultaneously to intensive antigenic stimulation in order to simulate conditions observed in developing nations. Mice were fed a diet low in total calories and protein for a 2-week period during the latter stages of postnatal development, and specific humoral and cellular immune responsiveness to transplantation antigens was assessed. A decreased capacity to develop cellular cytotoxicity in response to allogenic stimuli was seen in animals fed low-protein, low-calorie diets even 12 weeks after nutritional restitution had commenced. Protein deficiency alone had a similar effect, but by 12 weeks of age, the cell-mediated immune responsiveness had returned to normal. Lower levels of hemagglutinating antibodies were observed in deprived mice after 5 weeks of nutritional rehabilitation; beyond this time period, responses were within normal ranges (Jose et al., 1973). A reduced number of θ-positive lymphocytes was also observed in thymus, spleen, and lymph nodes of deprived animals after 5 weeks of nutritional rehabilitation; however, 12 weeks of such supplementation resulted in a normal profile of splenic θ-positive cells. Of particular interest was the fact that the animals subjected to simultaneous intense antigenic stimulation did not experience deficient immune function, despite being fed the low-protein diet (Jose et al., 1973) (Tables V–VII). Therefore, both depressed cell-mediated immunity and the relative lack of thymus-derived lymphoid cells present in thymus, spleen, and lymph nodes were directly related to the magnitude of early nutritional deprivation of protein and calories, both in terms of the extent of immunosuppression and the duration of such immune dysfunction.

When pregnant mice were fed a low-calorie, low-protein diet (6% protein during the first 14 days of lactation and then either 6 or 2% protein up to 40 days of age), the immune responsiveness of the first-generation offspring at 40 days of age was significantly compromised (Hook and Hutcheson, 1976). The direct plaque-forming cell response to heterologous erythrocytes from control animals was 93-fold and 3-fold greater than that

Table V
Long-Term Effects of Nutritional Depletion at Weaning on Lymphoid Cell Population in Spleen Lymph Nodes and Thymus[a]

Diets at weaning	Weeks on normal diet	Total number of lymphoid cells spleen[b]	Percentage θ positive[c]		
			Spleen	Lymph nodes	Thymus
28% casein	5	128 ± 8.2	36	52	79
	12	136 ± 7.3	34	48	76
6% casein	5	92 ± 5.2	16[d]	32[d]	57[d]
	12	114 ± 6.5	32	36[d]	77
6% casein half-calorie	5	76 ± 4.1	11[d]	21[d]	49[d]
	12	93 ± 4.8	26[d]	34[d]	72
6% casein pertussis	5	145 ± 8.3	33	46	77
	12	163 ± 8.7	29	49	79

[a]Reproduced with permission from Jose et al. (1973).
[b]Mean ± SD × 10^6.
[c]Calculated from the number of mononuclear cells per organ, the percentage of lymphocytes in stained smears, and the percentage reduction in mononuclear cells after treatment with anti-θ serum compared to reductions after normal AKR serum.
[d]Significantly different from normal animals ($p < .01$).

of mice fed the diets containing 2 and 6% protein, respectively. These differences between the dietary groups remained significant even after adjustment for decreased spleen size and total spleen cell number, which were significantly lower in the mice fed the protein–calorie–deficient diets during development. In addition, the mean titers of serum hemagglutinating

Table VI
Long-Term Effects of Nutritional Deprivation at Weaning on Hemagglutinating Antibody Titers Tested 12 Days after Primary Allogenic Tumor Cell Inoculation and after 5, 8, and 12 Weeks on a Normal Diet[a]

Diets at weaning	Mean log hemagglutination titer		
	5 weeks	8 weeks	12 weeks
28% casein	4.3	4.5	4.4
6% casein	3.6[b]	4.1	4.2
6% casein half calorie	2.7[b]	3.9	3.9
6% casein pertussis	4.8	4.9	4.7

[a]Reproduced with permission from Jose et al. (1973).
[b]Significantly different from normally fed mice ($p < .01$).

Table VII

Long-Term Effects of Nutritional Deprivation at Weaning on Cytotoxic Cellular Immune Responses Tested by *in Vitro* Assay after 5, 8, and 12 Weeks on a Normal Diet

Diets at weaning	Total calories/mouse day	Cell-mediated lysis					
		5 weeks		8 weeks		12 weeks	
		cpm ± SD[b]	Lysis (%)	cpm ± SD	Lysis (%)	cpm ± SD	Lysis (%)
28% casein	8.5	4178 ± 396	82	4036 ± 421	78	4294 ± 398	84
6% casein	8.0	1452 ± 189	18[a]	2058 ± 245	32[a]	4028 ± 476	78
6% casein half-calorie	4.0	707 ± 131	8[a]	1322 ± 141	15[a]	3057 ± 321	56[a]
6% casein pertussis	9.0	4170 ± 449	81	3962 ± 381	76	3763 ± 411	72
Nonimmune mice		674	0	668	0	584	0

[a] Reproduced with permission from Jose *et al.* (1973).

[b] Mean cpm and SD. ^{51}Cr released from DBA/2 mastocytoma target cells during 2-hr incubation with sensitized C_3H spleen cells at 1:100 ratio. Total releasable activity in each test was adjusted to 5000 cpm. There were 10 mice per group.

[c] Percentage specific lysis of target cells.

[d] Significantly different from values in normal diet mice ($p < .01$).

antibody to sheep erythrocytes reflected a similar trend, being markedly lower in the protein-energy malnourished mice (Hook and Hutcheson, 1976). It would therefore appear that in experimental animals, cell-mediated immunity and possibly humoral immunity may both be significantly affected by PEM. Similar observations have been made in inbred rats fed a diet whose protein and calorie content was 25% of that fed to controls prior to and during gestation but then returned to the control diet at parturition, thereby limiting the period of nutritional deprivation to fetal development (except for possible effects on lactation) (Chandra, 1975b). Such rats displayed a marked reduction in the plaque-forming cell responsiveness of spleen cells; direct IgM plaques and especially indirect IgG plaques were substantially reduced. Serum hemolysin titers to heterologous erythrocytes were also significantly reduced by nutritional deprivation. In addition, despite nutritional repletion of F_1 offspring beginning at birth, immunodeficiency persisted in the F_2 generation offspring of F_1 females mated with healthy control male rats (Chandra, 1975b).

Mechanisms that may account for the immunodeficiency observed in animals fed restricted amounts of protein and calories during development have been suggested (Srivastava et al., 1981). In particular, abnormal metabolism of nucleotides and nucleosides in both the thymus and spleen of neonatal offspring of rats who experienced such dietary deprivation has been seen. For example, thymocytes and splenocytes from the malnourished rats had altered intracellular levels of ATP, ADP, cAMP, 5'AMP, and adenosine, suggesting that such metabolic alterations may be fundamental to the immunodeficiency observed in animals deprived of essential nutrients during critical periods of development.

More recently, a different aspect of host defense has been studied, i.e., the development of gut IgA-forming plasma cells in both overnourished and undernourished mice produced by manipulation of litter size, a method commonly utilized in studies of postnatal nurture. These studies are of particular interest because defective secretory immunity in the gut and respiratory tract has also been reported in protein-energy malnourished children. This defect in IgA secretion may be the key factor in the increased incidence of gastroenteritis and upper respiratory tract infections in infants and children in less developed countries. In contrast, overnutrition, obtained by reducing litters to four pups, had no significant impact on the number of gut IgA plasma cells. Further, undernutrition, produced by increasing litters to 20 pups, resulted in fewer proximal gut IgA plasma cells only when mice were further restricted in food intake by being fed only every other day. When the offspring were so restricted, they experienced a 60% reduction in proximal gut IgA plasma cells. When they were fed *ad libitum* after weaning, these differences were no longer apparent. The authors caution that although undernutrition may have resulted in defective immunocompetence, there may have been sufficient antigenic stimulation to allow normal numbers of gut IgA plasma cells to appear.

STUDIES OF PROTEIN DEFICIENCY DURING IMMUNE ONTOGENY

Because protein is considered to be one of the essential nutrients frequently deficient in diets of socioeconomically deprived populations, a number of animal studies focusing only on protein deficiency have been reported. One of the most interesting studies was an attempt to simulate the synergistic interaction between nutritional deficiencies and increased risk of pathogenic challenge during the neonatal period (Cruz and Waner, 1978). These investigators studied the interactive influences on growth and immune development of concurrent sublethal cytomegalovirus infection in mice fed a low-protein diet introduced at the 21st day postpartum. Infection with cytomegalovirus resulted in stunted growth of offspring as well as immunosuppression, as reflected by impaired mitogen responsiveness and decreased direct plaque-forming cell responsiveness to sheep erythrocytes (Cruz and Waner, 1978) (Tables VIII, IX). However, when all nutritional requirements were met during the postnatal period, mice responded effectively to the cytomegalovirus infection; growth rates rebounded to normal levels within 28–42 days after infection. In neonatal mice, the effects on growth and immunosuppression in uninfected, protein-malnourished animals were similar to those of infected, well-nourished ones (e.g., decreased body weight, impaired T-cell function), leading the authors to suggest that protein malnutrition during the prenatal period "mimics" the detrimental influences of cytomegalovirus infection. When neonatal cytomegalovirus infection and undernutrition (protein deficiency) were introduced simultaneously, there was a synergistic negative impact on growth and immune function, resulting in a significantly more profound immunosuppression and a much greater delay in the response to cytomegalovirus challenge. This experimental model closely resembles the situation in less developed countries. In children, however, there is often more than a single agent involved and the infectious dose is sublethal. In addition, the diet of human populations would most likely be deficient in more than one nutrient. Similarly, such nutritional deprivation, to a variable degree, would have existed prenatally and during the immediate postnatal period, as well as during the later stages of postnatal development. Increased susceptibility to infectious agents after protein deficiency during gestation has been confirmed by other investigators (Watson et al., 1976).

There are many studies of immune function following gestational protein

Table VIII

Effect of MCMV Infection on the Growth of Well-Nourished and Undernourished Mice[a]

		Wt (g) at age (days):			
Nutritional status	Infection status	15	21	28	42
Well-nourished	Uninfected	8.88 ± 0.94[b] (55)[c]	12.44 ± 0.97 (55)	18.94 ± 0.56 (25)	25.24 ± 1.76 (16)
	MCMV	8.25 ± 1.44 (50)	10.28 ± 1.83 (50)	13.51 ± 1.41 (18)	23.97 ± 2.73 (8)
Undernourished[a]	Uninfected			14.73 ± 0.71 (21)	22.17 ± 2.45 (12)
	MCMV			11.32 ± 2.04 (22)	18.09 ± 2.91 (13)

[a]Reproduced with permission from Cruz and Waner (1978).

[b]Mean ± SD.

[c]Numbers in parentheses represent the number of animals in each group.

[a]Mice were infected with MCMV at <24 hr of age; the deficient diet was initiated at 21 days of age.

Table IX

Effect of Neonatal MCMV Infection on the Antibody Response of Well-Nourished and Undernourished Mice to T Cell-Dependent Antigen[a,b]

Nutritional and infection status	Number of direct anti-SRBC PFC at age (days)[c]:			
	12	21	28	42
Well-nourished				
Uninfected	4014 ± 547	8725 ± 1157	21,050 ± 2,792	29,360 ± 3,895
Infected	66 ± 8	1328 ± 176	2,405 ± 319	23,121 ± 3,067
Undernourished				
Uninfected			7,354 ± 975	10,568 ± 1,402
Infected			980 ± 130	2,338 ± 310

[a]Reproduced with permission from Cruz and Waner (1978).

[b]Mice were injected intraperitoneally 4 days previously with 0.1 ml of a 12% (vol/vol) SRBC suspension.

[c]Data for each group (mean ± SD) were obtained from the spleens of eight mice examined individually.

deficiency. Examination of lymphoid organ weights after protein deprivation *in utero* revealed that thymic weights were low at birth and tended to
remain significantly low at 5 months of age, even after nutritional rehabilitation at birth (Olusi *et al.,* 1976). Histological examination of such thymus
glands indicated that this form of IUGR is associated with a delay in thymic
development (Lansdown, 1977). Thymus tissue obtained from protein-deprived rats and mice contained fewer small lymphocytes and showed an
aberrant organization of the cortex and medulla. The clear distinction between cortex and medulla was lost in protein-deficient animals; there was
also a relative increase in epithelial cells in both structures. In contrast,
Hassall's corpuscles were largely absent (Lansdown, 1977).

The immune responsiveness of rodents deprived of protein during gestation was markedly altered. When rats were fed a protein-deficient diet for 4
days prior to mating and then throughout gestation, there was a delay in the
appearance of IgG_{2B} in malnourished offspring (Olusi *et al.,* 1976) (Table
X). Additionally, while serum levels of IgG_{2A} in well-nourished control
offspring began to increase on day 16 postpartum, no such increase occurred in protein-malnourished progeny. Moreover, even when offspring of
malnourished dams were rehabilitated nutritionally for 4 months with a
high-protein diet, their IgG levels in serum remained significantly lower

Table X

Effects of Intrauterine Malnutrition on the Serum Concentrations
of IgG Allotypes[a,b]

	Offspring of control dam		Offspring of malnourished dam	
Day	IgG_{2A}	IgG_{2B}	IgG_{2A}	IgG_{2B}
0	98.3	Not detectable	90.7	Not detectable
4	90.6	Not detectable	83.5	Not detectable
8	81.2	39.6	77.1	Not detectable
12	65.1	58.7	63.6	Not detectable
16	73.8	60.8	60.7	36.3
20	78.9	70.1	59.3	40.1
24	83.6	77.1	60.4	42.3

[a]Reproduced with permission from Olusi *et al.* (1976).
[b]The serum concentrations of both IgG allotypes are expressed as
percentages of a standard adult rat reference serum.

than those of well-nourished control offspring (Olusi *et al.,* 1976). Offspring born to dams who had been fed a diet deficient in protein for 3 months prior to and throughout gestation had a prolonged period of reduced immune function (Gebhardt and Newberne, 1974). Even when the progeny of such deprived dams were fed a high-protein diet for 4 months, there was decreased antibody response to antigenic challenge. For example, offspring of deprived dams formed only 58 ± 4 plaques per 10^6 spleen cells in response to SRBC immunization compared to 275 ± 13 plaques per 10^6 spleen cells in control offspring (Gebhardt and Newberne, 1974). In addition, *in vitro* mitogen responsiveness of splenic lymphocytes to phytohemagglutinin continued to show a 60% reduction even after months of nutritional rehabilitation. Thus, protein deficiency alone can impair immune responsiveness for prolonged periods, perhaps permanently, if imposed during critical periods of immune ontogeny.

Studies of the influence of protein deficiency during gestation on nonspecific immune functions have also been performed. Rats were fed an 8% casein diet between days 5 and 19 of gestation (compared with a 25% protein diet fed to control dams), thereby limiting the period of deprivation to the end of pregnancy. Serum complement levels were different in both groups of dams. The offspring of control dams developed normal CH_{50} levels by 35 days of age. At the same age, levels of serum complement in the protein-deficient offspring were only one-third those of controls. Even at 90 days of age, the progeny of protein-deficient dams had not attained the normal levels of complement. Protein-deficient dams also had significantly lower levels of complement in milk. Control dams had levels of milk complement approximately twofold greater than serum complement levels, whereas no such difference was seen in protein-deficient dams. This may explain the decreased complement levels in their respective offspring. Finally, a low-protein diet (8% protein) commenced 7 days prior to mating and continued during gestation and lactation resulted in altered levels of alveolar macrophage superoxide dismutase activity in both guinea pigs and rats (Watson *et al.,* 1976).

EXPERIMENTAL VITAMIN DEFICIENCIES DURING IMMUNE ONTOGENESIS

Vitamin deficiency during development and its influence on the ontogenesis of intact immune function has been investigated rather sporadically. It is difficult to generalize about vitamin deficiencies and their impact on any physiological parameter, since vitamins are a heterogeneous group of compounds. Nonetheless, the potential importance of such deficiencies is becoming apparent as methodology to detect marginal degrees of deficiency is developed.

One water-soluble vitamin that has been investigated more extensively than most is pyridoxine. Davis *et al.* (1970) first noted that when pyridoxine was withheld during gestation in rats, both dams and offspring experienced thymic involution. Other groups (Robson and Schwarz, 1975) utilized a diet devoid of pyridoxine fed from day 4 of pregnancy until birth, as well as a pyridoxine antagonist. There was an elevated mortality rate among the progeny of pyridoxine-deficient dams. Even after 3 months of a complete control diet, rats deprived of pyridoxine during gestation exhibited significantly low levels of mixed lymphocyte reactivity and a defective graft-versus-host reaction (Robson and Schwarz, 1975). This immunodeficiency was due to an impaired reactivity of individual lymphocytes, because the total number of lymphocytes was not decreased at 3 months of age. In offspring deprived of pyridoxine during both gestation and lactation, low levels of pyridoxine were found in the spleen and thymus. At 9 days of age, IgG levels in the sera of dams and pups were within normal ranges, indicating that passive transfer of antibodies was not altered by a dietary deficiency of pyridoxine. However, on day 35, the number of spleen cells in pups was decreased, and there was a marked reduction in plaque-forming cell responses to SRBC immunization; there was a 40-fold reduction in plaques per spleen and a 20-fold reduction in plaques per 10^6 spleen cells. Because pyridoxine deficiency has been shown to alter food intake levels, pair-fed controls were also included in this study. While plaque-forming cell responsiveness in these food-restricted controls was also affected, the influence was not nearly as great as that observed in the pyridoxine-deficient progeny. Therefore, if pyridoxine deficiency is induced during critical periods of development, whether by dietary or nondietary means, an apparently permanent alteration of immunocompetence can result.

Other water-soluble B vitamins have been investigated far less thoroughly; however, limited studies have underscored the possible importance of folate in immune ontogeny. Neonatal guinea pigs, which ordinarily are not susceptible to infection with *Shigella flexneri,* were fatally susceptible after consuming a folate-deficient diet for 13–15 days after birth: 89% of deficient animals died after challenge, 50% within the first 24 hr, indicating a nearly total inability to resist infection (Table XI) (Haltalin *et al.,* 1970). The presence of a virulent bacteremia in the folate-deficient animals correlated closely with a fatal outcome. In contrast to the frequently fatal outcome in folate-deficient guinea pigs, controls showed no evidence of infection. However, in contrast to the influence of pyridoxine deficiency, the increased susceptibility to *S. flexneri* induced in folate-deficient neonatal

Table XI

Mortality Following Oral Challenge with 10^9 *Shigella flexneri* 2a[a,b]

Time of death following challenge	Diet		
	Folic acid deficient (18)	Folic acid supplemented (18)	Optimal (16)
< 24 hr	9	0	0
24–48 hr	3	1	0
48–72 hr	2	0	0
16–31 days	2	2	0
Deaths not associated with *Shigella* infection	0	3	0

[a]Reproduced with permission from Haltalin *et al.* (1970).
[b]Numbers in parentheses are the numbers of animals in each group.

guinea pigs was reversible if, at 14 days of age, the surviving animals were refed the complete control diet and then challenged at 45 or 135 days of age (Nelson and Haltalin, 1972). Thus, the enhanced susceptibility to *S. flexneri* observed in these animals was reversible with nutritional supplementation. No information on parameters of immune function is available for animals subjected to folate deficiency during prenatal development.

Information regarding biotin and vitamin B_{12} deficiencies during development is available only through preliminary observations of individuals with congenital disorders involving the metabolism of these essential B vitamins. In children with biotin-responsive carboxylase deficiency, immunodeficiency of both B and T cell–mediated systems may be present in association with this metabolic disorder (Cowan *et al.,* 1979). However, in other instances, this biotin-responsive carboxylase deficiency may not be associated with deficient immunological function. Lymphocytes from such patients are deficient in the activity of three biotin-associated enzymes [propionyl-coenzyme A (CoA) carboxylase, 3-methylcrotonyl-CoA carboxylase, and pyruvate carboxylase]; these enzyme activities returned to normal levels, along with parameters of immune function, with biotin supplementation (Cowan *et al.,* 1979). Similarly, in infants with congenital transcobalamin II (a vitamin B_{12}–binding protein) deficiency, agammaglobulinemia occurs together with granulocyte dysfunction. Phagocytic cells from such patients exhibit a lack of intracellular bactericidal killing activity; other parameters of granulocyte function, e.g., nitroblue tetrazolium reduction, and phagocytosis appear to be normal. Therefore, studies of humans with disordered metabolism of biotin and vitamin B_{12} during the postnatal period indicate that both of these essential nutrients may play key roles in the development of an effective immune defense. Appropriate experimental models need be developed to investigate the role of these two B vitamins in immune ontogeny.

The only fat-soluble vitamin whose role during development has been investigated is vitamin E (Jackson *et al.,* 1978). When hens were fed diets supplemented with either 150 or 450 ppm vitamin E and then immunized with *Brucella abortis,* the offspring had significantly higher than normal levels of passively transferred antibodies at 2 and 7 days of age. Such passive antibody transfer in chicks takes place via the yolk sac. This finding is particularly impressive since dietary supplementation with vitamin E does not increase maternal serum antibody levels significantly (Jackson *et al.,* 1978). In contrast, supplementation with 90, 300, or 900 ppm vitamin E has no such positive influence on antibody transfer to offspring. Thus, one sees a biphasic dose-dependent response with two peaks of maximal effect; this biphasic pattern was also observed at other stages of the life cycle and in other species. Additionally, these results underscore the potential importance of nutritional immunological interactions in successful veterinary practice.

EXPERIMENTAL LIPOTROPE DEFICIENCY DURING IMMUNE ONTOGENY

Newberne and his colleagues have utilized diets deficient in lipotropes (e.g., choline, methionine) to investigate the influence of prenatal and postnatal nutritional deficiencies on the development of the immune response. Initial studies were conducted in dams deprived of lipotropes for 3 months, mated with healthy males, and fed the deficient diet throughout gestation. After parturition, the groups were differentially manipulated to investigate possible differences between lipotrope deficiency during prenatal and postnatal periods. The most dramatic effects were obtained in animals deprived of lipotropes, even with only a marginal deficiency, during both gestation and lactation (Newberne and Gebhardt, 1973). Even after 3 months of nutritional rehabilitation postweaning, animals deprived of lipotropes during development exhibited markedly increased mortality rates due to *Salmonella typhimurium* (Newberne and Gebhardt, 1973) (Table XII). The size of spleen and thymus in the deprived offspring was also reduced even after 3 months of nutritional supplementation; the cellular densities of these organs were also reduced. Such rats also exhibited decreased serum antibody titers to SRBC immunization. In addition, the direct plaque-forming cell response was only 37 ± 8 plaques per 10^6 spleen cells in deprived rats versus 275 ± 13 plaques per 10^6 spleen cells in controls. Spleen cell mitogen responsiveness to phytohemagglutinin was

Table XII

Effect of Lipotropes on Resistance to Infection with *Salmonella typhimurium*[a]

Dietary lipotropes		Cumulative mortality (days post-infection)		
Gestation and lactation	Postweaning	7	14	30
Marginal	Marginal	31/62	50/62	56/62
Marginal	Complete	26/65	47/65	60/65
Complete	Complete	6/60	12/60	15/60
Complete	Marginal	8/60	12/60	20/60

[a]Reproduced with permission from Newberne and Gebhardt (1973).

decreased markedly, but that of thymus cells was intact. This may have indicated a lack of normal thymocyte mobilization in lipotrope-deficient offspring. In addition, when animals were deprived during both gestation and lactation, a decreased skin test response to phytohemagglutinin and a substantially reduced response of nonimmune splenocytes in the one-way mixed leukocyte culture were also observed (E. A. J. Williams *et al.,* 1979). If rats were deprived of lipotropes during gestation only, a decreased primary response to SRBC was observed. If the deficient diet was imposed during lactation only, the offspring did not exhibit a reduced response to heterologous erythrocytes but did show decreased mitogen responsiveness and a reduced skin test response to phytohemagglutinin (E. A. J. Williams *et al.,* 1979). In all of the lipotrope-deprived groups, with repeated sensitization with alloantigen *in vivo,* no further differences between deprived and control groups were noted in either cell-mediated or humoral immunity. This may emphasize that one of the principal defects in such nutritionally depleted animals is an impaired ability to recognize an antigen as foreign.

EXPERIMENTAL MINERAL DEFICIENCIES DURING IMMUNE ONTOGENY

The most comprehensively studied dietary mineral, and possibly one of the best-studied of all nutrients with regard to its effect on the development of the immune response, is zinc. When a zinc deficiency was imposed on mice beginning at parturition and continuing throughout the postnatal period, profound abrogation of a number of immune functions was observed. These postnatally zinc-deprived mice experienced a selective retardation of lymphoid organ growth, most notably of the thymus (Beach *et al.,* 1979; 1980a,b). Moreover, a variety of immune parameters were altered by postnatal zinc deprivation, including a depressed *in vitro* blast transformation response to mitogens, especially those known to activate T cells specifically (concanavalin A and phytohemagglutinin) (Beach *et al.,* 1979), a decreased direct plaque-forming cell response (both per spleen and per 10^6 spleen cells) to SRBC immunization (Beach *et al.,* 1980b), and a highly aberrant serum immunoglobulin profile with elevated levels of IgG_1 and no detectable IgM, IgG_{2A}, or IgA (Beach *et al.,* 1980b). Even marginal dietary deprivation of zinc during postnatal development was associated with a significant impairment of immunological function, with a particularly altered response to T-cell mitogens and an abnormal serum immunoglobulin profile (Table XIII, Fig. 5) (Beach *et al.,* 1979).

Zwickl and Fraker (1980) have shown that when mice consumed a zinc-deficient diet for 7–11 days beginning at 2 weeks of age, they also experienced a profound depression of plaque-forming cell responsiveness to SRBC, forming only 7–35% as many plaques as controls. The response of postnatally zinc-deprived mice to dextran was also reduced to 40% of control levels (Zwickl and Fraker, 1980). Nutritional repletion for as little as 4 days returned the plaque-forming cell responsiveness to normal. Many similar observations, e.g., thymic atrophy, abnormal serum immunoglobulin profile, and impaired T-cell function, along with an increased incidence of infectious disease, have been observed in children with acrodermatitis enteropathica, a congenital disorder of zinc metabolism that tends to mimic postnatal zinc deficiency in humans (Rodin and Goldman, 1969; Chandra, 1980b). Children with acrodermatitis enteropathica also experience defective phagocyte chemotaxis, which, along with the other defects, can be corrected with zinc administration (Weston *et al.,* 1977). Finally, patients fed intravenously during the postnatal period are at risk of developing zinc deficiency unless they are specifically supplemented (Srouji *et al.,* 1978).

Most recently, experimental zinc deficiency only during the fetal period has been examined. Offspring of mice moderately deprived of zinc between days 7 and 20 of gestation experienced a profound suppression of serum IgM levels, along with an impaired direct plaque-forming cell responsiveness to heterologous erythrocytes early in life. This immunodeficiency persisted even at 6 months of age in F_1 progeny. Perhaps the most remarkable evidence from these experiments is that such immunodeficiency was passed on to F_2 and F_3 generations, although it was less than that seen in F_1 offspring (Beach *et al.,* 1982c). Similar observations were made by Chandra (1975b) when both F_1 and F_2 offspring experienced immunosuppression as a result of caloric restriction on F_0 dams. The mechanism whereby defective immunocompetence is passed on to subsequent generations after *in utero* deprivation of essential nutrients remains a mystery. However, intensive

Table XIII

Serum Immunoglobulin Concentrations of NIH Pups at 6 Weeks[a,b]

Diet	IgA	IgM	IgG_1	IgG_{2A}	IgG_{2B}	IgG_{total}	Ig_{total}
100 ppm zinc *ad libitum* fed (15)	76 ± 6	16.8 ± 2.3	379 ± 18	265 ± 12	61 ± 4	705 ± 34	797.8 ± 42.3
100 ppm zinc inanition controls (15)	55 ± 3	13.5 ± 1.1	290 ± 14[c]	150 ± 8[c]	53 ± 2	493 ± 24[c]	561.5 ± 28.1[c]
9.0 ppm zinc marginal deficiency (15)	N/D[c]	15.0 ± 1.7	382 ± 20	131 ± 8[c]	57 ± 4	570 ± 32[d]	585.0 ± 33.7[c]
5.0 ppm zinc moderate deficiency (14)	N/D[c]	N/D[c]	841 ± 27[c]	N/D[c]	58 ± 3	899 ± 30[c,e]	899.0 ± 30.0[d]
2.5 ppm zinc severe deficiency (12)	N/D[c]	N/D[c]	520 ± 26[c]	N/D[c]	50 ± 4[a]	570 ± 30.0[c]	570.0 ± 30.0[c]

[a]Reproduced with permission from Beach *et al.* (1979).
[b]Results expressed in mg/dl as means ± SEM. Number of animals shown in parentheses. N/D = none detectable.
[c]Significantly different from *ad libitum* controls at $p < .01$.
[d]Significantly different from *ad libitum* controls at $p < .05$.
[e]Significantly different from inanition controls at $p < .01$.

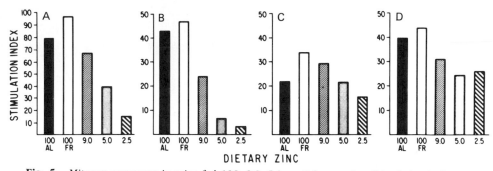

Fig. 5. Mitogen responses in mice fed 100, 9.0, 5.0, or 2.5 ppm zinc. Stimulation indices (total mitogen cpm/background (media) cpm) of splenic lymphocytes of mice to concanavalin A, phytohemagglutinin-P, lipopolysaccharide, and pokeweed mitogen at 4 weeks of age. AL, *ad lib;* FR, food restricted. Reproduced with permission from Beach *et al.* (1979).

investigation should focus on this mechanism; it may help to explain the persistent immune dysfunction in children of Third World countries.

Far less is known regarding the influence of other trace elements on the development of immune function. A copper-deficient diet from the time of parturition throughout the postnatal period resulted in a significant decrease in antibody production to SRBC in mice (Prohaska and Lukasewycz, 1981). This decrease was most notable in mice that experienced a marked drop in commonly measured parameters of copper status, e.g., ceruloplasmin, liver copper levels (Table XIV). However, even when these measures of copper status were not significantly low, there was a 36% reduction in antibody-producing cells per 10^6 splenocytes (Prohaska and Lukasewycz, 1981). Serum activity of ceruloplasmin was highly correlated with residual ability to produce antibodies to heterologous erythrocytes. Copper deficiency in neonates is distinct from zinc deficiency in that animals deprived of copper have normal or enlarged spleens and "apparently normal" thymuses (Prohaska and Lukasewycz, 1981).

When iron deficiency was imposed in rats for 30 days prior to gestation, throughout gestation, and then during lactation, an enhanced susceptibility to infection with *S. typhimurium* was noted (Baggs and Miller, 1973). Even rat pups exposed to iron deficiency during the suckling period alone, through cross-fostering experiments, were more than normally susceptible to such infections. The authors suggested that one possible mechanism that might account for such decreased resistance to infection is a reduced number of myeloperoxidase-containing cells, whose total number is too low to respond effectively to the infectious challenge (Baggs and Miller, 1973). Other parameters of immune function, however, many of which are

Table XIV
Effect of Dietary Copper Deficiency in Mice[a,b]

Parameter	Male			Female		
	+Cu (n = 12)	-Cu$_1$ (n = 6)	-Cu$_2$ (n = 5)	+Cu (n = 9)	-Cu$_1$ (n = 3)	-Cu$_2$ (n = 14)
Body weight (g)	23.2 ± 3.7	15.6 ± 2.3	17.8 ± 1.6	17.6 ± 2.2	13.1 ± 0.83	15.2 ± 4.2
Spleen weight (mg)	152 ± 44	291 ± 132	114 ± 17	120 ± 32	177 ± 63	115 ± 40
Hemoglobin (g/dl)	14.6 ± 0.4	7.14 ± 2.83	13.1 ± 1.2	14.7 ± 0.79	5.15 ± 1.68	13.3 ± 0.49
Ceruloplasmin (U/liter)	23.4 ± 2.6	0.72 ± 0.99	7.32 ± 5.60	22.8 ± 1.9	0.16 ± 0.27	10.9 ± 3.54
Liver Cu (μg/g)	5.86 ± 0.78	2.05 ± 0.49	3.13 ± 0.50	3.89 ± 0.75	1.58 ± 0.17	3.32 ± 0.24
Liver Fe (μg/g)	61.7 ± 13.1	255 ± 122	126 ± 49	86.3 ± 20.1	296 ± 51	76.4 ± 14.2
Antibody-producing cells per 10⁶ splenocytes	1004 ± 132	175 ± 96	644 ± 165	874 ± 254	23.3 ± 5.8	793 ± 315

[a]Reproduced with permission from Prohaska and Lukasewycz (1981).

[b]Effects of dietary copper deficiency in C58 mice. On the day of parturition, C58 mouse dams were switched from a nonpurified diet (Mouse Chow, Ralston Purina) containing 12 mg of copper per kilogram to a purified mouse diet formulated to omit copper from the salt mix (modified AIN-76, ICN Nutritional Biochemicals) and containing 0.5 mg of copper per kilogram. Approximately half the dams were given supplemental copper (20 μg/ml) in their drinking water, while the remaining dams were given deionized water to drink. The pups were weaned at 3 weeks of age and transferred to stainless steel cages. For 4 to 6 weeks they were maintained on the diets that had been given to their respective dams. Then the mice were injected with SRBC and decapitated 4 days later to evaluate humoral-mediated immunity; blood was collected in acid-washed tubes. A small portion was removed to measure hemoglobin as cyanmethemoglobin with Drabkin reagent; the remainder was allowed to clot and the serum was assayed in duplicate for ceruloplasmin activity, with o-dianisidine used as the substrate. The spleen was removed to determine the number of antibody-producing cells, and the liver was wet-washed in HNO$_3$ to determine total copper and iron by atomic absorption spectroscopy. Values are means ± standard deviations for the indicated number of supplemented (+Cu) and unsupplemented (−Cu) mice from seven individual experiments. Values in the same row for a given sex, not sharing a common superscript, are significantly different from one another at p < .01.

known to be altered by iron deficiency, were not measured in this study. Preliminary experiments with selenium deficiency indicate that while such a diet did not affect immunocompetence in F_0 mice, F_1 offspring did display a significantly depressed direct plaque-forming cell response to SRBC immunization (Mulhern *et al.,* 1981). It is thus clear that insufficient trace metals during critical periods of immune development can profoundly influence the ultimate ability of the host to respond to pathogenic challenge.

6

Caloric Intake

INTRODUCTION

The caloric or energy content of an individual's diet influences a variety of physiological processes including immunological function. The energy intake above caloric expenditure is stored largely in the form of body fat. Thus, even small increases in caloric intake can have a significant impact on physiological function and can lead to obesity, particularly over a long period of time. Likewise, caloric intake even marginally below caloric expenditure over extended periods can result in significant loss of body mass and altered physiological function. It is not unlikely, therefore, that immunological parameters might also be affected by the ratio of energy intake to energy expenditure. Indeed, both increased and decreased caloric intake have been demonstrated to affect some aspect of immunological function and/or the response to infectious challenge in both experimental animals and humans.

Initially, many studies conducted among children with PEM in Third World nations attributed compromised immune function to a predominant lack of calories and protein. Children with the ill-defined syndrome of marasmus were considered to suffer primarily from an insufficient caloric intake. Consequently, the immunological aberrations observed in these children were assumed to occur as the result of a total energy intake chronically below caloric expenditure. With increased understanding of the effect of various nutritional factors on immunological function, as well as the wide range of nutrient deficiencies frequently observed with marasmus and other forms of PEM, it was realized that children with marasmus did not represent a suitable model for studying the influence of total caloric intake on immune responsiveness. Thus, attention turned to controlled experiments in animal systems and detailed exploration of two types of clinical conditions:

(1) experimentally induced total energy deprivation for a defined and limited temporal period, and (2) pathological conditions such as anorexia nervosa (AN) and obesity.

A few cautionary comments are in order here. In studies of experimental animals, the term *dietary restriction* is frequently used; however, it does not have the same meaning to all investigators. In some studies, dietary restriction implies that the deprived animals were given less of the same diet given to the control animals, by limiting either the total amount of food or the time during which it was available. In such cases, the experimental group undergoing dietary restriction is consuming not only less total energy but also less of all other dietary constituents. More recently, a number of groups have given animals reduced amounts of food supplemented with protein, vitamins, and minerals such that the intake of these essential dietary constituents is equivalent in the control and food-restricted animals. This type of regimen is generally referred to as "undernutrition without malnutrition." While this experimental design shows significant progress in isolating caloric intake as a single variable, the fat content of these diets still differs and may contribute to alterations in immunological parameters.

The influence of excessive caloric intake on immune responsiveness in animals has generally been studied in the genetically obese (*ob/ob*) mouse. Such animals show many of the physiological features of genetically normal animals subjected to overnutrition, as well as those of obese humans. Nonetheless, although obesity in humans is considered to have a genetic component, there are also many other environmental influences. Consequently, it can be questioned how precisely analogous the *ob/ob* mouse model is to clinically observed cases of human obesity. This is of particular relevance to isolated observations of physiological parameters such as immunological function, which are also under some genetic regulation. However, the genetically obese mouse model, especially in conjunction with epidemiological and clinical data, can provide important information on the influence of caloric excess on immune function.

Studies of calorie deficiency and immune responsiveness in humans are generally limited to two types of situations: total deprivation of energy under carefully controlled conditions, and pathological situations such as anorexia nervosa (AN) wherein the patient has experienced self-induced semistarvation. Experimentally induced starvation has the disadvantage that, for ethical reasons, it must be limited to only short periods of time; therefore, only a short-term or acute deficit of calories can be studied. A superimposed stress response (which has a notable effect on a variety of immunological parameters) to such fasting can be minimized by the utilization of subjects who frequently fast for either religious or other reasons.

Patients with AN have been studied fairly extensively, since they provide certain advantages. Subjects with AN generally consume diets that, while being low in total energy content, contain sufficient amounts of protein, vitamins, and minerals. Thus, these patients have a relatively specific caloric deficit. Moreover, patients with AN have often undergone years of abnormal dietary intake, and therefore the longer-term (often many years of deprivation) consequences of energy deprivation can be investigated. However, AN patients are also characterized by marked psychological aberrations, self-induced vomiting, malabsorption, excessive consumption of laxatives, etc. Thus, while AN provides an unusual opportunity to monitor the influence of a relatively specific dietary deficit of total energy content, the precautions noted above certainly apply.

CALORIC DEFICIT AND IMMUNOLOGICAL FUNCTION

EXPERIMENTAL ANIMAL MODELS

A number of early studies indicated that starvation in both domestic and experimental animals may contribute to an increased resistance to certain forms of disease, notably viral diseases. In cattle, foot-and-mouth disease increases during the season of greatest forage availability and diminishes when food supplies become less abundant (Edwards, 1937). This situation was reproduced in experimental animals; when hibernating or anorectic, animals were significantly less susceptible to foot-and-mouth disease than in the full-fed state. The now classic observations of Rous regarding decreased susceptibility of undernourished chickens to sarcoma virus further support this contention (Rous, 1911). Additional observations indicated that animals subjected to undernutrition experienced significantly less disease when challenged with vaccinia, polio, or foot-and-mouth disease virus (Sprunt 1942; Foster *et al.,* 1944). However, the relatively unsophisticated nature of most of these studies makes any conclusion highly tentative. In most cases, the animals observed were consuming diets that contained substantially lower than normal levels of a variety of nutrients, total energy content being but one.

The past decade has witnessed many investigations of total energy as a dietary factor influencing immune function. These studies began to employ diets that had fewer than normal total calories but contained adjusted levels of protein, vitamins, and minerals, so that control and deprived groups of mice consumed the same amounts. In the initial studies of Jose and Good (1973), measurement of specific humoral and cellular immune responses to malignant tumors in allogeneic, syngeneic, and autochthonous murine systems showed that both types of immunity were adversely affected. However, these adverse effects were largely on the primary immune response and could be overcome by repeated exposure to antigenic challenge, i.e., by the tertiary immune response. Humoral immunity to these tumors appeared to be the more sensitive of the two systems in animals subjected to energy deprivation. Because these animals experienced an inhibition of tumor growth, the authors speculated that a decrease in serum-blocking antibody, which in adequately nourished control mice may partially or completely inhibit tumor destruction by cell-mediated immune mechanisms, may result from caloric insufficiency (Jose and Good, 1971, 1973) (Fig. 1, Tables I–IV). They suggested that the observed inhibition of tumor growth may, at least in part, be an immune-mediated phenomenon rather than simply a slowdown of tumor growth due to a lack of essential nutrients.

Further studies indicated that reducing caloric intake while maintaining the level of other essential nutrients completely prevented the development of spontaneous mammary adenocarcinoma in C3H/Umc mice (Fernandes *et al.,* 1976c) (Tables V, VI). These mice consumed a diet containing approximately 60% of the total energy content of the control diet from 4 weeks of age on. Along with the diminished incidence of cancer in these mice, a variety of alterations in immunological function were also noted. The response of spleen cells to the T-lymphocyte mitogens concanavalin A (Con A) and phytohemagglutinin (PHA) was significantly higher in the calorie-deprived mice at 3 months of age; in addition, the response to the B-

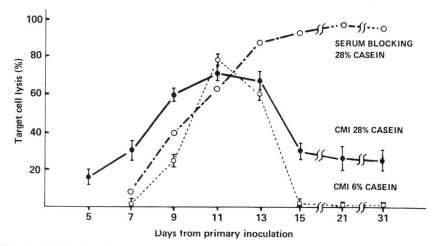

Fig. 1. Cell-mediated response of mice to tumor cells can be blocked with a serum factor. Reproduced with permission from Jose and Good (1973).

Table I

Allogenic System: Primary Cellular and Humoral Immune Responses of C57BL/6J Mice on Different Diets 11 Days After IP Inoculation with DBA/2 Mastocytoma[a,b]

Diets		Cell-mediated lysis		Serum		
Protein content as total calories (%)	Total calories/ mouse/day	Target cell[c] ^{51}Cr release (cpm)	Specific lysis (%)	Serum blocking specific lysis (%) (cells and serum)[d]	Mean log cytotoxic antibody titer	Mean log hemagglutin- ation titer
28	21	3085 ± 274	54	15	2.4	4.2
11	20	3002 ± 253	52	23	2.4	3.9
8	18	3249 ± 271	58	46[e]	1.6[e]	3.1[e]
8	9	3507 ± 286	64[e]	54[e]	1.5[e]	2.5[e]
5	18	3466 ± 293	63[e]	60[e]	1.2[e]	2.1[e]
5	9	3591 ± 301	66[e]	63[e]	0.9[e]	1.8[e]
3	15	1072 ± 123	10[e]	62[e]	0[e]	0[e]
Nonimmune		840 ± 63	0[e]	64[e]	0[e]	0[e]

[a]Reproduced with permission from Jose and Good (1973).

[b]Effect of lymphoid cells, lymphoid cells and serum, and serum with complement on ^{51}Cr-labeled mastocytoma cells *in vitro,* and serum hemagglutinating titer for DBA/2 red blood cells. Twenty mice per group, lymphocyte to target cell ratio: 100/1.

[c]Mean cpm ± SD of radioactivity released in each test after adjustment of total releasable activity to 5000 cpm.

[d]Percentage of specific lysis in each test with sensitized lymphocytes from mice on 28% casein diets and inactivated serum from each dietary group at 1/10 final dilution.

[e]Significantly different from 28% casein group ($p < .01$).

Table II

Serum Mediated Specific Lysis of ^{51}Cr-Labeled Mastocytoma Target (T) Cells with and without Added Complement[a]

Diet	T cells with inactivated serum from various groups		T cells with inactivated serum from various groups with complement added	
	cpm	Specific lysis (%)	cpm	Specific lysis (%)
Group 1: 30% protein	1552 ± 132	16	4261 ± 372	82
Group 2: 8% protein	1347 ± 87	11	1922 ± 143	25
Group 3: 22% protein half caloric	1511 ± 123	15	2578 ± 196	41
Unimmunized control	896 ± 96	0	1675 ± 121	19

[a]Reproduced with permission from Jose and Good (1971).

Table III

Syngeneic System: Primary Cellular and Humoral Immune Responses of C3Hf/Umc Mice in Different Dietary Groups 12 Days After IP Inoculation of C3H/Bi Mammary Tumor Cells[a,b]

Diets			Cell-mediated lysis		Blocking antibody	
Protein content as total calories (%)	Total calories/ mouse/day	Mean body weight (g)	cpm remaining in cultures	Inhibition of culture by spleen cells (%)	cpm remaining in cultures	Total inhibition of cultures by spleen cells and serum (%)
28	20	18.6 ± 1.6	1435 ± 86[c]	72	4885 ± 236[c]	2
11	19	16.4 ± 2.1	1594 ± 92	68	3221 ± 104	36[d]
8	18	12.8 ± 1.9	1659 ± 125	67	1914 ± 96	62[d]
8	9	11.2 ± 2.3	1322 ± 91	74	1593 ± 113	68[d]
5	18	9.8 ± 1.3	1417 ± 97	72	1615 ± 102	68[d]
5	9	8.8 ± 1.4	1147 ± 78	78	1231 ± 86	76[d]
3	13	7.6 ± 1.1	4413 ± 151	12[d]	1142 ± 88	78[d]
Nonimmune			4602 ± 163	8[d]	1211 ± 91	77[d]
Total incorporation			5000		5000	

[a]Reproduced with permission from Jose and Good (1973).

[b]Radioactivity remaining in microcultures of target cells after incubation with spleen cells or with spleen cells and serum from animals in different groups.

[c]Mean ± SD.

[d]Significantly different from 28% protein group ($p < .05$).

Table IV

Lysis of ^{51}Cr-Labeled Mastocytoma Target (T) Cells by Sensitized Spleen Lymphoid (L) Cells after 4-hr Incubation and Effect of Serum from Three Nutritional Groups[a]

Diet	T cells, 10% calf serum; L cells from various groups		Serum from different groups; T cells with L cells from group 1 animals	
	cpm	Specific lysis (%)[c]	cpm	Specific lysis (%)
Group 1: 30% protein	3398 ± 285	62	970 ± 282	5
Group 2: 8% protein	3650 ± 343	68	3667 ± 206	67
Group 3: 22% protein half caloric	3194 ± 224	57	1519 ± 182	17
Nonimmunized normal animal	781 ± 132	0	3573 ± 271	66

[a]Reproduced with permission from Jose and Good (1971).

[b]Mean cpm ± SD of 10 experiments after adjustment of maximum releasable radioactivity in each test to 5000 cpm.

[c] $\dfrac{\text{cpm of specimen} - \text{cpm with nonimmunized lymphocytes}}{\text{Total releasable activity} \times \text{cpm with nonimmunized lymphocytes}} \times 100\%$.

cell mitogen *Escherichia coli* LPS was maintained at normal levels (Fernandes *et al.,* 1976c). There was a marked depression of the direct (PFC) response to SRBC administration in low-calorie mice at 3 months of age; however, the secondary response was not significantly different from that of controls. When sensitized spleen lymphocytes from the low-calorie mice were injected into lethally X-irradiated recipients (950 R), they formed a

Table V

Rate of Appearance of Mammary Tumors (MT) and Mortality in C3H Female Mice Given a Diet with Normal or Restricted Calories[a]

Calories per day	Number of mice dead with tumors per total dead					Total dead MT/total	%
	101–200 days	201–300 days	301–400 days	401–500 days	501–600 days		
16	0	0	4/5	7/11	1/1	12/17	71
10	0/4	0	0/4	0/4	0/6	0/18	0

[a]Reproduced with permission from Fernandes *et al.* (1976c).

Table VI

Incorporation of ^{3}H-TdR with and without Mitogenic Stimulation of Spleen Cells from Normal
and Calorie-Restricted C3H/Umc 3-Month-Old Mice[a]

Calories per day	Cultures[b] (hr)	cpm of ^{3}H-TdR (at optimum concentration of mitogens[c])			
		Controls	+PHA (2.5 μg)	+Con A (0.5 μg)	+LPS (10 μg)
16	48	770 ± 240	100,164 ± 11,327	76,834 ± 16,825	42,018 ± 7,740
	72	467 ± 170	74,369 ± 4,597	101,274 ± 20,959	20,051 ± 4,669
10	48	1,636 ± 194	144,018 ± 11,087	103,752 ± 10,354	43,122 ± 734
	72	671 ± 226	80,712 ± 5,732	154,559 ± 6,218	21,360 ± 1,836

[a]Reproduced with permission from Fernandes et al. (1976c).

[b]0.5 × 10[6] spleen cells from four individual mice per group cultured in RPMI-1640 media (triplicates) with foetal calf serum (2%) for 48 or 72 hr at 37°C in CO_2 and humidity in 3.040 microtest II tissue culture plates. Cultures were labeled with tritiated thymidine ^{3}H-TdR (0.5 μCi per well) for an additional 16 hr.

[c]Source of mitogens—PHA (phytohemagglutinin) (HA17), Wellcome; Con A (concanavalin A), Sigma; LPS, Difco.

significantly greater number of secondary plaques per 10[6] cells than were generated by cells from spleens of mice fed the higher-calorie diet. It was suggested that the mechanism of these effects was related to a suppressor cell population (Fernandes et al., 1976c). Indeed, animals fed the low-calorie diet did exhibit increased lytic activity, as reflected by an increased capacity to suppress [^{125}I]UdR incorporation into DNA in vivo on injection with SRBC. Increased suppressor cell activity may be a critical factor in the suppression of spontaneous mammary adenocarcinoma, which occurred frequently in the well-fed mice. Endocrine hypofunction may contribute greatly to the observed alterations in immunological parameters.

The most comprehensive work in this area has been done by Walford and co-workers (1973). They have refined the experimental techniques necessary to induce significant undernutrition without malnutrition. Nonetheless, it should be noted that while adjustments for nearly all nutritional variables were included in these studies, the diets did differ in total fat content, and this parameter has clearly been demonstrated to affect immune function.

Initial investigations in this area involved diets containing approximately 60% of the total energy found in control diets, levels of protein, vitamins, and minerals being adjusted accordingly. The diets were introduced at the time of weaning and continued throughout the life span (Walford et al., 1973). In general, when such dietary restriction was imposed early in life, just prior to or just after weaning, it was found that both direct and indirect PFC responsiveness was depressed (Gebrase-DeLima et al., 1975). Responsiveness to both B- and T-cell mitogens (Con A, PHA, LPS, PPD, and PWM) was also significantly reduced early in life. Rates of skin allograft rejection were also compromised in dietarily restricted adult mice (7 months of age) compared to well-fed controls. However, later (20–22 months of age) the situation was reversed; the animals that had been restricted in caloric intake from the time of weaning showed significantly enhanced immune responsiveness compared with nonrestricted controls. This was particularly true of responsiveness to mitogens and PFC responsiveness (Gebrase-DeLima *et al.,* 1975). In contrast, rejection of skin allografts remained suppressed in dietarily restricted mice until quite late in life.

Further studies revealed that in mice 15 months of age or older, the absolute number of nucleated cells per spleen decreased two- to fourfold in the mice restricted at weaning (Weindruch *et al.,* 1982). In contrast, the proliferative response of spleen cells to PHA was significantly increased at both optimal and lower cell densities; such differences were not merely a reflection of an alteration in response kinetics. The response of spleen cells to Con A was affected to a variable extent, with a significantly enhanced response being observed in 33% of restricted mice. Dietary restriction commencing at weaning had no such effects on lymph node lymphocytes (Weindruch *et al.,* 1982). Of particular interest with regard to this experimental protocol was the fact that the duration of the fast had a substantial influence on the mitogen responsiveness of splenic and lymph node cells, e.g., a 48-hr fast decreased the response to Con A and PHA more than a 24-hr fast. Additional studies showed that there was a twofold increase in the percentage of splenic T cells in dietarily restricted mice (Weindruch *et al.,* 1982). However, because of the overall decrease in spleen cell number, there was up to a twofold decrease in the absolute number of splenic T cells. The proportion of PHA-stimulated blast cells obtained from restricted mice was nearly doubled (Weindruch *et al.,* 1982). These workers failed to demonstrate any suppression or synergy by cells from restricted animals in mixed cultures of cells from restricted and nutritionally replete animals. Thus, the increase in splenic T-cell phytohemagglutinin responsiveness due to dietary restriction could be attributed, at least in large part, to an increased proportion of T cells that are responsive to PHA.

Regarding possible mechanistic considerations, PHA-sensitive T lymphocytes seem to be Lyt-1$^+$ 2$^+$ 3$^+$, whereas Con A–responsive lymphocytes are Lyt 1$^+$ 2$^-$ 3$^-$ (Nakayama *et al.,* 1980). Dietary restriction is therefore consistent with an increase in the proportion of Lyt-1$^+$ 2$^+$ 3$^+$ cells, with few or no concomitant changes in Lyt-1$^+$ 2$^-$ 3$^-$ cells. In general, Lyt-1$^+$ 2$^+$ 3$^+$ T lymphocytes are thought to represent a less mature stage of T-cell development (Ledbetter *et al.,* 1980). Aging in mice has been associated with a decrease in the rate of T-cell migration from the thymus, and this is associated with a decreased cortex : medulla ratio in the thymus (Walford *et al.,* 1981). As reported earlier by these investigators, the cortex : medulla ratio was increased by dietary restriction and was correlated with elevated lympho-cyte blast transformation in response to PHA and Con A (Weindruch *et al.,* 1979; Weindruch and Suffin, 1980). Therefore, increased proportions of Lyt-1$^+$ 2$^-$ 3$^-$ cells, as reflected by elevated concanavalin A responsiveness, could also result from dietary restriction in certain strains of mice (Weindruch *et al.,* 1979). Thus, the enhancement of immunological function in these aged mice may be mediated in part by alterations in specific T-cell subpopulations, rates of thymocyte death, alterations in those subclasses of T lymphocytes scheduled to die, or alterations in their migratory behavior.

Natural killer (NK) cell function has been investigated in mice subjected to dietary restriction from the time of weaning (Weindruch *et al.,* 1983). In general, there was an age-related decline in the response of NK cells to YAC-1 target tumor cells in both groups of mice. Mice consuming the restricted diets exhibited significantly lower basal NK cell activity when tested at either 14–15 or 30–33 months of age. However, on injection of polyinosinic : polycytidylic acid (Poly I : C), which potentiates NK cell ac-tivity, mice fed the restricted diets responded more vigorously than did controls (Weindruch *et al.,* 1983). Indeed, the response to poly I : C in old restricted mice was comparable to that in young control mice. In addition, mice fed the restricted diets from weaning demonstrated an increased gen-eration of cytotoxic T lymphocytes (CTLs) in one-way leukocyte tumor (YAC-1 or P815) cell cultures when compared with age-matched controls (Weindruch *et al.,* 1983). CTL activity fell in both dietary groups of mice but was better maintained in restricted mice. The authors suggested that the mice fed the restricted diets may have had a higher resistance to tu-morigenic influences by having NK cells with accentuated responsiveness to signals of induction coupled with CTLs that were more efficient than those obtained from unrestricted controls. Possible contributory factors include alterations in NK cell subpopulations, altered responsiveness to interferon, or possibly an influence mediated through the thymus.

In general, when dietary restriction was introduced at weaning, the au-thors suggested that the immune system may have matured less rapidly and consequently may have "stayed younger" (i.e., remained more functional) for a longer period of time than was observed in well-fed controls. Longev-ity was also significantly prolonged in mice fed diets consistent with under-nutrition without malnutrition from the time of weaning. The differences in longevity could be related to alterations in the growth rates of mice sub-jected to different dietary regimens (Cheney *et al.,* 1980). Immunological parameters are not the only ones that are markedly affected by undernutri-tion; a variety of other physiological and endocrine functions are also altered by such early-onset, long-term dietary restriction (Nolen, 1972). Walford and colleagues (1981) feel it may also be related to the effects of dietary intake on DNA repairability and other life maintenance processes. Regarding the role of immunological factors, Meredith and Walford (1977, 1979) have suggested that the major histocompatability complex (MHC) may be an influential factor in controlling the lifespan, as has been shown using congenic strains of mice differing only at the *H-2* locus. As in undernourished mice, T-cell function, as reflected by responsiveness to mitogens, was better preserved in the long-lived strains of mice (Meredith and Walford, 1977). Nonetheless, the mechanism underlying the effects of lifetime restriction of dietary calories remains to be established.

Recent studies have begun to adapt such dietary manipulations to animals at midadulthood or even later (Weindruch and Walford, 1982; Weindruch *et al.,* 1982). When dietary restriction was instituted in later life, e.g., at 12 or 17 months of age, the body weight of the restricted animals stabilized at approximately 60–70% of that of unrestricted control animals, an observation of particular note because this is the approximate level of body weight observed in many patients with AN (see below). Many of the immunological parameters that were monitored indicated changes similar to those in animals that had consumed restricted diets from the time of weaning. Weindruch and colleagues (1982) found a significant decrease in the absolute number of splenic nucleated cells; however, the proportion of T cells in the spleen was significantly increased. Uptake of [^{3}H]thymidine by spleen cells in response to PHA stimulation was significantly increased in mice dietarily restricted at or after midadulthood (Weindruch *et al.,* 1982). In contrast, the response to Con A and B-cell mitogens was not significantly affected. The response to the injection of heterologous erythrocytes did not show major alterations in peak levels, but the kinetics were substantially altered. Finally, elevated cell-mediated cytotoxicity in response to DBA/2 mastocytoma cells in 27- to 29-month-old dietarily restricted mice was comparable to that of 5- to 6-month-old control mice (Weindruch *et al.,* 1982). Coincident with this preservation of immune function was an observed decrease in the incidence of spontaneous tumors and an increase in the mean and maximum life span by approximately 10–20% (Weindruch and Walford, 1982). Thus, this form of dietary restriction, i.e., undernutrition without malnutrition, commenced at midadulthood, resulted in a preservation of immune function into later life and was similar to the results obtained when consumption of the restricted diets began at weaning. Similar results were observed in strains of mice subject to autoimmune disease, i.e., the New Zealand and MRL/1 strains of mice (Fernandes *et al.,* 1976c, 1978a,b; Beach *et al.,* 1982a,b).

HUMAN STUDIES

As previously mentioned, two major types of energy deprivation and their impact on immunocompetence have been investigated in humans: (1) total fasting under carefully monitored conditions and (2) self-induced semistarvation known as anorexia nervosa (AN) (Dowd and Heatley, 1984). Due to ethical considerations, experimentally induced total energy deprivation must be acute, generally limited to 10 days or less. In Ancel Keys' landmark work on the biology of human starvation, he and others achieved a 25% reduction of body weight (over a 24-week period) in healthy young men and observed no increase in the incidence of infectious disease when compared with individually matched controls (Keys, 1950). However, because the experimental protocol did not include adjustments for complicating nutrient deficiencies, the results must be interpreted cautiously with regard to the precise role that total energy deprivation may have played.

More recently, Palmblad and colleagues developed a model of acute total energy deprivation that took place over a 10-day period (Palmblad, 1976). These experiments may also have reduced some of the complications introduced by stress-related factors, which are well known to influence immunological function, by using subjects who used fasting as part of their pattern of behavior. After 10 days of fasting, there was a significant decrease in serum levels of C3, orosomucoid, and haptoglobin (all acute-phase reactants); in contrast, serum levels of C4 were not significantly altered (Palmblad *et al.,* 1977). Titers of 2-mercaptoethanol–sensitive antibodies (most likely of the IgM class) to flagellin were significantly higher in the subjects starved for 10 days than they were in controls or in subjects starved but inoculated at the initiation of the deprivation period. Production of specific antibodies was therefore increased in response to refeeding, and this may have considerable significance for many earlier studies conducted in protein-energy malnourished children who were being refed while studied. There were no significant differences in 2-mercaptoethanol–resistant antibodies (of the IgG class) (Palmblad *et al.,* 1977). Moreover, levels of all classes (IgA, IgM, IgG, IgE) of serum immunoglobulins were not altered in acutely starved patients. In addition, while the levels of some acute-phase reactants were decreased by total energy deprivation, serum levels of α_1-antitrypsin and the capacity to produce interferon were no different in experimental subjects than in controls.

No changes in either circulatory T or B cells or monocytes were observed in starved subjects (Holm and Palmblad, 1976). There was a significant decrease in DNA synthesis of peripheral blood lymphocytes following stimulation with the mitogens PWA and PPD; however, there was no such influence on the response to concanavalin A. The delayed hypersensitivity response to both mumps antigen and PPD was not significantly altered when compared with controls. The authors also found a significant depression in neutrophil bactericidal capacity *in vitro* against *Staphylococcus aureus* (Palmblad, 1976). In addition, stainable activity of alkaline phosphatase showed a marked decrease in starved subjects. The decreased response to PWM may suggest a defect in B-cell function; granulocyte function likewise appears to be harmed by short-term total energy deprivation. In contrast, T lymphocytes seem to be largely untouched by acute starvation.

Immunohematological parameters in patients with AN have been under investigation for over 2 decades. The first indication that such individuals might have an aberrant hematological picture came from the studies of Carryer *et al.* (1959). Marked leukopenia (as defined by less than 5000 white cells/mm³ of blood) was observed in 9 of 26 patients with AN who had a mean body weight that was 68.1% of ideal body weight (IBW). In addition, 15 of 26 AN patients were found to have a relative lymphocytosis of 40% or greater (Carryer *et al.* 1959). Further studies by other groups of investigators confirmed these early observations and found that such patients also frequently exhibited neutropenia and thrombocytopenia (Gotch *et al.,* 1975). Bowers and Eckert (1978) found that patients with AN whose mean body weight was 63% of ideal body weight had not only markedly lower total white blood cell (WBC) counts but also lower absolute counts of lymphocytes, neutrophils, and monocytes (Fig. 2).

However, despite their aberrant immunological status, patients with AN seldom exhibit a marked increase in infectious disease (Dally, 1969; Bowers and Eckert, 1978). They rarely die from infectious disease, particularly viral infections; in fact, common colds and influenza are notably rare (Dally, 1969). Moreover, there is no correlation between the severity of leukopenia and the incidence of infection (Bowers and Eckert, 1978). The single disease entity that is described with increased frequency in AN is tuberculosis (Dally, 1969; Crisp *et al.,* 1976). In addition, and in occasional patients, recurrent episodes of infection have been observed; in general, dietary treatment alleviates the problem, and measures of immunological function return to normal simultaneously (Gotch *et al.,* 1975). The susceptibility of certain individuals to infective disease may be related to a drop in body weight below 60% of IBW, which may be of clinical significance (see below).

Specific aspects of immunity have also been studied in patients with AN. Serum levels of IgM and IgG have been reported to be significantly lower in patients with AN whose body weights were 59% of IBW than in age-matched controls, although they were not decreased to the same extent as

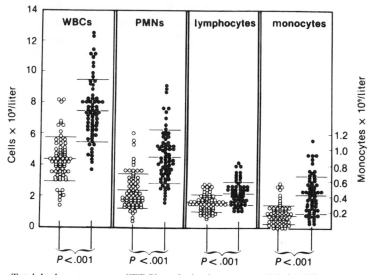

Fig. 2. Total leukocyte count (WBC) and absolute neutrophil (PMN), lymphocyte, and monocyte counts in 68 patients with anorexia nervosa (○) and 68 controls (●). Bar indicates mean (± SD). Reproduced with permission from Bowers and Eckert (1978).

other serum proteins such as those of the alternate complement pathway. Other investigators have found serum immunoglobulin levels to be within normal ranges, but this may be related to significantly higher body weight (75% of IBW) (Kim and Michael, 1975). Golla *et al.* (1981) found that patients with a body weight that was 75% of IBW had normal levels of B lymphocytes, and their mitogen responsiveness to PWM was actually higher than that of matched controls (Table VII). On treatment, this elevated responsiveness returned to values similar to those of controls (Table VIII). When humoral immunity was assessed by following the titer of antibodies to vaccination with influenza vaccine containing three different strains of the virus (A/England, A/Portchalmers, and A/Hong Kong), both control and AN subjects had similar initial hemagglutination inhibition titers against all three (Armstrong-Esther *et al.,* 1978). However, titers of antibody to A/Hong Kong influenza virus 2 months postvaccination were significantly higher in AN patients than in controls. Thus, it would appear that humoral immune function is not notably impaired and may actually, under some conditions, be enhanced by this form of self-induced semistarvation. Nonetheless, when body weight drops below approximately 60% of IBW on average, such patients may begin to experience compromised humoral immune responsiveness.

Table VII

Leukocyte Counts and Subpopulations in Patients with Anorexia Nervosa[a]

	Leukocytes (× 10³) (per mm³)	Polymorphonuclear leukocytes		Lymphocytes		T cells (%)	B cells (%)
		Number (× 10³)	%	Number (× 10³)	%		
Normal range	4.1–10.9	1.95–8.4	47–76	0.66–4.6	16–43		
Nadir 1	4.3	2.2	51.6	1.8	42.3	58	17
(control)						(69)	(14)
Nadir 2	4.3					48	20
(control)						(55)	(12)
Nadir 3	9.5	4.0	42	4.6	48.8	51	14
(control)						(59)	(17)
Nadir 4	2.1	0.75	35.5	1.2	55.5	64	17
(control)						(57)	(18)
Repletion 1	4.3	2.3	54.6	1.7	38.4	57	8
(control)						(64)	(24)
Repletion 2	4.4	1.9	42.7	2.0	46.1	54	15
(control)						(58)	(11)
Repletion 3	4.2	2.2	52.8	1.7	39.5	46	19
(control)						(59)	(13)
Repletion 4	2.0	0.8	39	0.9	46	56	16
(control)						(60)	(14)
Repletion 5	6.8	4.0	58.8	1.9	27.7	59	22
(control)						(59)	(13)

[a]Reproduced with permission from Golla *et al.* (1981).

Cell-mediated immune function has also been investigated in patients with AN. Peripheral blood of patients with a mean weight loss of 25% of IBW had normal numbers of T lymphocytes (Golla *et al.,* 1981). In addition, enhanced responsiveness to the T-cell mitogens concanavalin A and phytohemagglutinin was observed; they declined to normal levels with appropriate nutritional repletion (Golla *et al.,* 1981). Delayed-type hypersensitivity responsiveness has been examined by a number of groups, and variable results have been obtained. Golla *et al.* (1981) observed a mild impairment to the cutaneously administered antigens *Candida, Trichophyton,* SK-SD, PPD, and mumps. In contrast, Armstrong-Esther *et al.* (1978) showed no difference in delayed-type hypersensitivity responses between anorectics and controls. This group also found no significant effect of AN on the macrophage inhibition test (Armstrong-Esther *et al.,* 1978). An anergic response to the skin test antigens *Candida,* SK-SD, and mumps was found in 6 of 22 patients with AN. However, further examination of the results indi-

Table VIII

Weight Change, Complement Values, and Serum Proteins in Two Subpopulations of Patients
with Anorexia Nervosa[a]

	Percentage weight change	C total (units)	C3 (μg/dl)	C4 (μg/dl)	IgA (mg/ml)	IgM (mg/ml)	IgG (mg/ml)	Serum albumin (g/dl)
Normal value		41–90	88–252	12–72	0.3–3.0	0.2–1.4	6.4–14.3	3.3–4.5
Nadir group								
N1	25[b]	64	107	25	2.13	1.53	11.14	4.57
N2	32[b]							4.92
N3	18[b]		162	17	1.63	1.28	8.4	3.49
N4	27[b]	42	94	21	4.09	0.71	7.91	4.25
Repletion group								
R1	20[c]	61			2.42	1.54	13.7	
R2	14[c]	54	84	16	1.72	1.00	8.5	4.0
R3	13[c]	43	115	27	0.56	1.38	7.0	4.18
R4	51[c]	64	171	55	1.51	0.80	7.7	4.59
R5	12[c]	58	121	30	1.41	1.17	7.97	4.17

[a]Reproduced with permission from Golla *et al.* (1981).
[b]From usual.
[c]From nadir.

cated that when patients fell below 60% of IBW, they were frequently anergic, whereas at a higher body weight, this reaction seldom occurred. Thus, cell-mediated immunity was reasonably well preserved, or even enhanced, until weight loss was quite severe (below 60% of IBW). It was also found that anthropometric measures (weight for height, triceps skinfold thickness) correlated well with the observed anergy, whereas measures of visceral protein stores did not.

The generalized neutropenia frequently observed in anorectics has been suggested to be related to a number of factors. There is an overall bone marrow hypoplasia, underscoring a decreased production of granulocytes at that level. Such neutropenia is frequently associated with increased susceptibility to infection, e.g., in leukemia patients undergoing chemotherapy (Deinard *et al.,* 1974). However, patients with AN have a normal bone marrow reserve of neutrophils, as evidenced by normal release after hydrocortisone injection (Bowers and Eckert, 1978). This suggests a defect in the basic homeostatic mechanisms that control the distribution of PMNs between storage, marginated, and intravascular pools. In the majority of patients with AN studied, PMN bactericidal capacity was decreased, as reflected by a reduced rate of *in vitro* killing of *S. aureus* and *E. coli* (Gotch *et al.,* 1975; Palmblad *et al.,* 1977). In addition, PMN adherence was adversely affected in AN patients with a mean body weight approximately 73% of IBW (Palmblad *et al.,* 1977). In one study, mean values for PMN chemotaxis were not significantly different from those of controls, but 2 of 10 AN patients exhibited virtually no PMN chemotactic activity (Palmblad *et al.,* 1977).

Opsonic activity of serum obtained from AN patients toward *S. aureus* was within normal limits (Gotch *et al.,* 1975). Values for PMN intracellular alkaline phosphatase activity were significantly less than accepted reference values in most AN patients studied (Palmblad *et al.,* 1977). Metabolic activity of PMNs from AN patients under a variety of conditions has also been investigated. PMN production of $^{14}CO_2$ from labeled glucose was less in AN patients (63% of IBW) than in controls under both phagocytosing and nonphagocytosing conditions, but differences were more pronounced in nonphagocytosing cells (Kjosen *et al.,* 1975). Autologous serum failed to stimulate nonphagocytosing cells to the degree observed in controls; in fact, in two AN patients, an inhibition of $^{14}CO_2$ production was noted. Thus, the sera from AN patients seem to be defective in stimulatory capacity, and it is postulated that such serum factors most likely contribute to the observed impairment of glucose oxidation. Addition of latex particles to PMNs cultured in 50% autologous serum resulted in greater stimulation of glucose oxidation in AN than in control PMNs (Kjosen *et al.,* 1975). The high latent ability for phagocytosis in AN patients may help to account for their lack of increased infections.

The classic and alternate complement pathways have also been studied in patients with AN. In patients whose body weights averaged 59% of IBW, significantly lower levels of C1q, C2, C3, properdin, factor B, B1H, and C3b inactivator, as well as C4 binding protein and transferrin, were observed. In general, other groups have produced similar findings (Kim and Michael, 1975; Palmblad 1979). In contrast, levels of C4, C5, and C6 were all within noral ranges in most patients with AN (Kim and Michael, 1975; Palmblad, 1979). On treatment, there was a notable increase compared with pretreatment levels in C3, factor B, C3b inactivator, and BIH, as well as transferrin. In AN, levels of serum complement components and their regulatory proteins involved in the C3b amplification loop were disturbed more than were serum immunoglobulins or transferrin, and increased more following nutritional hyperalimentation. These findings suggest that the decreased synthesis of regulatory proteins (B1H and C3b inactivator) may represent the primary lesion and that because of this decrease there may be an increased turnover of the C3b loop of amplification, resulting in depletion of C3 and factor B. The authors also point out that the levels of proteins involved in the amplification loop provide a most sensitive index of nutritional/immunological status in AN, as well as a measure of the effectiveness of therapy.

Murray and Murray (1981) have proposed that immunological mechanisms adjust quite well to starvation and that during periods of famine, disease may be significantly curtailed (Figs. 3, 4). In addition, on refeeding and with a significant gain in body weight, there may be reactivation of disease processes such as malaria, tuberculosis, and brucellosis in famine victims. The authors observed this among victims of the Ogaden famine (Murray et al., 1976). While famine and pestilence have traditionally been considered to represent a synergistic interaction, the study of Murray and Murray (1977) in Third World countries experiencing famines led them to question this premise. According to these authors, if this synergistic hypothesis were true, populations subjected to repeated episodes of famine would perish; however, they do not, and this argues against a synergistic interaction. Murray and Murray (1981) have suggested that decreased food intake may lead to alterations in the levels of some hormones such as catecholamines and other substances that affect the rate of cellular growth such as chalones, interferon, and intracellular levels of cyclic nucleotides. All of these changes may help to slow the growth of not only the host tissues but also the pathogenic influences of those cells, especially intracellular infections and malignancy (Murray and Murray, 1981). This hypothesis is consistent with many observations in experimental animals as well as in human

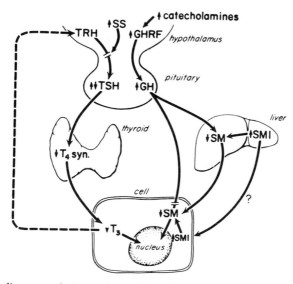

Fig. 3. Metabolic events during undernutrition that may favor increased resistance to tumorigenesis and intracellular infection. TRH, thyroid-releasing hormone; SS, somatostatin; GHRF, growth hormone-releasing factor; TSH, thyroid-stimulating hormone; GH, growth hormone; SM, somatomedin; SMI, somatomedin inhibitor; T_4, thyroxine; T_3, triiodothyronine; syn, synthesis. Reproduced with permission from Murray and Murray (1981).

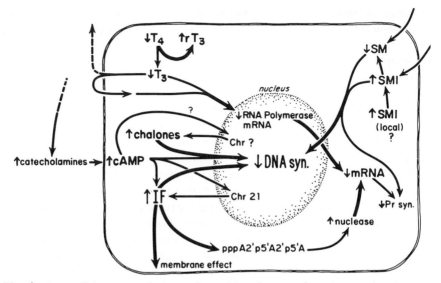

Fig. 4. Intracellular events during undernutrition that may favor increased resistance to tumorigenesis and intracellular infection. T_4, thyroxine; T_3, triiodothyronine; rT_3, reverse triiodothyronine; SM, somatomedin; SMI, somatomedin inhibitor; IF, interferon; Pr. syn., protein synthesis; Chr 21, chromosome 21; Chr ?, unknown chromosome; ?, uncertain. Reproduced with permission from Murray and Murray (1981).

patients with AN. The authors suggest that one of the most significant human defenses against infectious challenge may well be leanness. Anorexia may, in fact, represent an important component of the first-line host defense against infection. This raises important questions regarding the level of recommended dietary allowances and their impact on susceptibility to infectious disease. In addition, refeeding should be carefully considered in light of this information, with regard both to famine and to clinical situations requiring total parenteral nutrition. While this hypothesis is attractive for many reasons, much more evidence must be obtained before its validity can be ascertained. It is also important to remember that the effects of famine, undernutrition, or malnutrition on the immune system vary greatly depending on the specific nutrients that are deficient and the onset and duration of the deficiency.

DISORDERS OF CALORIC EXCESS

ANIMAL MODELS

The other extreme of imbalance in regard to caloric intake and expenditure, generally labeled *obesity* or *overweight,* results when caloric intake exceeds expenditures. As with the various types of caloric undernutrition, there are degrees of overnutrition, with an excess of greater than 20% of IBW representing obesity. Obesity is generally characterized by changes in multiple biochemical, hematological, and endocrine parameters. Consequently, there are two types of immunological alterations in obese organisms: (1) changes in the structure and function of immune system cells and (2) alterations in the microenvironment, e.g., serum, in which such immune reactions take place. As noted above, investigation of immunocompetence in overnutrition in experimental animals is largely focused on either over-fed animals or genetically obese strains of mice and rats.

Relatively little work has been done on immunological function in deliberately overfed animals. Newberne (1966) noted that the resistance of overfed dogs to distemper virus was decreased. More overfed dogs developed paralytic encephalitis than did normally fed or underfed counterparts. The metabolic and endocrine response to viral infection was notably affected by nutrition, as was evidenced by greater and more rapid loss of nitrogen and sharp elevations of serum cortisol and insulin in dogs subjected to overfeeding. Beyond this, little is known regarding the effects of overfeeding per se on immune function and response to infectious disease.

Genetically obese (*ob/ob*) mice have been characterized somewhat more fully in terms of immunological function than have experimentally overfed animals. Splenic and thymic weights were significantly lower in obese than in lean control mice (Chandra, 1980c; Chandra and Au, 1980b) (Table IX). In obese mice, both the spleen and the thymus contained significantly fewer than normal mononuclear cells, and the spleen also contained fewer Thy 1.2-positive cells (Meade *et al.,* 1979; Chandra, 1980c). Obese mice showed a decreased response to SRBC immunization; the indirect plaque-forming cell response, in particular, was sharply reduced in obese mice compared with lean controls when considered on the basis of total plaques per spleen (Chandra, 1980d). However, when considered as plaque-forming cells per 10^6 mononuclear spleen cells, the situation was reversed. The obese mice produced 401 ± 43 direct and 439 ± 51 indirect plaques per 10^6 cells, compared to 296 ± 27 direct and 348 ± 37 for lean controls (Chandra *et al.,* 1981d). It would therefore appear that the reduced plaque-forming cell responsiveness of *ob/ob* mice is due largely to a decreased number of responding cells in the spleen rather than a decrease in responsiveness per se.

NK cell activity was markedly increased in obese mice; a slight increase in antibody-dependent, cell-mediated cytotoxicity was also observed (Chandra, 1980d). Thymic hormone activity was elevated in most obese mice above levels observed in lean control counterparts (Chandra *et al.,* 1981b). Cell-mediated cytotoxicity of spleen cells obtained from obese mice immunized *in vivo* was substantially lower than that of lean controls

Table IX

Comparison of Obese Mice and Lean Controls with Regard to Organ Weights, Number of Mononuclear Cells, and PFC Response (Mean ± SE)[a]

Group	Body weight (g)	Thymus		Spleen		Direct PFC		Indirect PFC	
		Weight (mg)	Mononuclear cells × 10^6	Weight (mg)	Mononuclear cells × 10^6	Per spleen	Per 10^6 cells	Per spleen	Per 10^6 cells
Obese (n = 7)[a]	40.1 ± 1.72	73 ± 5.1 (0.182)[b]	142 ± 14	98 ± 8.3 (0.244)	176 ± 16	63,536 ± 6,921	361 ± 34	83,952 ± 5,251	477 ± 41
Control (n = 7)	21.0 ± 0.73	89 ± 6.3 (0.423)	225 ± 17	115 ± 7.9 (0.547)	288 ± 11	81,792 ± 5,193	284 ± 21	114,624 ± 7,814	398 ± 33
p	<.001	<.05	<.01	<.05	<.01	<.05	<.05	<.05	<.05

[a] Reproduced with permission from Chandra and Au (1980b).
[b] n = number of animals.
[c] Figures in parentheses refer to organ weight expressed as a percentage of body weight.

(Meade *et al.,* 1979; Chandra, 1980d). In contrast, the generation of CTLs against alloantigens (^{51}Cr-labeled chicken erythrocytes) following immunization *in vitro* was not impaired. This supports the hypothesis that genetically obese mice have a deleterious microenvironment in which such CTLs must operate. Similar differences between *in vivo* and *in vitro* cytotoxic responses to allogeneic antigenic stimuli have also been noted in the mutant diabetic mouse (C57Bl-Ks-db+) (Fernandes *et al.,* 1978a,c). It has also been noted that physiological levels of insulin, which are often elevated in obese animals, can have a direct effect on immune functions such as cell-mediated cytotoxicity (Strom *et al.,* 1975). Moreover, thymic lymphocytes from *ob/ob* mice have fewer insulin receptors than do controls, and consequently display a decreased responsiveness to insulin similar to that noted in liver and fat cells of *ob/ob* mice (Soli *et al.,* 1974). The dissociation between results obtained *in vivo* and *in vitro* in obese mice suggests that the numerous nutritional, metabolic, and endocrine alterations documented in these mice may be responsible for the observed changes in immune function (e.g., hyperedema; changes in circulating levels of hormones such as insulin, adrenocorticotropic hormone, growth hormone, progesterone, and thyroxin; or alterations in serum levels of other essential nutrients such as iron and zinc).

HUMAN STUDIES

The influence of obesity in humans on immunological function and the response to infectious disease is highly controversial. In fact, there continues to be considerable debate regarding the extent of the negative impact of obesity on human health in general. While some groups suggest that obesity has a significant impact on both morbidity and mortality for a variety of reasons (Marks, 1959; Mann, 1974a,b), others conclude that the evidence is weak at best (Fitzgerald, 1981). Because nearly all of the evidence utilized in these studies is epidemiological, it is quite difficult to establish cause-and-effect relationships. A complete discussion of the various views of obesity and its relationship to morbidity and mortality is beyond the scope of this volume. For the present purposes, it is sufficient to point out that there are cases in which obesity has been correlated with impaired response to infectious challenge. For instance, the incidence of wound infections among surgical patients was 18.1% in those considered to be obese versus only 7.1% in patients of normal weight (Meares, 1975). In another study of "clean" wounds, 13.5% of obese patients developed wound infections compared with only 1.8% of normal-weight individuals. Nonetheless, it is impossible at present to determine the quantitative impact of obesity on either susceptibility to infectious disease or the ultimate impact on mortality of such an interaction.

Preliminary investigations have focused on specific aspects of immunity in obese patients. In one study, 38% of adolescents considered to be obese on the basis of anthropometric data were found to have variably impaired cell-mediated immunity but normal levels of IgG, IgM, and IgA (Chandra and Kutty, 1980) (Table X). Cutaneous delayed-type hypersensitivity responsiveness to *Candida,* PPD, SK-SD, mumps, and tricophyton was depressed in many obese patients, as reflected by a significantly lower frequency of positive reactions when compared with controls matched for age and sex. Nonetheless, all obese patients did exhibit a delayed-type hypersensitivity response to at least one antigen. In addition, *in vitro* lymphocyte transformation in response to phytohemagglutinin stimulation was also decreased in 11 of 38 of these patients (Chandra and Kutty, 1980). In contrast, obese patients and normal controls had similar numbers of T and B peripheral blood lymphocytes, as well as similar levels of serum immunoglobulins of all classes and the C3 and C4 complement components (Chandra and Kutty, 1980). Additional studies of nutritional status in these obese patients revealed that serum levels of cholesterol, triglycerides, and lipoproteins were all within normal ranges. However, obese adolescents had a significantly higher incidence of iron and zinc deficiency, as reflected by deficient serum values of these micronutrients. Moreover, there was a significant correlation between these deficiencies and the observed immune dysfunction. Nutritional supplementation for 4 weeks with these micronutrients resulted in normalization of the immune parameters. Low plasma zinc levels are frequently observed in obese patients from all age groups (Atkinson *et al.,* 1978). However, the mechanism responsible for this condition remains obscure.

In addition to the above observations on cell-mediated and humoral immunity, the function of PMNs in obese patients has been examined. Morbid obese patients exhibited a significant decrease in PMN cytotoxicity against *Staphylococcus* in the presence of pooled serum (Palmblad *et al.,* 1977), despite an increase in the mean level of PMN adherence in these obese patients. In contrast, no significant influences of morbid obesity on chemotaxis or opsonic capacity of plasma were noted (Palmblad *et al.,* 1977). Moreover, the defective aspects of PMN function did not correlate with plasma levels of triglycerides, cholesterol, free fatty acids, or phospholipids, or with the degree of obesity (Palmblad *et al.,* 1977). Kjosen *et al.* (1975) have demonstrated decreased glucose oxidation by PMNs obtained from patients with morbid obesity. Such defective metabolism may contribute to the observed decrease in bacterial cytocapacity observed in PMNs obtained

Table X

Serum Concentrations of Immunoglobulins and Complement Components, PHA-Induced Lymphocyte Proliferation, and Bacterial Killing Capacity of PMN[a,b]

Group	Number	IgG (g/liter)	IgA (g/liter)	IgM (g/liter)	C3 (g/liter)	C4 (g/liter)	Lymphocyte stimulation index	Bactericidal capacity of PMN
Obese	28	10.86 ± 2.04	1.96 ± 0.23	1.02 ± 0.14	1.56 ± 0.12	0.27 ± 0.04	30 ± 9	19 ± 5
Control	28	11.91 ± 1.56	1.71 ± 0.21	1.15 ± 0.12	1.45 ± 0.13	0.33 ± 0.04	107 ± 15	2 ± 1
p		NS[c]	NS	NS	NS	NS	<.01	<.01

[a]Reproduced with permission from Chandra and Kutty (1980).

[b]Data are shown as mean ± SEM. Significance of differences was assessed by Student's t-test.

[c]NS, not significant.

from obese patients. In less obese patients, there were no observed indications of impaired PMN functions either before the institution of a nutritionally balanced diet containing 600 kcal/day or at any time during the 4-week dietary treatment (Palmblad *et al.,* 1980).

A number of investigators have also utilized various treatment regimens to study the influence of obesity and its magnitude and reduction on immunological competence. Palmblad *et al.* (1980) studied morbidly obese patients subjected to small intestinal shunt operations. These patients were investigated before surgery and then followed for 9 months postoperatively. Prior to surgery, they demonstrated an impaired bactericidal capacity of PMNs. Adherence of PMNs was also increased preoperatively. For the first 2–4 months after surgery, with steady weight loss, the patients showed a gradual increase in PMN bactericidal capacity (Palmblad *et al.,* 1980). After this period, the values for obese patients were somewhat similar to those of age- and sex-matched controls of normal weight. PMN adherence showed a transient decrease but then returned to the aberrantly elevated levels that had been observed preoperatively in morbidly obese patients. Therefore, with a small intestinal shunt operation, obese patients experienced a normalization of depressed PMN bactericidal capacity, while elevated PMN adherence remained essentially unchanged. Hallberg *et al.* (1976) investigated similar types of patients subjected to small intestinal shunt operations. Within 1 year of surgery, the authors saw an improved reactivity to both *Candida* and PPD in delayed-type hypersensitivity responses. In addition, they saw a significant rise in the responsiveness of peripheral blood lymphocytes to phytohemagglutinin stimulation. No concurrent changes in serum immunoglobulin levels, WBC count (total or differential), or rosetting T lymphocytes were observed (Hallberg *et al.,* 1976) (Tables XI, XII).

In pediatric and adolescent obese patients, a protein-supplemented fast and a carbohydrate-free diet for a 4-week period resulted in small but significant decreases in a large number of serum proteins (e.g., albumin, transferrin, retinol-binding protein), including the complement component β-1c (Merritt *et al.,* 1981). When 400 kcal of glucose was substituted daily for some of the protein (so that it was no longer a carbohydrate-free diet), levels of all serum proteins returned to normal except complement component β-1c. However, β-1c did increase, and differences between subjects given a maintenance diet and some of those fasting were no longer significant (Merritt *et al.* 1981). It may be that even higher levels of carbohydrates (more than 400 kcal glucose) or total calories (more than the 600 administered) are necessary to maintain normal levels of β-1c. These results also point out the importance of carbohydrates in addition to protein and calories as a key factor in serum protein homeostasis.

Table XI

Total White Blood Cell (WBC) Count and Percentage Distribution of Lymphocytes
and Different Granulocytes in Obese Subjects Before and at Intervals
After
Jejuno-Ileostomy Operation (mean ± SEM)[a]

	Preoperatively	4 months	8 months	12 months
Total WBC ±	8810 ± 874 (10)[b]	6665 ± 919 (9)	8133 ± 713 (9)	7140 ± 552 (10)
Lymphocytes (%)	34 ± 3 (12)	30 ± 3 (11)	37 ± 2.3 (12)	30 ± 3.4 (10)
Monocytes (%)	4.1 ± 0.9 (12)	3.4 ± 0.6 (10)	5.2 ± 0.7 (11)	3.9 ± 0.7 (10)
Neutrophilic granulocytes (%)	55 ± 2.5 (12)	62 ± 3 (11)	55 ± 2.5 (12)	54 ± 5.6 (10)
Eosinophilic granulocytes (%)	2.1 ± 0.5 (12)	1.7 ± 0.3 (11)	1.0 ± 0.4 (12)	1.8 ± 1.0 (10)
Basophilic granulocytes (%)	0.8 ± 0.3 (12)	0.3 ± 0.1 (11)	0.6 ± 0.3 (12)	0.5 ± 0.2 (10)
Nonsegmented granulocytes (%)	2.1 ± 1.0 (12)	2.5 ± 0.6 (11)	1.4 ± 0.5 (12)	1.9 ± 0.9 (10)

[a]Reproduced with permission from Hallberg et al. (1976).
[b]Numbers in parentheses indicate number of subjects.

The mechanisms leading to compromised immune function in obese patients remain obscure. Plasma from patients with disorders of lipoprotein metabolism, as might be exhibited by a large number of obese patients, has been shown to alter the function of lymphoid cells (Waddell et al., 1976). Uptake of tritiated thymidine in response to phytohemagglutinin stimulation was sharply reduced in mononuclear leukocytes cultured in the presence of plasma from patients with type 4 and type 5 hyperlipidemia. The specific function of suppression has been attributed to the very low density lipoprotein and chylomicron fractions of the blood (Waddell et al., 1976). However, other investigators have been unable to confirm these observations. Chandra and Kutty (1980) observed abnormally low PMN adherence with hyperglycemia (which may also be observed in obese patients), in this case due to poorly controlled diabetes. In fact, there was an inverse correlation between PMN adherence and blood glucose concentrations. Therapy with insulin resulted in rapid recovery of PMN adherence. PMNs obtained from normal patients also exhibited decreased adherence in vitro when glucose was added to the culture medium. However, once again, these observations have not been confirmed by all investigators. As noted above,

Table XII

Skin Reactions to PPD and *Candida albicans* Antigen[a,b]

Antigen	Preoperatively	4 months	8 months	12 months
PPD	13.2 ± 1.1	21.3 ± 1.7[c]	285. ± 6.2[d]	33.2 ± 9.1[d]
Candida albicans (delayed reactions)	9.3 ± 1.5	32.2 ± 14.4[d]	30.7 ± 6.7[d]	25.2 ± 6.8[d]
Candida albicans (immediate reactions)	2/11	1/6	6/11	8/8
n	11	6	11	11
				(*Candida*: 8 patients)

[a] Reproduced with permission from Hallberg *et al.* (1976).

[b] Values given are mean values ± SEM within the test group (mm diameter), except for the immediate reactions to *Candida*, which are number positive/number tested.

[c] $p < .001$.

[d] $p < .05$.

specific deficiencies of iron and zinc may also contribute to the immune dysfunction observed in obese patients. In addition, many of these nutritional effects may be mediated by alterations in levels of specific hormones such as adrenocorticosteroids, insulin, and growth hormone. Any or all of these may have a substantial impact on immune responsiveness.

7

Protein

INTRODUCTION

Protein has been the nutrient most widely studied in clinical and laboratory evaluations of nutritional immunological interactions. As noted in Chapter 4, the major nutritional shortage facing the Third World was once considered to be protein insufficiency. Because many individuals with PEM experience significant immune dysfunction, a basic premise developed in the 1960s that protein deficiency resulted in impaired immunological function. As knowledge of the nature of the major nutritional problems facing Third World populations increased, it was found that deficiencies of total calories and a wide range of specific nutrients was far more common than protein deficiency. In addition, protein requirements were revised downward in the early 1970s, which meant that the number of individuals supposedly consuming protein-deficient diets was far fewer than had been surmised. This also implied that the immunodeficiency observed in many individuals with PEM might be related to other, often multiple, nutrient deficiencies rather than to protein.

Experimental animal models were developed to examine protein deficiency in isolation. Such studies demonstrated that while deprivation of adequate dietary protein did result in impaired immunological function under certain circumstances, in others, depending on the degree and duration of deprivation and the parameters of the immune response being monitored, immunocompetence might actually be potentiated by protein deficiency. The relationship between dietary protein intake and immunological function has turned out to be far more complex than was originally suspected. In general, deficiencies of single amino acids have effects similar to those of protein deficiency as a whole, since for maximum utilization of dietary protein or amino acids for protein synthesis, all of the essential amino acids must be available to the body at approximately the same time. Thus, it can be said that in general, omission of single essential amino acids from the diet produces effects similar to those of protein deficiency. However, there have been relatively few studies on the effects of specific amino acid deficiencies on the immune system.

While we have been able to gain a better perspective on the role of protein nutriture in host immunocompetence, much more information is needed. In addition, caution must be exercised in interpreting the results obtained to date, largely due to the variability of experimental protocols. Further, there has been no agreement on the amount of dietary protein that constitutes deficiency. Diets have been employed with a protein content ranging from essentially none to 8%, all labeled "low protein" or "protein deficient." In addition, control diets have ranged from 20 to 35% protein and have employed different sources of protein, with a dramatic influence on biological availability. Some studies have been conducted in rapidly growing animals, whereas others used adult animals; little distinction is made of the concomitant differences in most studies. The duration of the dietary protein deprivation is also a major consideration. The periods of deprivation employed have ranged from a few days to a few months. Once again, little distinction is made on the basis of these differences in many studies. Protein deficiency, particularly if severe, has been noted to result in some inanition, as reflected by decreased food intake measurements and loss of body weight. Yet, very few studies have provided pair-fed controls, allowing differentiation between protein deprivation and the inadvertent deficiency of total calories or even of a wide range of nutrients due to a reduction in dietary intake.

It is hoped that in future studies, these variables will be treated more carefully. It should be possible to utilize protein deficiency as a model to study precise interactions with the immune response. In addition, because protein is required in large amounts, its intake can be manipulated under clinical conditions. Finally, while there may not be as many protein-deficient individuals as was once supposed, inadequate protein intake is a problem for many and may well be a factor compromising immunocompetence.

PROTEIN AND THE RESPONSE TO INFECTIOUS DISEASE

A diet containing low levels of protein has long been suspected to reduce host resistance to a variety of infectious processes. Particular emphasis was placed on the role of inadequate protein nutriture in the pathogenesis of tuberculosis and upper respiratory tract infections (Tui *et al.,* 1954). It was repeatedly pointed out that *Mycobacterium tuberculosis* appeared to be a particular problem among those consuming poorly balanced diets. Morbidity seemed to be much more severe and mortality rates were frequently elevated in inadequately nourished hosts (Long, 1941). The major problem with these studies, of course, was the multiplicity of potentially contributory factors involved. For instance, the individuals most likely to consume nutritionally deficient diets also had the greatest exposure to other highly correlated risk factors such as crowding and poor sanitation. As our knowledge of health conditions in the Third World has increased, it has become apparent that tuberculosis is not the only infectious process that might have an intimate relationship with malnutrition and poor sanitation. It was suspected that inadequate intake of specific nutrients such as protein might also set up a similar synergistic interaction with a wide range of pathogens, especially the enteric infections.

To clarify the nature of this interaction between protein and the response to infectious disease, many experimental protocols were used in animal models. The pathogenesis of *M. tuberculosis* in a variety of species such as rabbits, hamsters, guinea pigs, and a variety of avian species was affected by the level of protein nutriture (Ratcliffe and Merrick, 1957a,b). Such animals showed persistent lesions due to the invasive pathogen and frequently were unable to mount an effective response against the disease. In addition, infection with tuberculosis was found to have a major negative impact on the nutritional status of the host animal, especially that of protein/nitrogen. Patients with tuberculosis had markedly negative nitrogen balances, and these correlated with the substantial weight loss observed in many. However, as has been pointed out in Chapter 6, this may be part of a natural host defense mechanism. With regard to this point, a reactivation tuberculosis has been seen under conditions of famine and sudden refeeding in the refugee camps of East Africa (Murray and Murray, 1977).

Perhaps the most pertinent study on this subject emphasized that protein deficiency can indeed influence susceptibility to tuberculosis (Bhuyan and Ramalingaswami, 1973). To investigate the nature of this influence, infected guinea pigs were deprived of protein (2% protein diet for 5 weeks), and their response to intradermal BCG vaccination was monitored. It was found that in those consuming the low-protein diet, there was a fundamental inhibition of both systemic and local immune responses to the tubercle bacillus. Tuberculin sensitivity was markedly impaired in 20% of the animals fed the low-protein diet; in the remainder, the response to bacteria was absent (Bhuyan and Ramalingaswami, 1973), suggesting a depression in macrophage-mediated and T cell—mediated immunological responses. The localized dermal nodules were poorly formed in response to the intradermal infection, which correlated with a marked delay in macrophage mobilization. In addition to the observed retardation, far fewer macrophages were attracted to the site of the lesion. The lymph node that drained the site of the injection appeared to be atrophic and indicated very little lymphoid cell proliferation in the paracortical region (Bhuyan and Ramalingaswami, 1973). In the draining lymph node, accumulation of macrophages did occur, but was late and became quite diffuse and marked, in contrast to the paucity of macrophages seen in the lesion itself. Epithelioid cell transformation was markedly retarded at both sites, and at no time were mature, well-formed granulomas observed. In addition, there was long-term persistence of bacteria in both the dermal lesions and the draining lymph nodes, emphasizing the protein-deprived host's inability to eliminate the offending pathogen. As will be pointed out below, however, this delayed-type hypersensitivity response in protein-depleted animals may reflect a variety of immune cell dysfunctions.

A number of other infectious agents have also been studied in relation to level of dietary protein. When staphylococcal bacteremia was induced in rabbits, it was found that a marked deviation in response to this pathogen occurred in animals fed a low-protein diet. Clearance of the invading organisms from the blood was markedly impaired (Bhuyan and Ramalingaswami, 1972) (Table I). In addition, there was a pronounced persistence and multiplication of bacteria in both tissues and blood; correlated with this ineffective response to the pathogen was a poor and transitory neutrophilic response and the formation of focal necrotizing lesions rather than well-characterized abscesses. These conditions were associated with an elevated rate of mortality, which tended to occur very early after infection (Bhuyan and Ramalingaswami, 1972). This very high and early rate of mortality in the protein-deficient rabbits could be attributed to a fulminating septicemia,

Table I

Persistence and Multiplication of *Staphylococcus aureus*
(Average Count Per Milliliter of Blood, Showing Positive Growth)[a]

Study groups	3 hr	6 hr	1 day	2 days	3 days	4 days	5 days	10 days
				Time after intravenous inoculation				
High protein								
Count	<100	<100	350	<100	<100	120	<100	0
Positivity	9/12	6/12	6/12	2/7	2/7	1/5	1/4	0/2
Low protein								
Count	<100	<100	1300	530	210	0	0	0
Positivity	11/12	11/12	12/12	2/3	2/2	0/0	0/0	0/0

[a]Reproduced with permission from Bhuyan and Ramalingswami (1972).

which was due, in part, to the rapid and essentially unimpeded growth of the bacteria as well as the excess production of bacterial toxin.

Price and Bell (1975) also noted an impaired resistance to heat-inactivated *Escherichia coli* (as well as its purified endotoxin), *Enterobacteriae, Salmonella tymphimurium,* and *Bacillus licheniformis* in mice raised from weaning on a diet containing 4% protein. Protein-depleted mice appeared to be particularly sensitive to gram-negative bacteria (e.g., *E. coli* and other related enterics) (Price and Bell, 1975). The presence of the endotoxin alone could not explain the toxicity of such bacterial infections, but it did seem to interact synergistically with all the cell mass that was injected to produce death in many of the animals. The response to bacterial infections with streptococcus was also found to be markedly depressed in mice fed a low-protein diet (Cooper *et al.,* 1974). It thus appears that bacterial infections are in general greatly aggravated in protein-deprived hosts.

In contrast to the results obtained with bacterial infections, there was an enhanced immune response to pseudorabies virus in protein-deficient mice. Indeed, the titer of virus necessary to attain 50% mortality in protein-deficient mice was 100-fold larger than that required for well-nourished control mice (Cooper *et al.,* 1974) (Fig. 1, Tables II, III). In addition, the immune response to the fungal infection coccidiosis was also better in chicks fed low levels of dietary protein (5% protein diet for 2 weeks prior to inoculation of the coccidia) (Britton *et al.,* 1964) (Table IV). The disparity between the response to infection with bacteria and the responses that were noted on challenge with viruses or fungi established an important distinction that characterized much later work. Because bacterial infection is frequently neutralized via humoral immune mechanisms (particularly extracellular bacterial infections), it was suggested that the greater incidence and severity of such infections indicated an impaired humoral immune response. In contrast, it was believed that the cell-mediated immune function remained essentially intact or was actually enhanced by protein deprivation, as exemplified by increased resistance to viral and fungal infections.

DIETARY PROTEIN AND THE HUMORAL IMMUNE RESPONSE

Dietary protein has a potent effect on the development of humoral immune responses. A number of factors have contributed to this conclusion. If protein deficiency affects the response to infectious disease, then it must be exerting this influence by acting on one of the two immune mechanisms,

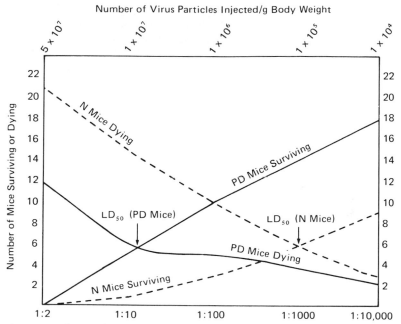

Fig. 1. Accumulation of deaths and survivals in mice infected with pseudorabies virus. The volumes of inocula of the five virus dilutions were adjusted so that each mouse received the indicated number of virus particles per gram body weight. N mice, control mice (C-2 mice); PD mice, CPI mice (PI-2 mice). (Reproduced with permission from Cooper *et al.,* 1974.)

Table II

Enhancement of Resistance to a Virus (Pseudorabies) by Chronic Dietary Protein Insufficiency in Mice[a]

		Diet-related mortality (%)		
Dilution of virus	Number of virus particles/ml	8% casein (depletion)	27% casein (normal)	Number of mice used/dilution of virus
1:2	$0.5 \times 10^{6-7}$	100	100	6
1:10	$1.0 \times 10^{5-6}$	55[b]	94	6
1:100	$1.0 \times 10^{4-6}$	33	77	6
1:1000	$1.0 \times 10^{3-4}$	22	50	6
1:10,000	$1.0 \times 10^{2-3}$	10	25	6

[a]Reproduced with permission from Cooper *et al.* (1974).
[b]Under scored numbers indicate LD_{50} values.

Table III

Lack of Effect of Chronic Protein Insufficiency on the Primary
and Secondary Antibody Response to *Brucella abortus*[a]

Dietary treatment, % casein	Number of mice and designation[b]	Total number of mice	Log$_2$ titers[c]	p[d]
Primary response				
8	8 PI-1	20	6.8 ± 0.7	ns
	7 PI-2			
	5 PI-3			
27	8 C-1	20	7.4 ± 1.0	
	7 C-2			
	5 C-3			
Secondary response				
8	8 PI-1	20	11.1 ± 1.3	ns
	7 PI-2			
	5 PI-3			
27	8 C-1	20	10.9 ± 0.8	
	7 C-2			
	5 C-3			

[a]Reproduced with permission from Cooper *et al.* (1974).
[b]See Fig. 1. The decreasing numbers of mice in successive generations were a result of mice deaths consequent to initial bleeding.
[c]Means ± SE. The first dilution of serum was 1:10.
[d]This reflects Student's *t* test compared with the response of control mice fed 27% casein diets. ns, not significant.

Table IV

Mortality of Chicks from Coccidiosis When Starved, Fed a Protein-Free Diet,
or a 20% Protein Diet[a]

Diet	Days postinoculation				
	5	6	7	8	9
	Cumulative % mortality[b]				
Starved[c]	3	10	27	27	27
Protein free[d]	0	17	29	29	29
20% protein[d]	32	45	50	55	55

[a]Reproduced with permission from Britton *et al.* (1964).
[b]Mean value of 2 groups of 12 chicks each.
[c]Starved for 48 hr before and 96 hr after inoculation.
[d]Diets fed for 48 hr before and 1 week after inoculation.

humoral or cellular. Moreover, antibody molecules consist largely of protein, with only a small fraction of carbohydrate; therefore, a deficiency of protein can very likely affect the synthesis and secretion of immunoglobulins. Indeed, during diet-induced protein deficiency, there was an overall decline in serum proteins, and it seemed logical to assume that there would be a proportionate decline in the serum concentrations of immunoglobulins. However, the observation that PEM in children was only infrequently accompanied by a decline in serum immunoglobulins, and in fact often occurred with elevated levels of circulating antibody molecules, tended to compromise this hypothesis. While such children could have experienced excessive antigenic stimulation that accounted for their increased levels of serum immunoglobulins, it was also possible that protein deficiency, at the levels experienced by human populations, did not coincide with impaired production of immunoglobulins.

This subject was further studied by Cohen and Hansen (1962). In a series of labeling studies, they showed that patients with kwashiorkor did not experience a reduction in the synthesis of γ globulins. In contrast, the synthesis of albumin was depressed. In fact, the authors suggested that the synthesis of γ globulins might be maintained preferentially in the face of protein deficiency, to the ultimate detriment of the host (Cohen and Hansen, 1962). These findings certainly did not agree with the hypothesis that humoral immunity is depressed in dietary protein deficiency.

As our understanding of the immune response has expanded and its complexity and the multiplicity of interactions have become established, such seeming paradoxes have become better understood. It is now known that one cannot speak of humoral immunity as a single phenomenon. Antibody responses are the product of the interaction of numerous cell populations. Some antigens require more cell interactions than others. Given the tremendous number of interactions, protein deficiency may influence the humoral immune response in various ways, depending on what type of antigen is administered, in what dosage, as well as the number of times the animal is challenged; secondary antibody responses require different types of interactions from primary responses.

EFFECT ON LYMPHOID TISSUE

Before discussing the effects of protein deficiency on antibody production per se, we will consider the general influence of dietary protein deprivation on lymphoid tissues throughout the body. The specific influence of dietary protein restriction on lymphoid tissue has been addressed by a number of investigators. As with many other nutrient deficiencies, in wean-

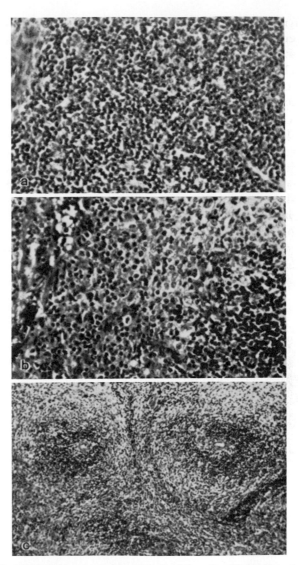

Fig. 2. The spleen of BALB/c mice fed the 20% diet (a) or the 4% diet (b and c). (a) and (b) show the loss of mature small mononuclear cells in the outer follicular areas. In both figures the arteriole is to the right. There is an even distribution of small lymphocytes in the follicle of high-protein mice that is replaced in the low-protein mice by a lower density population of larger immature cells. The clustering of mature small lymphocytes around the arteriole is evident in the lower right of (b) and is shown at lower magnification in (c). The existence of mature lymphocytes in the periarteriolar T-dependent areas indicates persistent long-lived recirculating T-cell function in protein-deprived mice. [H & E; magnification, (a) and (b) × 280; (c) × 112.] (Reproduced with permission from Bell *et al.,* 1976b.)

ling mice thymic tissue seemed to be particularly sensitive to protein deficiency. Spleen and mesenteric lymph nodes were also affected by protein
deficiency (4% protein diet), but to a lesser extent than was thymus (Bell *et
al.,* 1976a) (Figs. 2–4). It was found that the decreased lymphoid organ
weights reflected impaired growth due to lack of protein for cell division, as
well as an adrenal steroid–mediated lympholysis resulting in the death of
certain cells (and possibly specific cell populations) (Table V). Mice fed the
low-protein diet had 10–20% of the total number of lymphoid cells of mice
fed complete diets (Bell *et al.,* 1976a) (Figs. 5, 6). Resident B lymphocytes
and the pool of circulating T lymphocytes were not notably affected by a
lack of dietary protein. In marked contrast, nonmigratory T cells, stem cells,
and other cells in the reticuloendothelial system were most severely altered
by the protein deficiency (Bell *et al.,* 1976a). While no effects of protein
deficiency on the capacity to form germinal centers was noted at any point,
there was a significant elimination of cell recruitment to specific nodes

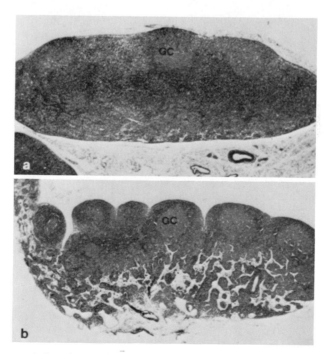

Fig. 3. Mesenteric lymph node (MLN) of BALB/c mice fed the 20% diet (a) or the 4% diet
(b) for 2 weeks. Note the formation of germinal centers (GC) in deprived MLN but somewhat
reduced cellularity. (H & E; magnification × 28.) (Reproduced with permission from Bell *et
al.,* 1976b.)

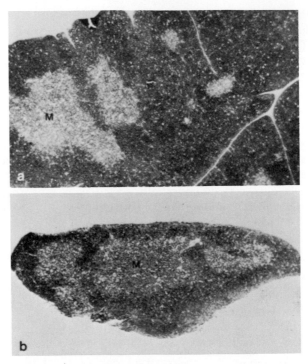

Fig. 4. Thymus of BALB/c mice fed 20% protein diets (a) or 4% protein diets (b) for 10 days after weaning. There is a gross reduction in the size of the cortex in deprived mice. The medulla (M) persists with little reduction in size and occupies a relatively larger proportion of thymic volume. (H & E; magnification × 28.) (Reproduced with permission from Bell *et al.,* 1976b.)

Table V

Effect of Adrenalectomy on Lymphoid Organ Weight in Mice Fed a 4% Protein Diet[a]

	Body weight (g)	Spleen (mg)	Thymus (mg)	Mesenteric lymph node (mg)
Adrenalectomized 1 week deprived	9.1	53	47	27
Sham 1 week deprived	10.3	47 (ns)	47 (ns)	27 (ns)
Adrenalectomized 2 weeks deprived	9.7	58	38	29
Sham 2 weeks deprived	9.3	24 ($p < .001$)	8 ($p < .001$)	16 ($p < .005$)

[a]Reproduced with permission from Bell *et al.* (1976b).
[b]ns, not significant.

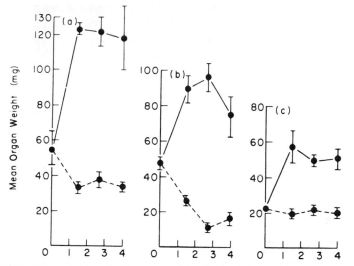

Fig. 5. Changes in major lymphoid organ weights during the first 4 weeks after weaning on 4% (●- - -●) and 20% (●———●) protein diets BALB/c mice. (a) Spleen, (b) thymus, (c) mesenteric lymph node. (Reproduced with permission from Bell *et al.,* 1976b.)

following antigenic stimulation (Bell *et al.,* 1975). Long-term nutritional rehabilitation with normal levels of dietary protein restored the immune response in these mice even after a 2-month period of nutritional deficiency.

Many studies have examined the effects of protein deprivation on antibody formation in experimental animals. For example, adult male rats were

Table VI

Peak Splenomegaly Responses Induced by *Brucellus abortus*[a]

Strain of mice	Diet	Antigen dose Primary	Antigen dose Secondary	Stimulation Index Primary	Stimulation Index Secondary
Balb/c	Normal	10^8	10^8	3.82 ± 0.09	1.95 ± 0.05
	4% albumin	10^8	10^8	0.91 ± 0.16	1.21 ± 0.15
	4% casein	10^8	10^8	1.59 ± 0.12	0.78 ± 0.05
C_{57} Bl	Normal	10^8	10^8	2.74 ± 0.12	1.59 ± 0.11
	4% albumin	10^8	10^8	0.79 ± 0.08	0.93 ± 0.11
	Normal	10^7	10^8	0.56 ± 0.05	2.71 ± 0.10
	4% albumin	10^7	10^8	0.31 ± 0.04	0.97 ± 0.08
	Normal	10^7	10^7	—	0.55 ± 0.05
	4% albumin	10^7	10^7	—	0.58 ± 0.06

[a]Reproduced with permission from Price and Bell (1977).

fed a very-low-protein diet for 5 weeks; the spleens of these animals were hypocellular and markedly reduced in weight. This weight reduction correlated with notably diminished titers of antibodies in response to heterologous erythrocyte immunization (Kenney *et al.,* 1968). In animals depleted of protein, the number of antibody-forming cells (AFC) and the titers of antibodies to specific antigens were diminished to approximately one-third the level observed in animals fed the control diet (containing approximately 25% protein). Levels of γ globulin were also substantially reduced, but not as greatly as levels of specific antibody titers (Kenney *et al.,* 1968). Since these animals appeared to be producing the same levels of antibodies, it was suggested that the reduction in antibodies was due to a decrease in the number of cells capable of producing them, especially in light of the markedly depleted splenic weights. However, because of the severe protein depletion in this study, the clinical significance of this finding is not clear.

In another study, animals fed a diet containing 3% protein for 3–4 weeks produced significantly lower antibody responses to an intraperitoneal dose of 10^9 SRBC (Mathur *et al.,* 1972). Protein deficiency resulted in a 70–80% reduction in the number of plaques obtained in a Jerne direct plaque-forming cell system, and an even greater reduction when assessed per 10^6 spleen cells. This is a particularly critical index to monitor in such mice, because splenic as well as thymic weights were dramatically reduced in protein-depleted animals. Finally, injection of thymocytes from syngeneic animals at the time of SRBC immunization allowed a major restitution of immunological capability in these protein-depleted animals (Mathur *et al.,* 1972). This observation is consistent with the thymic dependency of antigens such as heterogeneous erythrocytes and might be explained by defective T helper cell function.

The importance of the antigen dosage used to challenge protein-deficient animals was first emphasized by Price and Bell (1977). They showed that depending on the level of antigen administered to mice, there was either an increased or decreased response, as reflected by the resulting reciprocal mean hemagglutination titers. Specifically, antibody responsiveness to *Brucella abortus* immunization was slightly lower in mice fed a diet containing 4% protein when high doses of antigen were administered. However, when a lower dose of antigen was employed, antibody responsiveness was either normal or frequently increased (Price and Bell, 1977). Moreover, the splenomegaly generally observed following challenge with *B. abortus* was markedly less severe. While the results utilizing SRBC were generally less dramatic, they produced many similar trends (Price and Bell, 1977) (Tables VI, VII). However, the observations in response to SRBC immunization most likely reflected the effects of protein deficiency on the population of helper T cells. In general, in mice deprived of dietary protein, antibody production

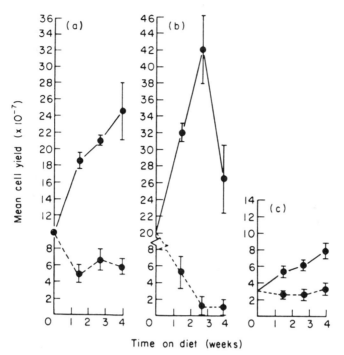

Fig. 6. Major lymphoid organ cell yields during the first 4 weeks of feeding 4% (●- - -●) and 20% (●——●) protein diets, BALB/c mice. (a) Spleen cell yield, (b) thymus cell yield, (c) mesenteric lymph node cell yield. (Reproduced with permission from Bell *et al.*, 1976b.)

was often short-lived and involved high levels of circulating IgM, consistent with defective function in the T helper cell population, most likely due to the greater thymic dependency of antibody response to heterologous erythrocytes.

Sequential administration of multiple antigens, particularly those with shared or similar determinants (e.g., vaccines prepared from *B. abortus* and *E. Coli* or red blood cells from various species) can result in increased responsiveness to the last antigen administered. It has been suggested that such "sequential competition" represents a T cell–dependent phenomenon that is mediated by a soluble humoral factor, perhaps immunoglobulin. Mice fed a diet containing 4% protein exhibited a much broader range of conditions under which immunization with diphtheria toxoid (both primary and secondary infections) significantly impaired the response to administration of tetanus toxoid when compared with mice fed a diet containing 18% protein (Price, 1978b). This was in contrast to the finding of no significant differences between protein-deprived and control mice with respect to

Table VII
Secondary Responses to SRC[a,b]

Antigen dose		Total agglutinins[c]		2ME-resistant agglutinins[d]	
Primary	Secondary	N	D	N	D
5×10^6	5×10^6	5.66	5.73 ns[e]	4.07	3.51 ns
5×10^6	5×10^7	6.38	7.93 ($p < .05$)	5.25	5.41 ns
5×10^6	5×10^8	7.93	6.39 ($p < .05$)	7.37	4.33 ($p < .01$)
5×10^7	5×10^7	8.83	7.76 ns	8.44	6.04 ($p < .001$)
5×10^7	5×10^8	8.71	7.82 ns	8.38	6.56 ($p < .01$)
5×10^8	5×10^8	8.87	5.97 ($p < .001$)	8.44	3.81 ($p < .001$)

[a]Reproduced with permission from Price and Bell (1977).
[b]Pooled $\log_2$ reciprocal geometric mean titres produced by groups of three normally fed (N) and protein-deficient (D) mice primed and rechallenged with SRC 1 and 3 weeks after weaning, respectively, and bled 2, 6, or 12 days after rechallenge.
[c]Agglutination titers recorded with untreated sera (IgG and IgM).
[d]Agglutination titers recorded with 2ME-treated sera (IgG only).
[e]Significance level for the difference between N and D mice, calculated from LSD values. Groups where the difference was not significant at $p < .05$ are marked ns.

simultaneous administration of a battery of antigens; all mice, irrespective of their nutritional status, demonstrated an intact response to all antigens administered simultaneously.

These findings have potential importance for vaccination programs throughout the world and may assist in explaining reduced seroconversion rates in Third World children who receive multiple antigen vaccines (Ruben *et al.,* 1973) (Tables VIII–X). In this respect, it is interesting that supplementation of New Guinean school children with 25 g of dietary

Table VIII
Measles Seroconversions by Age Groups[a]

Age group (months)	SMY[c]			SMYT[d]		
	Total	Converters Number	%	Total	Converters Number	%
6–8	22	14	63.6	22	13	59.1
9–24	66	59	89.4[b]	55	39	70.9[b]

[a]Reproduced with permission from Ruben *et al.* (1973).
[b]Significant difference, $p < .025$; $\chi^2 = 5.51$.
[c]Small pox–measles–yellow fever vaccine.
[d]Tetanus, diptheria, and pertussis vaccine.

Table IX

Major Reaction Rates to Smallpox Vaccination and Seroconversion Rates in Susceptible Subjects[a]

| | | | | Percentage positive | | | | | |
| | | | | Pertussis | Tetanus | | Diphtheria | | |
Group	Vaccination scar	Measles (HI)[b]	Yellow fever (neutralization)	$\geq 1:8^c$	$>0.01^d$	$>0.1^d$	$>0.01^d$	$>0.1^d$
O[e]	4.6	2.1	5.3	12.7	9.0	1.7	12.4	3.4
SMY	97.6	83.0	96.6					
SMYT	97.3	67.6	94.8	70.1	100.0	100.0	87.3	77.8
T[f]				79.7	97.4	94.9	89.1	76.5

[a]Reproduced with permission from Ruben et al.
(1973).
[b]Titer ≥ 1:5.
[c]Agglutination titer.

[d]Antitoxin units.
[e]Group O received a placebo.
[f]Group T received diptheria, pertussis, and tetanus vaccine.

protein (in addition to the approximately 10 g found in the normal diet) resulted in a significant enhancement of antibody production in response to immunization with monomeric flagellin prepared from *Salmonella adelaide* (Mathews *et al.,* 1972).

To determine whether chronic protein deficiency produced a shortage of competent precursor cells (either cells directly responsible for antibody production or the requisite "helper" cells) or a deficiency of nonspecifically activated accessory cells and factors (e.g., nonspecific splenic phagocytic cells), transfer experiments in irradiated mice were employed. Direct PFC responsiveness and antibody production in response to SRBC immunization were elevated in irradiated adult mice fed a control diet (18% protein) and reconstituted with spleen cells obtained from mice fed a low-protein diet (4% protein) for 1–3 weeks (Price, 1978a). In this case, the effect was not influenced by the duration of the original protein deficiency, the period of time after immunization when the assay was performed, or the number of cells transferred. Furthermore, time course experiments revealed that enhancement of cellular proliferation within the initial 3- to 5-day period after spleen cell transfer resulted in heightened responsiveness (Price 1978a). On the basis of these observations, it was concluded that the depressed responsiveness frequently reported in protein-deficient mice might be attributed to impaired reticuloendothelial cell function and deficient levels of protein synthesis not directly related to the spleen.

To investigate further the mechanism whereby protein deficiency alters the antibody response to various antigens, Price (1978a) studied the ability of various strains of protein-deficient mice to respond to T cell–indepen-

Table X

Postvaccination Serologic Titers in Susceptible Subjects[a]

Measles (HI)

	Titer levels								Percentage
Group	<5	5	10	20	40	80	160	320	Total	positive
Saline	92	0	1	0	0	1	0	0	94	2.1
SMY	15	0	6	2	4	16	21	24	88	83.0
SMY DPT[b]	25	0	3	3	9	8	10	19	77	67.5

Yellow fever (neutralization)

Group	Positive	Negative	Total	Percentage positive
Saline	5	89	94	5.3
SMY	85	3	88	96.6
SMY DPT	73	4	77	94.8

Pertussis (agglutination)

	Titer levels								Percentage
Group	<8	8	16	32	64	128	256	512	Total	positive
Saline and SMY	41	5	1	0	0	0	0	0	47	12.8
SMY DPT	23	11	8	8	10	10	5	2	77	70.1
DPT	16	11	10	8	10	9	13	2	79	79.7

Tetanus (antitoxin)

				Percentage	
Group	≥0.01	≥0.1	Total	≥0.01	≥0.1
Saline and SMY	16	3	176	9.1	1.7
SMY DPT	78	78	78	100.0	100.0
DPT	77	75	79	97.5	94.9

Diphtheria (antitoxin)

Group	≥0.01	≥0.1	Total	≥0.01	≥0.1
Saline and SMY	18	5	145	12.4	3.4
SMY DPT	55	49	63	87.3	77.8
DPT	57	49	64	89.1	76.6

[a]Reproduced with permission from Ruben *et al.* (1973).
[b]DPT, diptheria, pertussis, and tetanus vaccine.

dent antigens, e.g., polyvinyl pyrillodine (PVP) and type III pneumococcal polysaccharide (S III). While both can elicit a primary IgM response without T helper cells, the production of significant levels of serum IgG and appropriate immunological memory does not follow S III administration, and serum levels of IgG remain distinctly low after PVP administration.

The response to intraperitoneal injection of S III was substantially more depressed than was the response to intravenous injection (Price, 1978a). Because macrophage uptake and processing of antigens administered intraperitoneally are particularly critical in generating an effective immune response to S III, this difference in the rate of injection underscores the importance of impaired phagocytic cell function in protein deprivation.

Protein deficiency also greatly facilitated the development of tolerance to a variety of antigens, particularly (although not exclusively) the T-independent antigens (Price and Bell, 1977; Price, 1978a). Dietary protein deficiency decreased the minimum dosage of PVP, S III, and SRBC required to induce tolerance (Price, 1978b). Because the mechanism of tolerance is not well understood, it is difficult to speculate on the significance of these findings. It is possible that the impaired function of reticuloendothelial system cells allows prolonged circulation of lower levels of antigen, thereby promoting tolerance. A variety of abnormalities in the regulatory activity of both B- and T-cell subsets could also contribute to the enhanced induction of tolerance.

Experimental protein deficiency has been used as a model in which to study the possibilities of nutritional rehabilitation and its effects on immunological phenomena. When mice that had previously been fed a protein-deficient diet of 4% protein were transferred to a diet containing 18% protein, rapid proliferation of splenic B cells relative to other hematopoietic cells was noted (Price and Bell 1976). Thymic growth underwent a similar although more delayed spurt (Bell *et al.,* 1976b).

It is possible that the depression of antibody responses reflects the markedly altered function of phagocytic cells (e.g., macrophages responsible for antigen processing and presentation) during protein deprivation. When nutritional rehabilitation is initiated, it is conceivable that immunologically specific macrophages are rendered unresponsive for a temporary period due to the shunting of cell populations into a rapid proliferative phase. A similar role could be attributed to any lymphoid cell line responsible for inducing or regulating antibody responses to this variety of antigens. Another possible explanation might involve a rapid expansion of the T-suppressor population following restitution of normal dietary protein. In any case, it is quite likely that during protein deprivation, the reduced availability of protein results in a new balance between the various subsets of immune system cells. When nutritional rehabilitation is suddenly initiated, a new form of homeostasis must be achieved. The different results obtained with variations in the type, dosage, and sequence of antigen administration emphasize the fine-tuned nature of the homeostatic mechanism.

Elegant studies have examined the differential response of protein-malnourished mice to immunization with alloantigens (i.e., cells from a strain of mice that differed in the *H-2* locus from the recipient's cells) (Malave and Layrisse, 1976). Weanling mice fed a low-protein diet containing 8% protein experienced either primary or secondary stimulation, and the titers of serum antibodies were monitored. Primary responses were assessed by titrating serum hemagglutinin responses and quantitating the direct PFC response. It was found that in addition to a marked production increase of spleen cells, the number of IgM-producing plaques was reduced only slightly (Malave and Layrisse, 1976). However, the number of direct alloantibody-producing plaques per 10^6 spleen cells was actually increased, a finding consistent with other studies employing primarily T-independent antigens in protein-deficient experimental animals. As with other studies, these normal or elevated IgM responses may represent the ineffective activity of T-suppressor populations involved in controlling the magnitude of immunological reactions. In addition, serum hemagglutination titers obtained during the primary response were normal or elevated when compared with those of well-nourished, age-matched controls (Malave and Pocino, 1980). In contrast to this increase in the IgM response, IgG was depressed in both primary and secondary responses. Because the secondary response is largely composed of an IgG response, IgG-forming plaques were most notably depressed in this phase of the immune response. It appears that one of the cell populations involved in the production of IgG responses is markedly altered in protein deficiency, whereas the IgM-producing apparatus continues to function largely intact. This would be consistent with the degree of thymic dependency if responses such as adequately functioning T helper cells are critical for the normal production of a secondary antibody response, which is generally composed of large amounts of IgG.

PROTEIN AND CELL-MEDIATED IMMUNE FUNCTION

As is evident in the preceding section, it is not possible to analyze the influence of protein nutriture on the humoral immune response without examining concomitant changes in cell populations considered to belong to the cellular immune system. As with many other nutrients, the major influence of protein nutriture on antibody production involves alterations in subpopulations of regulatory T cells.

In one of the first studies to examine the role of protein nutriture in cell-mediated immune function, Cooper *et al.* (1974) found an enhanced graft-versus-host reaction (GVHR) utilizing the Simonsen assay of spleen weights following inoculation with donor cells in mice fed an 8% protein diet. While this is an unsophisticated assay, the study did provide some initial insight into the possible mechanism that might produce an enhanced response to viral pathogens. Moreover, other data indicated that protein-deprived mice also exhibited an accelerated rate of skin allograft rejection. The response of splenic lymphocytes to PHA, a T cell mitogen, was also enhanced substantially by a dietary protein deficit (Cooper *et al.,* 1974). All of these findings tend to indicate that cell-mediated immunity in the protein-deprived host either remains intact or is enhanced. Purkayastha *et al.* (1975) examined the rate of homograft rejection in rats fed different levels of dietary protein. Nonetheless, and in contrast to earlier studies, feeding a 3% protein diet did not significantly alter the mean survival time of skin homografts. Indeed, protein deficiency did not alter either first- or second-set graft rejection in these animals.

Cooper *et.al.* (1974) and Bell and Hazell (1975) found a pronounced increase in graft-versus-host (GVH) activity in mice fed a 4% protein diet compared to mice fed a control diet containing 20% protein (Fig. 7). In addition to the increased responsiveness, the slope of the curve reflecting GVHR capacity was also altered for cells from thymus and from Peyer's patches, indicating changes in the populations of reactive cells (Figs. 8, 9). In contrast, while an increased GVHR capacity was also noted (up to four-fold) in mesenteric lymph nodes and spleen, there was no similar alteration in the slope of the curve, indicating that there was no fundamental alteration in responsive cell populations (Bell and Hazell, 1975). The authors suggested that the observed changes might reflect the fact that T cells, which are the key effector element in GVHR, have a longer life span than do circulating B cells, thus possibly contributing to their retention of functional reactivity in the face of specific nutritional insults. One must note, however, that pair feeding also increased GVH (Table XI), thence our emphasis in the early part of this chapter on the use of controls.

Because spleen weight was used as the index of GVHR in many previous studies (Cooper *et al.,* 1974; Bell and Hazell, 1975), Malave *et al.* (1978) attempted to utilize a more precise method of quantifying allograft rejection. In their studies, in response to alloantigen administration, lymphocytes obtained from the spleen, thymus, and lymph nodes of protein-deficient mice (8% protein diet) incorporated a significantly greater amount of ^{125}IUDR than did lymphocytes obtained from control animals fed a diet containing 27% protein (Malave *et al.,* 1978). These results indicate that mice fed a moderately protein-deficient diet for 3–5 weeks have a greater ability to cause lymphocyte proliferation in response to alloantigen admin-

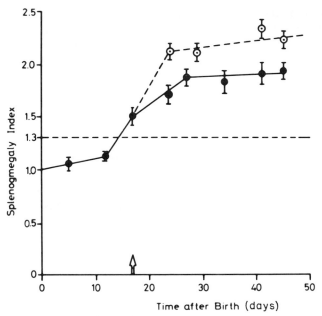

Fig. 7. The development of GVH reactivity in spleen cells in normal and deprived mice. (●——●), Spleen cells from normal mice; (⊙- - - -⊙), spleen cells from deprived mice. The arrow at 17 days represents the day of weaning and the first day of feeding normal and deprived diets. Positive responses (spleen index greater than 1.3) are not detected until the day of weaning but deprived mice rapidly exceed the capacity of normal controls to initiate GVH reactions. (Reproduced with permission from Bell and Hazell, 1975.)

istration than do normal mice. This may indicate normal or enhanced cellular immunity in such moderately malnourished animals, and may reflect either an increased proportion of reactive cells or alterations in the ratios of the various cell subpopulations.

Further studies by Kramer and Good (1978) indicated that while *in vitro* cell-mediated immunity was indeed enhanced, *in vivo* testing revealed little or no change. In these studies, guinea pigs were fed various protein-deficient diets (3, 6, 9, and 27% protein) (Kramer and Good, 1978). While antibody responsiveness was reduced in proportion to the reduction in protein intake, such animals continued to manifest normal or elevated levels of cell-mediated immunity, as reflected by *in vitro* testing. Guinea pigs fed the lowest level of protein produced (*in vitro*) levels of MIF equal to those produced by lymphocytes obtained from animals fed 24% protein. Moreover, lymphocytes obtained from animals fed 6 and 9% protein actually had significantly higher levels of MIF. The response of splenic lymphocytes to

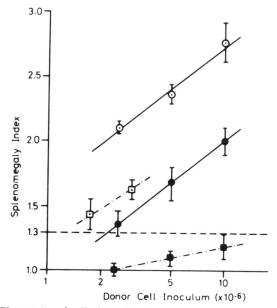

Fig. 8. The GVH capacity of cells from the spleen and Peyer's patches of normal and deprived mice. (●), Spleen cells from normal mice; (⊙), spleen cells from deprived mice; (■), Peyer's patch cells from normal mice; (□), Peyer's patch cells from deprived mice. Broken line at 1.3 represents the baseline of a positive GVH response. Each point represents the mean ± SE of a minimum of four recipient litters. Peyer's patch cells fail to induce significant splenomegaly even at the highest dose (10^7 cells) injected, whereas deprived Peyer's patch cells were active at a dose as low as 1.75×10^6 cells. Dose response lines for spleen cells were parallel and deprived cells were significantly more active at all doses tested. (Reproduced with permission from Bell and Hazell, 1975.)

mitogenic stimulation with phytohemagglutinin showed no significant differences between control animals and their counterparts fed low-protein diets (Kramer and Good, 1978). However, when the various groups of animals were tested for delayed-type hypersensitivity, the protein-depleted animals showed very little evidence of intact cellular immunity, as reflected by failure of induration after intradermal administration of BCG vaccine. Moreover, those indurations that did occur were quantitatively reduced and showed a variety of histological abnormalities. One possible explanation for the variance in these observations is that individual cells involved in cellular immunity may be hyperactive in protein deficiency, but in the whole animal, there may be a severe reduction in cell number due to an inability to undergo clonal expansion given the appropriate stimulus. This hypothesis is also consistent with the numerous aberrations in regulatory function that

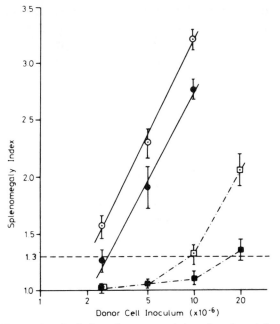

Fig. 9. The GVH capacity of cells from the mesenteric lymph node and thymus of normal and deprived mice. (●), Mesenteric lymph node cells from normal mice; (☉), mesenteric lymph node cells from deprived mice; (■), thymocytes from normal mice; (☐), thymocytes from deprived mice. Broken line (- - - -) represents the baseline of a positive GVH response. Each point represents the mean ± SE of a minimum of four recipient litters. The regression coefficients of deprived and normal mesenteric lymph node cells were equal, indicating parallel lines whereas the degree of splenomegaly was significantly higher for all doses of deprived spleen cells. Dose response lines for thymocytes were not parallel and differed significantly only at a dose of 2×10^7 cells. (Reproduced with permission from Bell and Hazell, 1975.)

Table XI

Effect of Quantity Restriction (Pair Feeding) of a Normal Diet
on Capacity to Initiate GVH Reactions[a]

Treatment	Spleen index	Significance[b]
Pair-fed spleen 5×10^6	2.05 ± 0.09	
Normal spleen 5×10^6	1.68 ± 0.13	Pair-fed versus normal ($p < .05$)
Deprived spleen 5×10^6	2.36 ± 0.06	Pair-fed versus deprived ($p < .005$)
Pair-fed thymus 2×10^7	1.39 ± 0.09	
Normal thymus 2×10^7	1.37 ± 0.09	Pair-fed versus normal (NS)
Deprived thymus 2×10^7	2.06 ± 0.14	Pair-fed versus deprived ($p < .01$)

[a]Reproduced with permission from Bell and Hazell (1975).
[b]Significance assessed by Student's t test.

have been noted in protein-deprived animals, which may also fail to undergo clonal expansion under conditions of insufficient dietary protein.

In order to compare the influences of protein restriction on cell-mediated immune function at different stages of the life cycle, inbred mice were fed low-protein diets (4% protein) at either 6 weeks of age (immature) or 35 weeks of age (mature) (Watson and Haffer, 1980). It was found that in immature mice there was a notable decrease in the proportion of θ-bearing cells and a significant depression of lymphocyte transformation in response to PHA (Figs. 10, 11). The mixed lymphocyte reaction (MLR) of spleen cells obtained from protein-deprived immature mice was also significantly depressed. These alterations in immunocompetence occurred after only 2 weeks on the diet and persisted for up to 8 weeks (Watson and Haffer, 1980). While θ-bearing cell populations were not altered by protein restriction in the mature mice, there was a significant suppression in both MLR and mitogen responsiveness after 7 weeks of the low-protein diet; this

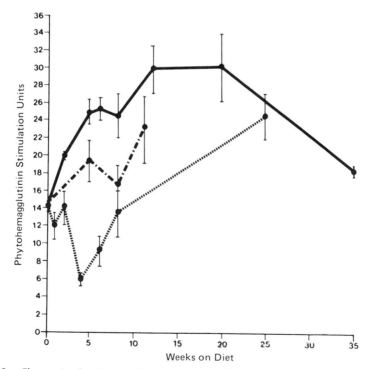

Fig. 10. Changes in phytohemagglutinin responses of immature BALB/c mice on low-protein diet. ▬▬, 20% protein diet at 5 weeks; ·····, 4% protein diet at 5 weeks; ·▬·▬, 4% protein diet at 6 weeks. (Reproduced with permission from Watson and Haffer, 1980.)

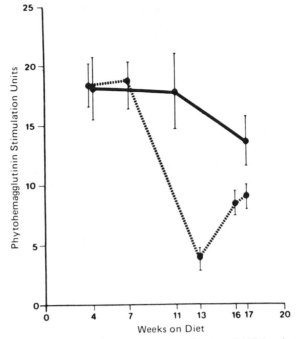

Fig. 11. Changes in phytohemagglutinin responses of mature BALB/c mice on low-protein diet. ▬, 20% protein diet at 35 weeks; ····, 4% protein diet at 35 weeks. (Reproduced with permission from Watson and Haffer, 1980.)

persisted for an additional 6 weeks. Thus, there are substantially different effects of dietary protein restriction on immunological function, depending on the stage of the life cycle in which the deprivation occurs. The authors suggest that the immature immune system is more susceptible to protein deficiency than is the immune system of older mice. However, it would appear that the influence consists of a delay in maturation rather than a permanent impairment in immunocompetence.

PROTEIN NUTRITURE AND OTHER IMMUNE MECHANISMS

Protein malnutrition also influences a variety of processes that are involved in effective host defense but that do not possess the specificity of humoral and cell-mediated immunity. The reduction in phagocytic activity and the resultant increased susceptibility to infectious disease have already been pointed out (Bhuyan and Ramalingaswami, 1973, 1974). In fact, a reduction in the number of observed peritoneal macrophages was noted in several other studies (Price and Bell, 1975); their paucity correlated with an impaired capacity to clear ^{125}I-labeled *E. coli* from both peripheral blood and spleen.

Feeding rabbits a protein-free diet for 8 weeks resulted in a marked retardation of the normal granulomatous response to secondary systemic challenge with *M. tuberculosis*. The reduction in granuloma formation was correlated with a substantial reduction in the mobilization of macrophages at the site of infection (Bhuyan and Ramalingaswami, 1974). The response of macrophages in bone marrow and spleen was particularly poor, and in the lung only a patchy, diffuse granulomatous response was seen. The increased and prolonged pathogenicity of the tubercle bacillus in protein-deprived animals may reflect either decreased numbers of macrophages available to fight the infection or a reduced ability of those present to respond. Further studies have shown that macrophages obtained from protein-deficient animals have an impaired ability to eliminate PVP (Coovadia and Soothill, 1976). It appears that the reduced rate of clearance may be due to defective antibody affinity. Weanling rats deprived of protein also show evidence of a depressed inflammatory response when injected with suspended latex particles (Slonecher and Osmanlhi, 1974) (Fig. 12). In addition, a defective type I hypersensitivity response has also been demonstrated in mice fed a 4% protein diet (Rose and Turner, 1978).

Perhaps the most important study on the influence of protein deficiency upon immunocompetence concerns the effects on secretory immunity. An earlier study conducted in malnourished children indicated that nasopharyngeal secretory antibody responses were reduced in PEM after administration of live virus vaccines against measles or polio (Chandra, 1975a,b). This is of particular concern, since gastroenteritis and diarrheal diseases are the leading causes of morbidity and mortality among children in the Third World. A principal host defense mechanism against such pathogens is the local secretory immune response. Additionally, such infections exemplify the synergistic and reciprocal nature of malnutrition and infectious disease in the Third World; malnutrition increases susceptibility to enteric infections, and such enteric infections then further impair nutritional status through means such as inanition, malabsorption, and increased intestinal transit time. The study of secretory immunity is also of interest because it represents a mix of humoral and cell-mediated immunity; the production of IgA is particularly thymic dependent (Guy-Grand *et al.,* 1975).

Barry and Pierce (1979) have investigated the effects of protein deprivation (3.2% versus 24% protein diet) on the secretory IgA response to *Vibrio cholerae* toxin in the intestinal lamina propia of mice. It was found

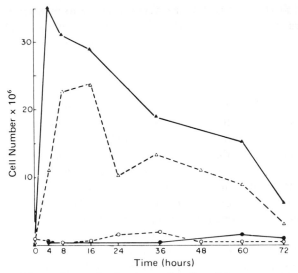

Fig. 12. Neutrophils are the predominant granulocytic cell type present in the acute peritoneal exudates of rats. Protein deficiency causes a reduction in the average numbers of granulocytes in these exudates but also produces an earlier eosinophilic response to this irritant. The average cell number in each cell class was determined in five animals at each experimental interval. The averages were calculated from the total cell population in the exudate harvest and the percentage of each cell type present. The latter was determined by differential counts on exudate smear preparations. ▲, neutrophils (18% diet); △, neutrophils (0.5% diet); ●, eosinophils (18% diet); ○, eosinophils (0.05% diet). (Reproduced with permission from Slonecker and Osmanski, 1974.)

that if protein deprivation was initiated 2–4 weeks prior to enteric priming with cholera toxin, a markedly depressed mucosal antibody response occurred (Barry and Pierce, 1979). The degree of impairment was correlated with the duration of deprivation prior to enteric priming. A significantly shorter period was required to compromise markedly the secondary response compared with the primary response. This most likely points to a defective population of T helper cells, which have been shown to be particularly sensitive to nutritional manipulation. These investigators further found that populations of antigen-specific T suppressor cells were also deficient (Barry and Pierce, 1979). Analysis of thoracic duct lymphocyte populations confirmed the defective responses occurring in the intestinal lamina propria. In addition, these alterations were not confined to the cholera toxin; impaired production of specific memory cells and suppressor cells was noted in additional antigens studied (Barry and Pierce, 1979). Protein deprivation may directly impair the ability to generate clonal expansion of all immune cell populations or may specifically affect the clonal expansion of populations of cells necessary for the generation/expansion of other critical interacting cells.

AMINO ACIDS

While the influence of protein deprivation on immunological function has been reasonably well investigated, considerably less is known regarding the effects of dietary deficiencies of individual amino acids, both essential and nonessential. The difference between protein deficiency and amino acid deficiency may not be notable, since the shortage of a single amino acid limits the biological value and consequently the dietary level of available protein. However, the levels of amino acids may be of concern not only in deficiency but also in terms of an excess of either essential or nonessential amino acids. They may also be important if there is a relative imbalance of two or more amino acids.

The study of amino acids and their influence on immunocompetence is of particular importance for two reasons. First, many foods that comprise major dietary staples in the Third World (e.g., corn, beans) are frequently lacking in a specific amino acid (e.g., lysine, methionine). Second, manipulation of the serum levels of specific amino acids may possibly provide an important avenue of therapeutic intervention in a variety of pathological processes.

Most work has involved the essential amino acids, tryptophan being the amino acid most widely studied. Over 30 years ago, it was shown that the antibody response to heterologous erythrocyte immunization, as assessed by hemagglutination titer, was significantly depressed in rats fed a diet deficient in tryptophan (Lubovici and Axelrod, 1951). In addition, experimental animals fed tryptophan-deficient diets had significantly lower hemolysin titers of IgM and IgG following SRBC immunization (Kenny *et al.,* 1970). Such immunodepression is readily reversible on dietary restoration of tryptophan. The response to specific antigen administration has also been shown to be depressed in the dietary deficiency of tryptophan (Jose and Good, 1973). In contrast, cell-mediated immune function, as reflected by cytotoxic spleen cell responses, remained intact in mice fed diets deficient in tryptophan (Jose and Good, 1973). When diets deficient in both phenylalanine and tryptophan were fed to mice, they exhibited atrophic lymphoid organs and had impaired clearance of radiolabeled PVP (Coovadia and Soothill, 1976) (Fig. 13). The authors postulated that defective reticuloendothelial cell function might be due to poor antibody affinity, which altered the phagocytosis of the foreign material.

Other essential amino acids have also been studied, although less exten-

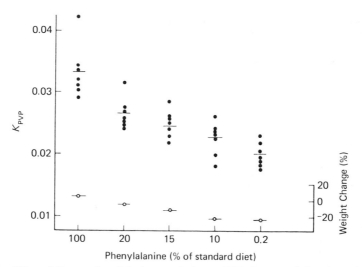

Fig. 13. Effect of dietary phenylalanine restriction on PVP clearance (K) and weight change in male Ajax mice. (Reproduced with permission from Coovadia and Soothill, 1976.)

sively. Rats deprived of phenylalanine alone showed defective responsiveness to both SRBC and a variety of synthetic peptides administered in conjunction with complete Freund's adjuvant (Gershoff *et al.*, 1968). One of the most profound impairments observed was a combined deficiency of tyrosine and phenylalanine, resulting in a marked depression of antibody responses while failing to alter cell-mediated immunocompetence (Jose and Good, 1973). Combined deficiency of methionine and cysteine also caused a marked depression in humoral immune function, while specific deficiencies of lysine, histidine, or arginine produced more moderate reductions in antibody response (Jose and Good, 1973). Deficiency of methionine has also been suggested to affect the ability of PMNs to damage phagocytosed microorganisms oxidatively (Tsan and Chen, 1980) (Tables XII, XIII, Figs. 14, 15).

Interest has been generated in utilizing a depletion of specific serum amino acids in the treatment of leukemias (Crowther, 1971). One of the major problems with this treatment protocol is the concomitant immunosuppression that results from administration of L-asparaginase obtained from *E. coli* and *Vibro succinogenes* (Distasio and Niederman, 1976; Distasio *et al.*, 1977; Durden and Distasio, 1980). In contrast to many other essential amino acids at least, lysine deficiency was shown in one study to have no apparent influence on antibody production against heterologous erythrocytes (Kenney *et al.*, 1970).

As a group, branched chain amino acids (BCAA) have also been studied

Table XII

Effect of D_2O on the Oxidation of Methionine
by Human PMN and Granular Fractions[a,b]

		Methionine sulfoxide		Mean stimulation[c] (%)
		Experiment 1 (%)	Experiment 2 (%)	
Human PMN				
Resting	H_2O	2.5	0	
	D_2O	1.8	0	—
Phagocytosing	H_2O	22.6	16	
	D_2O	53.1	59.7	192
Granular fraction				
Alone	H_2O	1.4	0	
	D_2O	0	0	—
+ H_2O_2 (0.2 mM)	H_2O	18.8	15.9	
	D_2O	46.3	57.9	200

[a]Reproduced with permission from Tsan and Chen (1980).

[b]Concentration of methionine was 102 μM. When D_2O was used, its final concentration was 60%.

[c]Percent stimulation of methionine oxidation in D_2O over H_2O.

Table XIII

Oxidation of Methionine
by Human PMN[a,b]

	Methionine sulfoxide (%)
Resting cells	
Intracellular (5%)[c]	1.0 ± 0.6 (3)[d]
Extracellular (95%)	1.1 ± 0.6 (9)
Phagocytosing cells	
Intracellular (1.5%)	77.0 ± 0.6 (3)
Extracellular (98.5%)	80.0 ± 6.1 (9)
+1 mM n-ethylmaleimide	1.0 ± 0.4 (4)

[a]Reproduced with permission from Tsan and Chen (1980).

[b]The results are expressed as mean ± 1 SEM of the percentage of methionine oxidized to methionine sulfoxide. PMN (1.5 × 10[7]) were incubated with 0.1 μCi of [^{14}C]methionine (22 μM) in the presence or absence of latex particles or n-ethylmaleimide for 30 min at 37°C.

[c]Percentage of the total radioactivity at the end of incubation.

[d]Number of experiments.

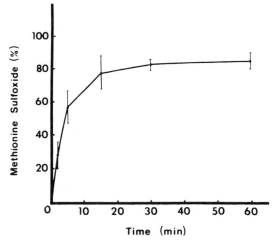

Fig. 14. A time course of the oxidation of methionine by human PMN during phagocytosis. Human PMN (1.5×10^7) were incubated with methionine (22 μM) for 2–60 min in the presence of latex particles. The results are expressed as a percentage of methionine oxidized to methionine sulfoxide in the final media (mean ± SEM of three experiments). (Reproduced with permission from Tsan and Chen, 1980.)

relatively extensively. Diets limited in each of the BCAA, initiated at weaning, resulted in impaired host resistance to *S. typhimurium* and depressed antibody titers, but no effect on cellular immune responsiveness were seen (Petro and Bhattacharee, 1981) (Tables XIV, XV). Moderate deficiency of valine caused a marked depression of antibody responses while failing to alter cell-mediated immunity (Jose and Good, 1973). In contrast, a diet moderately deficient in leucine failed to depress antibody responsiveness and actually enhanced the cytotoxic activity of immune spleen cells directed against tumor cell antigens (Jose and Good, 1973).

Excessive BCAA such as leucine also altered immune function when fed in conjunction with low levels of dietary protein. When such conditions were met, reduced antibody responses were observed, along with decreased PFC responsiveness to heterologous erythrocyte immunization and a depletion in the number of T rosette–forming cells (Chevalier and Ashkenasy, 1977). This is of interest because diets that contain substantial amounts of corn, such as those seen in Latin America, may contain high levels of leucine in conjunction with low levels of dietary protein. Indeed, in these experiments, it was noted that the interactive effects of high dietary leucine, along with the protein-deficient diet, produced an immunodepression as severe as that caused by complete removal of protein from the diet (Chevalier and Ashkenasy, 1977); of particular interest was the abrogation

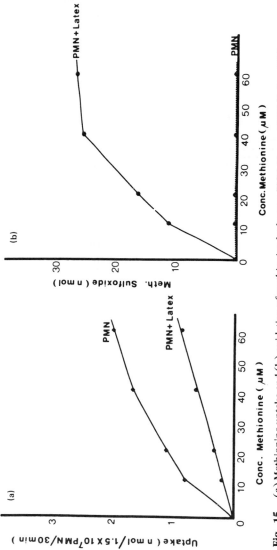

Fig. 15. (a) Methionine uptake and (b) oxidation of methionine by human PMN. Human PMN (1.5×10^7) were incubated with methionine at various concentrations (conc) ($12–62 \mu M$) for 30 min in the presence or absence of latex particles. The amount of methionine uptake by the cells or the amount of methionine oxidized to methionine sulfoxide in the final media were then determined. Each point represents the mean of two experiments. (Reproduced with permission from Tsan and Chen, 1980.)

Table XIV
Effects of Dietary Essential Amino Acid Limitations on the
Responsiveness of Murine Spleen Cells to PHA[a]

	[³H]thymidine incorporation (cpm, $\times 10^3$)[b]	
Dietary limitation	With PHA	Without PHA
None	22.2 ± 17.6^c	1.00 ± 0.33
Leucine	27.3 ± 26.4	2.20 ± 1.31
Isoleucine	44.4 ± 21.6^d	2.99 ± 2.23
Valine	44.3 ± 28.8	3.36 ± 1.04
Lysine	46.5 ± 16.4^d	2.93 ± 1.46

[a]Reproduced with permission from Petro and Bhattacharjee (1981).

[b]The spleens of mice from each dietary group were homogenized to a cell suspension and adjusted to 2×10^6 cells per millimeter in RPMI 1640 medium containing 10% fetal calf serum and 10µg of PHA-P per millimeter. The culture was incubated for 4 days, and the incorporation of [³H]thymidine into DNA was measured for the last 24 hr.

[c]Mean $\pm$ SD.

[d]Significantly different than mice fed the control diet ($p \leq .05$).

Table XV
Effects of Dietary Essential Amino Acid Limitations on the Ability of Mice
to Clear *Salmonella typhimurium* SR11 from the Peritoneal Cavity[a]

		S. typhimurium remaining (% of cells injected) in:[b]	
Dietary limitation	Number of *S. typhimurium* cells injected per mouse	Intracellular fluid	Extracellular fluid
None	1.01×10^6	3	69 ± 10
Leucine	0.94×10^6	4	90 ± 10^c
Isoleucine	1.20×10^6	4	59 ± 32
Valine	1.01×10^6	3	54 ± 16
Lysine	1.31×10^6	4	$39 \pm\ \ 5^c$

[a]Reproduced with permission from Petro and Bhattacharjee (1981).

[b]A minimum of five mice per dietary group were injected ip with 10^6 *S. typhimurium* cells. After 5 min each peritoneal cavity was washed with Hanks balanced salt solution, and the number of *S. typhimurium* cells associated with peritoneal cells was determined by lysing the peritoneal cells with water and rapid freezing and thawing. The numbers of CFU in the extracellular fluids were determined by a quantitative plate count technique.

[c]Significantly different than mice fed a control diet ($p \leq .05$).

of such immunosuppression by the inclusion in the diet of 0.2% isoleucine (Aschkenasy, 1979). This points to the significance of amino acid imbalances and emphasizes the importance of the relative levels of single amino acids in addition to their absolute levels.

Finally, a number of studies have focused on the effect of diets deficient in lipotropic amino acids (lipotropes are considered to be methionine and choline, along with folate and vitamin B_{12}). As with many of the other amino acids, dietary deficiency of choline and methionine results in thymic involution (Griffith and Wade, 1939) and an impaired antibody response (Jose and Good, 1973). Depressed responses of splenic lymphocytes to the mitogens Con A, PHA, and pokeweed mitogen, as well as allogeneic lymphocytes, were observed in addition to depressed resistance to challenge with *S. typhimurium* (Gebhardt and Newberne, 1974; E. A. J. Williams *et al.,* 1979). Moreover, combined deficiencies of these amino acids with concurrent deficiencies of vitamin B_{12} or folate also resulted in marked impairment of immune functions (E. A. J. Williams, *et al.,* 1979).

These results are limited in scope but are sufficient to imply that manipulation of serum amino acids through dietary or other means may prove useful in the modulation of host defense mechanisms. Selective depletion of dietary amino acids has been utilized to slow the progression of autoimmune disease in experimental animals (Gardner *et al.,* 1977) as well as in the treatment of various neoplastic disorders (Durden and Distasio, 1980). Selective elevation of the serum levels of specific amino acids has not been carefully investigated and may merit systematic consideration.

8

Trace Elements

INTRODUCTION

The interaction of humans with their environment is extremely complex and intricate. While many chemicals are essential for survival, more than 96% of the human body is composed of oxygen, carbon, hydrogen, and nitrogen. Yet there are at least 14 trace elements that are now considered essential, at least for some animal species. Because these elements are present only in minute quantities in animal tissues, their critical role in the metabolic processes fundamental to life are not yet fully understood. With increasingly sensitive analytical techniques, we are now able to investigate the function of essential metals present in animal tissues in only trace quantities. The induction of deficiency syndromes in both humans and experimental animals has allowed the elucidation of many of the reactions in which trace elements such as copper, manganese, and zinc are involved. However, even among those elements already demonstrated to be essential, the full range of their action is not clear. In addition, the essential nature of other trace elements that have not been as well investigated needs further research (Underwood, 1977). In general, trace elements may interact both with other essential and nonessential trace metals and with nutrients such as proteins and various vitamins (Beach et al., 1982d).

Trace metals influence physiological, genetic, and psychological parameters of development, from prenatal stages through periods of growth, maintenance, and aging (Gershwin et al., 1983). In addition to evidence of trace metal deficiencies in malnourished children of underdeveloped nations (Fig. 1) (Golden et al., 1977, 1978; Hansen and Lehmann, 1969), studies have suggested that trace element deficiencies occur in technologically advanced countries as well (Fig. 2) (Klevay et al., 1979; Zook et al., 1973). Some epidemiological studies have shown that there may be a correlation

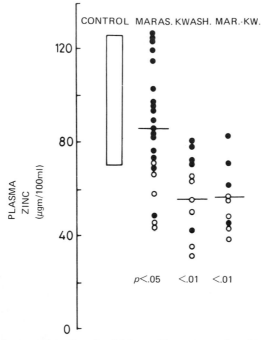

Fig. 1. Plasma zinc concentrations in children with marasmus, kwashiorkor, and marasmic-kwashiorkor defined by the Wellcome criteria. ●, children without skin ulceration; ○, children with skin ulceration. (Reproduced with permission from Golden and Golden, 1979.)

between the level of certain elements in the environment (e.g., land, water, and air) and the incidence and type of disease, particularly chronic, degenerative diseases such as cardiovascular disease and cancer. Thus, it is not surprising that interest has increased in utilizing the knowledge of trace element metabolism to understand better, to treat, and possibly to prevent a wide variety of human neoplasia (Gershwin *et al.,* 1983).

Both essential and nonessential metals may participate in neoplasia in a number of ways. First, in certain cases, the metal itself may act as a carcinogen. Several trace metals have been shown to be carcinogenic in both experimental animals and humans. Trace metals have produced a wide range of tumors by initiating the transformation of host cells to a malignant state and then by promoting the spread of the transformed tissue. Many metals, while not ordinarily carcinogenic per se, may become so in certain chemical forms (Schwartz *et al.,* 1975). Second, trace elements can also function more subtly as carcinogens; in this case, the metal promotes neoplastic growth by another factor acting in concert with the trace metal (Schwartz *et al.,* 1975). The interaction between a number of trace ele-

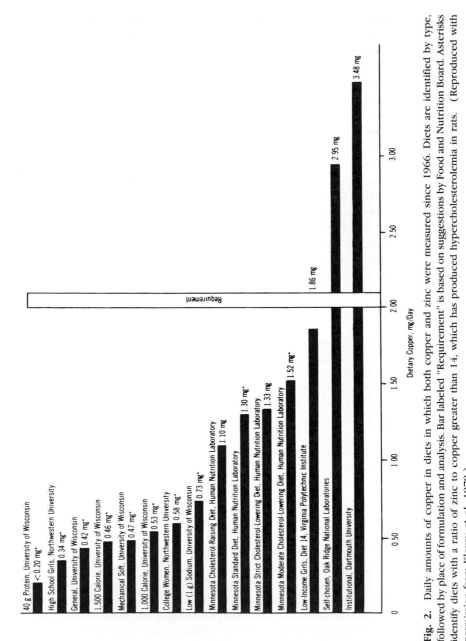

Fig. 2. Daily amounts of copper in diets in which both copper and zinc were measured since 1966. Diets are identified by type, followed by place of formulation and analysis. Bar labeled "Requirement" is based on suggestions by Food and Nutrition Board. Asterisks identify diets with a ratio of zinc to copper greater than 14, which has produced hypercholesterolemia in rats. (Reproduced with permission from Klevay *et al.,* 1979.)

ments and asbestos carcinogenesis is a good example of this phenomenon. A number of trace metals are capable of activating the potent carcinogen benzopyrene on incubation with asbestos fibers (Schwartz et al., 1975). A third example of cocarcinogenesis is the alteration of host immunosurveillance, which may result from trace element deficiency, with subsequently increased susceptibility to a known carcinogen (Gershwin et al., 1983). Fourth, the trace metal may act as a carcinostatic agent by slowing or halting the progression of an already established neoplastic lesion. Finally, the trace element may act in an anticarcinogenic capacity, thereby working antagonistically against an already established neoplasm by causing a reduction in its size or, in some cases, total regression. Complexes involving the noble metals are particularly promising in this capacity; for example, platinum compounds are already being employed therapeutically in clinical situations. The latter two types of compounds, i.e., carcinostatic and anticarcinogenic agents, hold promise for treating established neoplastic lesions, whereas the former two types of compounds, i.e., carcinogens and cocarcinogens, are of greater interest in the detection of possible carcinogenic agents in the environment.

TRACE ELEMENTS AND IMMUNITY

In recent years, great interest has been generated regarding the influence of nutrition on host immunocompetence (Good et al., 1976; Katz and Steihm, 1977; Suskind, 1977). Most studies have focused on protein and energy nutriture and their role in immune responsiveness (Fernandes et al., 1976a; Malave et al., 1980). In contrast, trace metals, many of which are critical for mammalian survival and reproduction, have only recently begun to be investigated in this connection. There is now concern that marginal deficiency of trace elements may represent a public health problem in developed nations (Fig. 2) (Klevay et al., 1979, 1980; Sandstead et al., 1967; Schlage and Wortberg, 1972a,b). Consumption of highly refined and heavily processed foods, in which the trace element content may be reduced significantly (Zook et al., 1973), might contribute to marginal trace element status in countries such as the United States (Hambidge et al., 1976).

Of those trace elements essential to humans, zinc has been studied more extensively than most. Human zinc deficiency was first described in the Middle East (Fig. 3) (Prasad et al., 1961) and has recently been found to be a factor in PEM (Hansen and Lehmann, 1969) and the immunodeficiency associated with it (Golden et al., 1978) (Fig. 4). Increased requirements for zinc during periods such as pregnancy, lactation, growth, development, and infectious or chronic disorders may contribute to marginal zinc status among

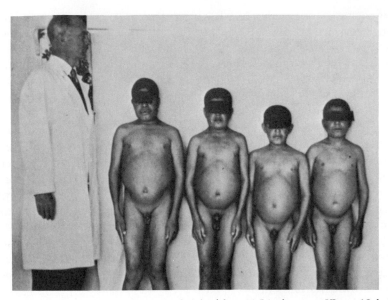

Fig. 3. From left to right: case V, age 21, height 4 feet, 11.5 inches; case VI, age 18, height 4 feet, 9 inches; case III, age 18, height 4 feet, 6 inches; case I, age 21, height 4 feet, 7 inches. Staff physician at left is 6 feet in height. (Reproduced with permission from Prasad *et al.,* 1961.)

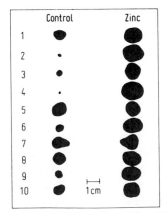

Fig. 4. Paired tracings of the area of induration from delayed-hypersensitivity skin reactions to *Candida* antigen in children with PEM. (Reproduced with permission from Golden *et al.,* 1978.)

specific subpopulations (Hambidge *et al.,* 1976, 1979a,b; Sandstead *et al.,* 1976). Observations of marginal zinc status coupled with experimental findings of altered immunocompetence and impaired response to pathogenic challenge in zinc-deprived animals (Beach *et al.,* 1980a,b; Chandra and Au, 1980a; Fernandes *et al.,* 1979; Fraker *et al.,* 1977) underscore the importance of studies designed to ascertain the effects of marginal or moderate zinc deficiency on all aspects of organismal function (Table I) (Figs. 5, 6).

Although there is now some understanding of the role in host metabolism of copper and manganese, considerably less is known concerning their role in normal immune function. Preliminary observations suggest that deprivation of these trace elements likewise leads to an alteration of immune responsiveness (McCoy *et al.,* 1979; Newberne *et al.,* 1968). Furthermore, some observations suggest that marginal copper deficiency may occur in human populations in the United States (Fig. 2) (Klevay *et al.,* 1979, 1980). This possibility has been emphasized by the demonstration of frank copper deficiency in premature, small-for-date, and malnourished infants (Al-Rashid and Spangler, 1971; Ashkinazi *et al.,* 1973; Blumenthal *et al.,* 1980; Cordano, 1978; Cordano *et al.,* 1964; Griscom *et al.,* 1971; Hekker *et al.,* 1978; Lahey *et al.,* 1952; Seely *et al.,* 1971; Tanaka *et al.,* 1980) and in patients receiving total parenteral nutrition (TPN) (Fleming *et al.,* 1976; Karpel and Peden, 1972; Solomons *et al.,* 1976; Vaughn and Weinberg, 1978). Although we do not believe that severe deprivation of zinc, copper, or manganese occurs to any significant extent among Western populations (not receiving TPN), there is now concern that marginal deficiency may occur and, in addition, may be compounded by increased requirements due to acute and chronic conditions noted earlier.

Table I

Survival of Zinc-Deprived Mice[a]

	Dietary treatment				
	100 ppm zinc, *ad libitum* fed (100)[b]	100 ppm zinc, food restricted (132)	9 ppm zinc (160)	5 ppm zinc (184)	2.5 ppm zinc (196)
Mice (%) surviving to:					
1 week of age	94.0	93.7	76.9	60.5	53.8
2 weeks of age	93.2	93.4	73.8	59.0	31.9
3 weeks of age	92.9	85.8	72.7	56.1	17.9
4 weeks of age	92.7	84.9	69.6	37.9	8.6
6 weeks of age	92.6	84.6	67.8	28.2	0
8 weeks of age	92.5	82.2	65.9	25.7	0

[a]Reproduced with permission from Beach *et al.* (1980a).
[b]Number of mice.

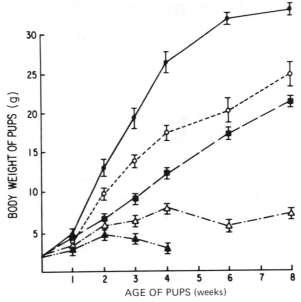

Fig. 5. Body weight of pups from birth to 8 weeks of age. Growth curves during the first 8 weeks postpartum indicated that dietary zinc deficiency was associated with a marked growth retardation, the degree of stunting being directly related to the degree of zinc deprivation. Caloric deficiency equal to the level of inanition observed in moderately deprived offspring (5 ppm zinc), while causing significant depression of growth rate, could account for only a portion of the marked stunting observed in the zinc-deprived pups. ●, 100 ppm zinc *ad libitum*; ○, 100 ppm zinc pair-fed; ■, 9.0 ppm zinc; △, 5.0 ppm zinc; ▲, 2.5 ppm zinc. (Reproduced with permission from Beach *et al.,* 1980a.)

A substantial number of studies in a variety of species have now shown that limiting or increasing the intake of trace metals can result in significant changes in response to a range of artificially induced oncogenic challenges and spontaneous malignancies (Beach *et al.,* 1982d; Carleton and Price, 1973; DiPaolo, 1964; Pories *et al.,* 1978a,b; Shimkin *et al.,* 1978). Additionally, altered trace element metabolism during malignancy occurs in clinical situations as well as in experimental animal models (Alexander *et al.,* 1972; Prasad *et al.,* 1969; Ranade *et al.,* 1979; Schuhmacher *et al.,* 1979). Some preliminary epidemiological studies suggest a possible relationship between the intake of some trace elements and the incidence of various types of cancer (Pories *et al.,* 1978b; Schrauzer, 1976). Copper, manganese, and especially zinc merit particular attention with regard to their potential role in the treatment and prevention of many different types of malignancy. Selenium likewise deserves special investigative attention in this regard; however, the information on this trace metal is scanty.

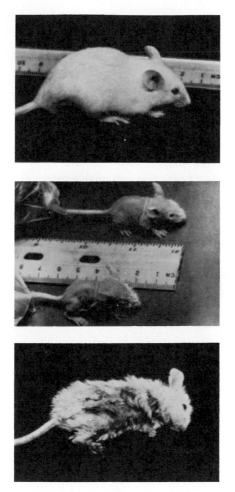

Fig. 6. General appearance of zinc-deprived mice. (a) *Ad libitum*-fed control pup at 4 weeks of age (top) was approximately twice the size of the severely deprived animals (below). Moderate and severe deprivation of zinc was associated with total alopecia. (b) Extensive dermatitis seen in a moderately zinc-deprived dam after 6 weeks on diet. Many pups fed the moderately and severely deficient diets exhibited a similar dermatitis. (Reproduced with permission from Beach *et al.,* 1980a.)

MANGANESE

While to date there has been only one report of a manganese deficiency in humans (Doisy, 1972), a considerable amount of research has been carried out on the metabolic role of manganese and the consequences of dietary manganese deficiency in animals. The deficiency syndrome that develops in animals fed insufficient manganese can be characterized in five basic ways: (1) somewhat impaired growth (Kemmerer *et al.,* 1931; Hurley *et al.,* 1958; Everson *et al.,* 1959), (2) skeletal abnormalities (Asling and Hurley, 1963; Leach and Lilburn, 1978; Hurley, 1981), (3) disturbed and/or depressed reproductive function (Hurley *et al.,* 1958; Everson *et al.,* 1959, Hurley, 1981), (4) congenital, irreversible ataxia in the newborn (Hurley, 1981), and (5) defects of carbohydrate and lipid metabolism (Hurley, 1982; Baly *et al.,* 1984a,b; Hurley *et al.,* 1984). While manganese deficiency is not accompanied by severe inappetance (as it is with zinc deficiency), the reduced rate of growth observed in manganese-deprived animals is the result of both decreased food consumption and reduced efficiency of food utilization (Underwood, 1977).

Skeletal abnormalities and ataxic behavior are the most visible manifestations of manganese deprivation. The precise nature of the alterations in bone structure depends on the species in which the deficiency is induced. Anomalies that have been noted include leg deformities, disproportionate bone growth, poorly formed joints, lameness, chondrodystrophy, perosis ("slipped tendon"), epiphyseal dysplasia, shortening and doming of the skull, and anomalous ossification of the inner ear (Hurley, 1981, Asling and Hurley, 1963). In most manganese-deficient animals, retarded skeletal maturation occurs because of inhibited endochondral osteogenesis at the site of the epiphyseal cartilages. These features of deficient animals point out the critical role of manganese in organic matrix synthesis, a function largely of deficient mucopolysaccharide synthesis (Hurley, 1981; Leach and Lilburn, 1978).

The congenital ataxia that has been observed in manganese-deprived offspring (rats) is characterized by lack of equilibrium, which is frequently accompanied by tremors, head retraction, and a delay in the development of reflexes necessary for body righting (Hurley, 1981; Erway *et al.,* 1970; Hurley and Everson, 1959). These alterations can be traced to a structural defect in the inner ear, leading to impaired vestibular function, most notably of the otoliths (Erway *et al.,* 1966). This altered vestibular function is a result of deficient mucopolysaccharide synthesis (Shrader *et al.,* 1973). A mutant strain of mouse (pallid) also demonstrates ataxic behavior as a consequence of defective otolith formation, which can be prevented by adequate dietary supplementation with manganese during gestation (Erway *et al.,* 1971).

From the study of deficient animals, limited information on the biochemical function of manganese has begun to accumulate. Like other essential transition elements, manganese is involved largely with enzyme function. Manganese functions in enzyme reactions either as part of the metalloenzymes or as a cofactor in metal–enzyme complexes (Underwood, 1977; Keen *et al.,* 1984). There are only three known manganese-containing metalloenzymes: arginase, pyruvate carboxylase, and manganese-superoxide dismutase (manganese-SOD). However, several types of enzymes are activated by manganese, including certain kinases, hydrolases, decarboxylases, and transferases (Keele *et al.,* 1970; Scrutton *et al.,* 1972; Underwood, 1977). Often these enzymes require a nonspecific metal so that manganese may be replaced, at least partially, by other divalent cations (e.g., magnesium), but in many cases other metals are less efficient than manganese in enzyme activation (Scruton *et al.,* 1972).

Manganese appears to play a critical role in three basic aspects of metabolism: (1) glycosaminoglycan synthesis, (2) carbohydrate metabolism, and (3) lipid metabolism (Leach and Lilburn, 1978; Keen *et al.,* 1984). For glycosaminoglycan metabolism, manganese is essential for the activation of glycosyltransferases (Underwood, 1977); thus, many of the lesions characteristic of manganese deficiency (e.g., skeletal abnormalities, congenital ataxia, and impaired eggshell formation) can be attributed directly to altered glycosyltransferase activity (Underwood, 1977). The alterations in mucopolysaccharide formation, which are largely responsible for many of the most apparent manifestations of manganese deficiency, can be attributed to depressed activity of xylosyl transferase. This enzyme is responsible for the transfer of xylose in the formation of the linkage between the polysaccharide and protein portions of the cartilaginous matrix (Leach and Lilburn, 1978). In addition to reduced glycosaminoglycan biosynthesis, the rate of glycosaminoglycan degradation is accelerated, as reflected by an increase in ^{35}S turnover in the cartilage of manganese-deprived animals (Leach and Meunster, 1962). In conclusion, it appears that many of the tissue lesions found in manganese deficiency are related to altered levels of glycosaminoglycans, which reflect the lack of manganese ions that are needed to activate glycosyltransferases (Leach *et al.,* 1978).

Carbohydrate metabolism involves manganese in two basic ways: (1) stabilization and/or activation of gluconeogenic enzymes and (2) the relationship between manganese and diabetes-like symptoms (Everson and Shrader, 1968; Leach and Lilburn, 1978). Some of the key enzymes involved in carbohydrate metabolism that require manganese for activation and/or stabilization include pyruvate carboxylase (PC), phosphoenolpyruvate carboxykinase (PEPCK), isocitrate dehydrogenase, and some forms of glycogen synthetase (e.g., placental forms). In some instances, it appears that magnesium may substitute for manganese, e.g., in PC (at least in chickens) and isocitrate dehydrogenase; in other cases, the manganese requirement may be quite specific. Several manganese-dependent enzymes require the action of other essential ions, such as iron, copper, zinc, or sulfate.

Guinea pigs deprived of manganese showed diabetes-like symptoms, as demonstrated by a decreased utilization of glucose. The latter was assessed by diabetes-like oral glucose tolerance curves. The diabetes-like response appeared to be related to the effect of manganese on pancreatic islet tissue. Histological examination of the pancreas, a tissue that contains a high local concentration of manganese, indicated hypertrophied islet tissue, with de-granulated β cells and an increased number of α cells in manganese-deficient guinea pigs. With adequate manganese supplementation, the glucose tolerance test curve returned to normal (Everson and Shrader, 1968).

Recent studies have demonstrated that manganese-deficient rats also show diabetes-like glucose tolerance curves. Plasma insulin levels were not commensurate with the high glucose levels. Insulin output from the pan-creas (due to the release of both stored and newly synthesized hormone) was lower than normal in deficient rats (Baly et al., 1984b). The activity of two key gluconeogenic enzymes, PC and PEPCK, was also affected by man-ganese deficiency. In newborn offspring, the activity of PC and PEPCK was higher in manganese-deficient rats than in controls for the first 3 days of life, and then dropped so that it was lower than in controls 8–30 days of age. The plasma glucose concentration was lower than normal in deficient pups. These results suggest that manganese deficiency impairs gluconeogenesis in the neonatal period at least partially through its effects on PC and PEPCK. Since neonatal mortality is very high during the first 4 days of postnatal life in manganese-deficient rat pups, impaired gluconeogenesis may be an important factor.

Lipid metabolism also involves manganese in several ways. Adequate manganese content in the diet prevents excess fat deposition in the liver (Barak et al., 1971; Bell and Hurley, 1973). This lipotropic action of man-ganese deficiency is accentuated when the choline content of the diet is reduced simultaneously. Additionally, manganese has been implicated in steroid biosynthesis. Through activation of the enzyme farnesyl pyrophos-phate synthetase, manganese is involved in the synthesis of squalene, an important precursor of cholesterol, and therefore of steroid hormones. Like many gluconeogenic enzymes, farnesyl pyrophosphate synthetase has an absolute metal requirement; magnesium may substitute for manganese, but is far less effective in activating or stabilizing the enzyme (Doisy, 1972). Such impaired biosynthesis of steroid hormones may account for the re-productive problems observed in manganese-deficient animals.

Altered lipid metabolism may also help to explain the aberrations in membrane integrity seen in manganese deficiency (Bell and Hurley, 1973). These fundamental alterations in membrane structure may produce marked abnormalities in subcellular organelles, such as swollen mitochondria, irreg-ular endoplasmic reticulum, and elongated and stacked cristae. These changes undoubtedly affect cellular function and may cause some of the gross manifestations observed in manganese-deficient animals.

However, alterations in membrane integrity may also be related to changes in SOD activity. SOD catalyzes the reaction of the superoxide anion to hydrogen peroxide, which is then acted on by catalase to produce oxygen and water. Two types of SOD have been found in mammalian liver. One contains copper and zinc and is located primarily in the cytosol. The other contains manganese (Mn SOD) and occurs primarily in the mitochondrial matrix (Fridovich, 1975). Offspring of manganese-deficient rats showed lower levels of liver Mn SOD activity than controls by 15 days of age. By day 60, their activity level was 25% less than that of controls. The reduced activity of Mn SOD appears to be of functional significance, since lipid peroxidation in isolated mitochondria from manganese-deficient rats was greater than that of controls by 15 days of age and was 50% higher by day 60 (Zidenberg-Cherr et al., 1983). Membrane damage of mitochondria was also apparent by electron microscopy by day 60 (Zidenberg-Cherr et al., 1983). It has been suggested that SOD may play a key role in many biological and pathological processes, such as aging and cancer; manganese nutrition and status may therefore be an important factor.

While preliminary studies have confirmed a number of specific roles of manganese in mammalian metabolism, many of its functions remain unclear. A good example of the latter is the putative role that manganese may play in nervous system function (Hurley et al., 1963). Such a role in the brain and central nervous system was postulated initially because of the similarity of symptoms between manganese toxicity and Parkinson's disease (Cotzias et al., 1976). Similarly, treatment with L-dopa alleviates these symptoms in both conditions (Hurley et al., 1963). Studies have indicated that cyclic nucleotides (e.g., cAMP) may provide the crucial link in the relationship between manganese and nervous system function (Papavasilou et al., 1979). Finally, additional confirmatory evidence has been provided by the Pallid mutant mouse, which has been shown to have disordered manganese metabolism (Erway et al., 1971). On further investigation, these mutant mice were found to have faulty metabolism of L-dopa. Manganese supplementation ameliorated faulty L-dopa metabolism and its consequent neurological manifestations (Cotzias et al., 1972).

Human requirements for manganese have been extrapolated largely from balance studies, although the few studies that exist are of questionable precision and in general have proven difficult to undertake (MacLeod and Robinson, 1972; Schlage et al., 1972b; Hurley, 1984). The Food and Nutrition Board of the National Academy of Sciences has estimated the "safe and adequate" daily intake of manganese to be 0.5–5.0 mg/day for adults. Another report suggested that the manganese requirement for girls between 6 and 10 years of age is approximately 1.25 mg/day, which is in keeping with the estimate above. Only a single case of human manganese deficiency has been reported. It was induced accidentally, coincidentally with vitamin K deficiency (Doisy, 1972). Symptoms in this subject included an inability to elevate depressed levels of clotting proteins in response to supplementation with vitamin K, severe hypocholesterolemia, slowed growth of nails and hair, dermatitis, reddening of the hair and beard, and moderate body weight loss (Doisy, 1972). The similarity between these symptoms ascribed to manganese deficiency (simultaneous with vitamin K deficiency) and those of kwashiorkor have been noted and warrants further investigation, particularly in light of evidence of altered metabolism of other trace elements such as zinc, copper, and iron in PEM (Golden and Golden, 1979, 1981; Golden *et al.,* 1977, 1978; Hansen and Lehmann, 1969). The best dietary sources of manganese are plant materials because the manganese content of animal tissues is usually very low.

A high incidence of manganese toxicity has been reported in miners who have been exposed to industrial contamination after prolonged work with manganese ores. Excess manganese was shown to enter the body as an oxide dust inhaled into the lungs, although contamination via the gastrointestinal tract is also possible. Manganese poisoning was characterized by locura manganica, a neuropsychiatric condition resembling schizophrenia, which subsequently develops into a permanent, crippling neurological disease with clinical manifestations similar to those of Parkinson's disease. The presence of elevated levels of manganese in the tissues is not essential for continuation of these neurological manifestations, and metal chelation therapy is not thought to have any beneficial therapeutic effects.

Very little is understood about the role of manganese in immunological function. The first information on manganese and the immune response came in 1949, when rats fed increased levels of manganese were shown to have a heightened susceptibility to pneumococcal infection. More recently, manganese-supplemented horses, goats, hens, and rabbits produced elevated antibody titers and maintained them over extended time periods. In addition, manganese supplementation resulted in increased levels of other nonspecific resistance factors, although the significance of these elevated proteins was not specified (Antonova *et al.,* 1968; Bazhora *et al.,* 1974; McCoy *et al.,* 1979). Unfortunately, much of this work has suffered from methodological inconsistencies. For example, the work done with hens included supplementation with cobalt and iodine simultaneously with the manganese supplementation, and also utilized a basal diet in which the levels of all trace elements were not specified. More recent experimentation has done little to reduce these basic inconsistencies. One study demonstrated that in rats fed marginally deficient levels of manganese, IgG agglutinins and the 19 S fraction of γ globulin were reduced, but the hemoly-sin titer was significantly elevated 9 days after intraperitoneal injection with SRBC. Addition of three times the manganese requirement resulted in a depression of both agglutinating and hemolyzing antibody responses in rats (McCoy *et al.,* 1979). To stress the interaction between manganese and other trace elements, it was shown that addition of copper, magnesium, or iron simultaneously with the elevated intake of manganese prevented this depression of antibody titer (Antonova *et al.,* 1968).

Interaction of manganese-containing metal salts with neutrophils and macrophages has also been demonstrated (Attramadal, 1969; Rabinovitch and Destefano, 1973). In the case of neutrophils, manganese-containing salts were shown to inhibit chemotaxis and were associated with a de-creased uptake and incorporation of labeled amino acids (Attramadal, 1969). A similar effect of manganese salts on fibroblast function was also observed (Attramadal, 1969; Rabinovitch and Destefano, 1973). In general, it was hypothesized that metal cations, such as in manganese salts, may interfere with the pathways of protein synthesis; the integrity of plasma, organelle, and nuclear membrane function; and the chemotactic function of leukocytes, thus suggesting that these compounds may possess anti-inflam-matory potential (Attramadal, 1969; Bryant, 1969). Manganese is known to alter the process of coagulation via the inhibition of glycosyltransferase activity, which is necessary for the synthesis of glycoproteins such as pro-thrombin (Doisy, 1972). In addition, manganese may also affect coagulation via a direct effect on the plasma membrane of the platelet (Bryant, 1969). These interactions with the plasma membrane have been suggested as a possible model for the effects of manganese on the membranes of cells employed in the immune response. Manganese may also act as a cofactor in an enzyme possibly associated with the stimulation of macrophage spread induced by glass-bound antigen–antibody complexes. Manganese was found to be the most potent divalent cation of those capable of inducing macrophage spread on such glass surfaces (Bryant, 1969; Rabinovitch and Destefano, 1973). All cells induced to spread by manganese were still capa-ble of phagocytosis (Attramadal, 1969; Bryant, 1969; Rabinovitch and De-stefano, 1973). These findings may help to delineate the precise role of manganese and similar divalent cations in cellular interactions, particularly those of cells involved with immunocompetence.

During the past decade, the presence of manganese in the concanavalin A molecule has been confirmed, although the precise mode of interaction between manganese and concanavalin A remains unclear. At physiological pH, concanavalin A exists largely as a tetramer, with each protomer (MW 27,000) containing one calcium and one manganese atom, both of which are octahedrally coordinated and share two aspartate ligands. It had been generally accepted that the binding of manganese was a necessary prelude to the binding of calcium and the subsequent interaction between concanavalin A and cell surface carbohydrates, which it must bind to exert its influence on cellular processes. More recently, however, it has been shown that this is more likely to occur at pH 5.5 and below, and that at physiological pH there may not be a requirement for the prior binding of manganese (R. D. Brown *et al.,* 1977). The biological significance of these facts is not yet clear, but to appreciate fully the interaction of manganese and such mitogens, it will be necessary to outline their precise nature and significance.

In vitro evidence has indicated that manganese may inhibit stimulation of lymphocytes by mitogens, most notably concanavalin A and phytohemagglutinin P. No such effect was observed in the response of lymphocytes to stimulation by the B-cell mitogen, *Escherichia coli* lipopolysaccharide (LPS) (Hart, 1978a) (Table II). This alteration of lymphocyte stimulation by mitogens seems to occur at the site of the cell membrane.

There may also be an interaction between manganese and calcium. More specifically, calcium ions are intimately involved in many aspects of lymphocyte activation (e.g., blast transformation in response to mitogens), and manganese may interact with calcium at many of these steps. Calcium and manganese are known to compete in a number of biological systems, and manganese can interfere with a number of calcium-dependent processes by competitive inhibition.

ZINC

A useful method for studying the role of trace metals in mammalian biology is to induce a deficiency by feeding a diet significantly or totally devoid of a specific element. Insufficient zinc intake causes a wide spectrum of metabolic changes in all animal species studied. Zinc is necessary for normal keratogenesis, and animals deprived of adequate dietary zinc demonstrate alopecia, a variety of epidermal and mucosal membrane lesions, and impaired wound-healing ability (Beach *et al.,* 1980a; Swenerton and Hurley, 1968; Wacker, 1978). With insufficient dietary zinc, endocrine parameters are markedly altered; hallmarks of zinc deficiency in humans include hypogonadism, sexual dysmaturity, infertility, and deranged adrenal steroid and human growth hormone secretion (Elcoate *et al.,* 1955; Failla and Cousins, 1978; Henkin, 1976; Sandstead *et al.,* 1967). While a relationship between zinc and insulin storage and secretion from β cells in the pancreas has been postulated, the precise nature of this interaction has not been characterized (Araquilla *et al.,* 1978). Animals deprived of zinc also exhibit behavioral disorders (Halas and Sandstead, 1975) and manifest hy-

Table II

Effect of Mn^{2+} on Mitogen Stimulation of Hamster Lymphoid Cells
Expressed As Stimulation Index (SI)[a,b]

	MnSo$_4$ (μM)[c]				
	0	1.0	10	100	200
Spleen					
Expt 1					
Control	1.0		0.7	0.6	0.5
2 µg Con A	34.2		73.4	12.2	3.0
50 µg PHA	10.2		13.3	0.9	0.4
25 µg LPS	10.0		22.0	17.1	21.1
Expt 2					
Control	1.0	1.1	1.3	1.1	
2 µG Con A	61.5	77.7	111.4	8.1	
25 µg LPS	6.4	9.7	12.6	14.6	
50 µg DxS	15.9	26.3	39.3	25.3	
Lymph node					
Expt 1					
Control	1.0		0.8	0.5	
2 µg ConA	41.7		59.3	9.0	
50 µg PHA	10.0		11.0	3.5	
Expt 2					
Control	1.0		1.1	0.6	0.3
2 µg Con A	45.9		60.1	9.8	1.2

[a]Reproduced with permission from Hart (1978a).

[b]Stimulation index is the ratio of the mean cpm [^3H]TdR incorporated into triplicate 72-hr cultures of 5 × 10^6 viable cells/mean cpm [^3H]TdR incorporated in the unstimulated control cultures. Variation from the mean incorporation was less than 10%.

[c]The cultures were equilibrated with the indicated concentrations of Mn^{2+} for 1 hr prior to addition of the mitogens.

poguesia, or an inadequate sense of taste (Catalanatto, 1978). As noted below, marked changes in the immune system and immunological responses have also been found (Beach *et al.,* 1979; Beach *et al.,* 1980c,d; Chandra and Au, 1980a; Fernandes *et al.,* 1979; Fraker *et al.,* 1977) (Table III).

During periods when the requirements for essential constituents of metabolism are greater than normal, experimental animals as well as humans are particularly affected by deprivation of zinc. Evidence of this phenomenon has been found in animals experiencing liver regeneration after partial hepatectomy (Weser *et al.,* 1973) and in animals undergoing the healing of experimentally introduced wounds (Wacker, 1978). A strong

Table III

PFC Response in C57BL/Ks Mice Maintained on Various Diets[a,b]

Diet[c]	Duration, weeks	Direct PFC per spleen	Indirect PFC per spleen
Zn⁻	2	29,127 ± 9,682	23,149 ± 8,402
Zn⁺PF	2	25,428 ± 1,276	19,699 ± 920
Zn⁻	4	18,502 ± 5,606	14,913 ± 5,446
Zn⁺PF	4	38,392 ± 9,902	31,934 ± 8,549
Lab chow	6	64,281 ± 7,152	53,294 ± 3,144
Zn⁻	6	8,278 ± 2,651	5,128 ± 2,312
Zn⁺PF	6	80,983 ± 2,772	69,071 ± 6,749
Zn⁺ *ad lib*	6	117,968 ± 15,858	95,446 ± 7,393
Lab chow	8	104,662 ± 18,937	74,647 ± 6,202

[a]Reproduced with permission from Fernandes *et al.* (1979).

[b]At least four mice were immunized with SRBC in each group. Data are shown as mean ± SEM.

[c]PF, pair-fed.

response to trace metal deficiency has been demonstrated repeatedly. In experimental studies of pregnant and lactating animals and their developing offspring, diets deficient in zinc have a particularly severe effect. Animals deprived of zinc during gestation experience high rates of fetal resorption and wastage, and produce fewer and less viable offspring (Hurley and Swenerton, 1966; Hurley *et al.,* 1971; Hurley, 1981). A wide variety of congenital anomalies have been noted in such deprived progeny; chromosomal aberrations have been observed in severely deprived animals (Bell *et al.,* 1975). Development of the central nervous system is especially affected by insufficient zinc (Hurley and Shrader, 1972; Beach *et al.,* 1980a; Golub *et al.,* 1983). Indeed, offspring deprived either prenatally or postnatally of adequate dietary zinc experience severely retarded growth (Hurley, 1981; Beach *et al.,* 1980a); such stunting is due, in part, to the inanition and consequent caloric deprivation that accompany zinc deficiency (Chesters, 1972). In addition, the observed effects of zinc deprivation may be due to the importance of zinc for the effective digestion, absorption, and metabolic utilization of a wide range of other nutrients, e.g., vitamin A (Smith *et al.,* 1973), vitamin E (Bettger *et al.,* 1980), proteins (Hardy-Muncy and Grasmussen, 1979), and copper (O'Dell *et al.,* 1976).

Appreciation of the fundamental role of zinc in mammalian structure and function has increased since the 1930s, when its essential nature was first established (Todd *et al.,* 1934). Much attention has centered on the role of zinc as an essential cofactor in the activity of over 100 enzymes. Zinc can function as a tightly bound moiety, termed a *metalloenzyme,* or as a more loosely bound entity, as in metal–enzyme complexes (Vallee, 1976). Zinc has also been shown to be critical in stabilizing the tertiary structure of nucleic acid and protein macromolecules (Vallee, 1976). The effects of zinc deficiency on any animal are most likely mediated by factors such as decreased enzyme activity, altered membrane structure, and aberrant DNA transcription and RNA translation. Experiments showing decreased activity levels of enzymes such as thymidine kinase and DNA polymerase (Dreosti and Hurley, 1975; Dreosti and Duncan, 1975; Falchuk *et al.,* 1975; Swenerton *et al.,* 1969), as well as altered binding of F_1 and F_3 histones to the DNA molecule, thereby affecting the synthesis of RNA (Andrews, 1979), help to substantiate such theories. A further possibility involves a direct interaction between zinc and the cell cycle, particularly during the progression from the G_1 to the S phase (Falchuk *et al.,* 1975; Vallee, 1976). The precise role of zinc in all aspects of cellular metabolism and replication remains to be fully elucidated.

Until relatively recently, little was known regarding the effect of trace element nutriture on immune responsiveness, and while the data now available can only be characterized as preliminary, a significant appreciation of the essentiality of zinc for intact immunological function exists. The first indication of this interaction came from human epidemiological surveys; patients with low levels of serum zinc had increased susceptibility to a variety of infectious disorders (Prasad *et al.,* 1961, 1963; Sandstead *et al.,* 1967); further investigation revealed that such individuals presented with hypogammaglobulinemia (Sandstead *et al.,* 1977), abnormal proportions of the immunoglobulin classes (Caggiano *et al.,* 1969), and defective cell-mediated immunity (Caggiano *et al.,* 1969). In addition, patients with the genetic (autosomal recessive) disorder of zinc metabolism, acrodermatitis enteropathica, have an increased incidence of infectious maladies (Endre *et al.,* 1975), a profoundly altered cellular immune response, including decreased mitogenic response to phytohemagglutinin (Table IV) (Oleske *et al.,* 1979), impaired response to a battery of skin test antigens (Oleske *et al.,* 1979), decreased numbers of circulating T lymphocytes (Oleske *et al.,* 1979), defective neutrophil chemotaxis (Weston *et al.,* 1977), and profound thymic atrophy at autopsy (Julius *et al.,* 1973). Zinc administration leads to nearly complete amelioration of the immunodeficiency syndrome in these patients (Oleske *et al.,* 1979; Weston *et al.,* 1977).

More recently, protein-energy malnourished children have been shown to have low levels of serum zinc (Golden and Golden, 1979), and the immunodeficiency syndrome observed in such patients (Golden *et al.,* 1977, 1978) is corrected, at least in part, by zinc administration (Golden and Golden, 1981b) (Table V and Fig. 9). Both infant (Srouji *et al.,* 1978) and

Table IV

Correlation of T- and B-Cell Variables and Plasma Zinc Levels in Acrodermatitis Enteropathica, 1974–1977[a]

Age (years)	Date	T Cells/mm³ (%)	B Cells/mm³ (%)	Mitogen stimulation indexes			Immunoglobulin (mg/dl)			Plasma zinc (µg/dl)
				PHA	Con A	PWM	IgG	IgM	IgA	
Normal values		1500–2500 (65–80)	240–500 (10–20)	>30	>15	>15	—	—	—	70–120
4	12/74	4030 (65)	248 (2)	11	11	2	—	—	—	—
		710 (42)	777 (46)	4	7	1	210	30	<6	22
5	12/75	197 (18)	208 (19)	60	55	9	300	30	<6	30
		2287 (64)	180 (4)	—	—	—	165	15	<6	60
		457 (15)	548 (18)	66	82	6	165	30	<6	78
		3388 (80)	466 (11)	—	—	—	740[c]	44	<6	82
6	12/76	—	—	—	—	—	530[c]	28	7	100
		4205 (90)	140 (4)	105	66	3	640[c]	35	7	160
7	12/77	—	—	—	—	—	560[c]	16	<6	—

[a]Reproduced with permission from Oleske *et al.* (1979).

[b]PHA indicates phytohemagglutinin; Con A, Conconavalin A; PWM, pokeweed mitogen.

[c]IgG, κ monoclonal spike.

208

Table V

Clinical Characteristics, Plasma Zinc, and Thymic Assessment Before and After Supplementation of Recently Malnourished Children with Zinc Acetate[a]

Patient number	Age (months)	Sex	Diagnosis on admission	Plasma zinc (µg/dl)		UMD/CD ratio[b] (× 100)		Thymus size[c]		Rank order		Sign[a]	
				Before	After	Before	After	Before	After	Before	After	Before	After
1	15	M	Marasmus	48	97	17	31	S	M	2	11	−	+
2	9	M	Marasmus	51	72	31	35	M	L	8	15	−	+
3	15	F	Marasmus	55	103	17	19	S	S	3	4	−	+
4	15	M	Marasmus	34	95	27	28	M	L	7	14	−	+
5	17	M	Marasmus	88	111	21	24	S	M	6	12	−	+
6	13	M	Kwashiorkor	75	115	21	26	S	M	5	13	−	+
7	10	M	Marasmus	80	156	23	30	S	L	1	16	−	+
8	16	M	Marasmus	76	90	34	37	M	L	9	10	−	+
					$p < .02$		$p < .02$		$p < .02$		$p < .01$		$p < .01$

[a]Reproduced with permission from Golden *et al.* (1977).
[b]UMD, upper mediastinal diameter; CD, chest diameter.
[c]S, small; M, medium; L, large
[d]−, smaller thymus; +, larger thymus.

209

adult patients (Pekarek *et al.,* 1979) undergoing long-term parenteral alimentation also have impaired immunological function, particularly in cell-mediated immune responses, which are corrected in large part by adequate zinc supplementation (Pekarek *et al.,* 1979). TPN has been shown to reduce both plasma zinc and copper significantly (Solomons *et al.,* 1976) (Fig. 7, Table VI). Patients with immunodeficiency diseases present with severe hypogammaglobulinemia, depressed response to mitogens and antigens, and decreased levels of thymopoietin and serum thymic factor, along with low levels of serum zinc; zinc repletion is associated with the restoration of many of these immune functions (Cunningham-Rundles *et al.,* 1980). The immunodeficiency complicating a number of other disorders has been shown to be associated with low levels of plasma zinc; the disorders include Down's syndrome (Bjorksten *et al.,* 1980), sickle-cell disease (Brewer *et al.,* 1976), and obesity (Chandra *et al.,* 1980). Also affected are patients responding to trauma such as infectious disease (Beisel, 1976) and severe burns (Lennard *et al.,* 1974). Finally, a hallmark of the physiological response to invasion by pathogenic microorganisms or their toxins is a transient decline in serum zinc, with a concomitant sequestering of zinc in the liver (Beisel, 1976). These alterations related to infections are apparently mediated, at least in part, by adrenal steroid hormones (Falchuk, 1977) and a serum protein referred to as leukocytic endogenous mediator (LEM) (Beisel, 1976). The full implications of this decline in serum zinc in response to infectious challenge remain to be understood. While all of these observations suggest a possible interplay between zinc and the immune response, well-controlled studies in appropriate animal models, involving both *in vitro* and *in vivo* systems, will be required to substantiate the nature of this interaction.

The first major information concerned the essentiality of zinc for blast transformation of lymphocytes (Alford, 1970; Chesters, 1972; Ruhl and Bochert, 1971). This interaction was a reasonable extension of the conclusive evidence that zinc was required for DNA synthesis (Dreosti and Duncan, 1975; Falchuk *et al.,* 1975; Swenerton *et al.,* 1969), a central feature of blast transformation of lymphocytes. The stimulation of blast transformation by mitogens such as phytohemagglutinin was inhibited by metal-chelating agents such as disodium EDTA (Alford, 1970); this inhibition was overcome by appropriate addition of zinc (Alford, 1970; Chesters, 1972. Zinc must be present for the entire period of blast transformation, with maximum stimulation of DNA synthesis (and therefore lymphocyte transformation occurring after 6 days of incubation) (Ruhl and Bochert, 1971). A soluble factor produced by monocytes seems to be required for the stimulation of peripheral blood lymphocytes by zinc (Ruhl and Kirchner, 1978). Zinc itself acts as a mitogen for both T cells (Ruhl and

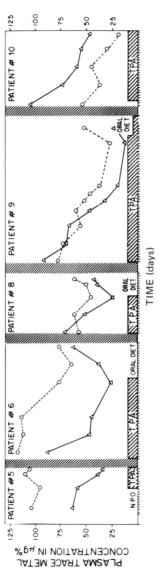

Fig. 7. Serial plasma zinc (○) and copper (△) values during TPN in five patients. (Reproduced with permission from Solomons *et al.*, 1976.)

Table VI

Plasma Zinc and Copper Before and After TPN

Patient number	Plasma zinc (µg/dl)			Plasma copper (µg/dl)			Duration of TPN (weeks)
	Before	After	Δ	Before	After	Δ	
1	45	15	−30	45	15	−30	7½
2	60	67	+7	65	35	−30	7
3	70	55	−15	140	78	−62	3
4	50	45	−5	125	30	−95	5½
5	95	106	+11	58	30	−28	1¾
6	119	79	−40	87	26	−61	4½
7	36	51	+15	132	76	−58	3
8	56	46	−10	74	26	−48	2
9	78	28	−50	91	12	−79	7
10	54	16	−35	105	46	−59	4
11	53	12	−42	15	4	−11	7½
12	38	14	−24	54	10	−44	3
13	98	64	−34	150	58	−92	3

[a]Reproduced with permission from Solomons et al. (1976).

Bochert, 1971) and B cells (Hart, 1978b); the degree of responsiveness depends on the age of the animal (Rao et al., 1979). Inhibitors of DNA, RNA, and protein synthesis can inhibit the effects of zinc on lymphocytes, indicating that zinc acts on specific metabolic pathways in these cells. Work has shown that transferrin may be intimately involved in this interaction, since lymphocytes have been reported to possess receptors for zinc–transferrin (Phillips, 1976). Binding of the zinc–transferrin complex precedes blast transformation (Phillips and Azaki, 1974) and is followed by a rapid uptake of zinc by lymphocytes, which in turn is followed by a rapid increase in DNA and RNA synthesis (Phillips and Azaki, 1974). Various agents such as poly-L-ornithine are capable of stimulating zinc uptake by lymphocytes and may represent a potential avenue of immunopotentiation (Phillips et al., 1979). It is possible that lymphocytes may represent an appropriate model for the investigation of the possible role of zinc in processes of cell division and in the transition process by which the cell progresses from a resting state to active proliferation.

Attention has now shifted to the investigation of the ways and the potential reversibility in which altered levels of dietary zinc affect immune responsiveness (Beach et al., 1983). As with human patients, the initial indication of an interaction between zinc and immunological function in experimental animals was that animals deficient in zinc are unable to respond effectively to pathogens of bacterial (Pekarek et al., 1977), viral (Tennican et al., 1979), and parasitic origin (Flagstad et al., 1972). As with acrodermatitis enteropathica in humans, a heritable disorder of zinc metabolism in cattle, Lethal Trait A46, provided initial information on the possible importance of zinc for intact immunological function; such cattle showed particularly aberrant cell-mediated immune functions and generally died of infection at an early age (Brummerstedt et al., 1974). Subsequent tests for immune function in a variety of zinc-deficient animals showed that in postnatal life those immune events mediated by T lymphocytes seemed to be most profoundly affected by zinc deprivation. Animals showed thymic involution (Chandra et al., 1980); depressed PFC responses, particularly the indirect or IgG-mediated aspect, in response to sheep erythrocyte immunization (Chandra et al., 1980; Fernandes et al., 1979; Fraker et al., 1977); depressed response to mitogens, especially the T-cell mitogens concanavalin A and phytohemagglutinin, which could be partially restored by immunopotentiation with levamisole; depressed cytotoxic response of spleen cells after in vivo immunization with EL 4 lymphoma tumor cells (Chandra and Au, 1980; Fernandes et al., 1979); low levels of natural killer (NK) cell activity (Fernandes et al., 1979); low levels of circulating thymic hormones (Iwata et al., 1979); and normal or elevated levels of antibody-dependent, cell-mediated cytotoxicity (Chandra and Au, 1980a; Fernandes et al., 1979).

A progressive appearance of autologous rosette-forming cells, a property of a specific subset of immature T cells present in zinc-sufficient animals only at low levels, also occurs in mice deprived of zinc (Nash et al., 1979). Simultaneously, there is a progressive loss of Thy-1.2+ cells and a proportional increase in the number of cells bearing F_c receptors (Fernandes et al., 1979). Fraker and associates have suggested that the immune defect in zinc deprivation may be localized, at least in part, at the level of T helper cell function. Transfer experiments have shown that appropriate administration of thymocytes derived from immunologically competent, zinc-sufficient mice can partially restore antibody responses to SRBC immunization (Fraker et al., 1978).

While the effects of zinc deprivation seem to be focused on the thymus and T cell–mediated functions, evidence indicates that B cells may also be affected by zinc availability. In vitro experiments utilizing human B lymphocytes have shown that when zinc is added to the culture medium, it activates lymphocytes to undergo blast transformation, as do also pokeweed mitogen, PPD, and diphtheria toxoid, all of which are B-cell mitogens; zinc is also capable of acting synergistically with some of these established mitogenic agents (Cunningham-Rundles et al., 1980). In most cases, restitution of zinc in the diet resulted in at least partial, and at times complete, restoration of immune function in humans (Golden et al., 1978) and experimental animals (Fraker et al., 1978; Zwickl and Fraker, 1980).

If deprivation of zinc was imposed during fetal or early postnatal development, the immune dysfunction that resulted was even more profound than that at later stages; while growth and development of zinc-deprived offspring were markedly retarded (Beach *et al.*, 1980a), growth of lymphoid organs, most notably the thymus, was more severely altered than that of other organs (Beach *et al.*, 1979). Immune function was also shown to be altered, as indicated by a depressed response to mitogens, especially concanavalin A and phytohemagglutinin (Beach *et al.*, 1979); altered the direct PFC response to sheep erythrocyte immunization, whether assessed per spleen or per 10^6 spleen white cells (Beach *et al.*, 1980c,d); and a markedly altered serum immunoglobulin profile, with no detectable serum IgM, IgG$_{2a}$, or IgA, and notably elevated levels of IgG$_1$ (Beach *et al.*, 1980c,d). One of the most remarkable observations of the studies in developing mice was the finding that even marginal deprivation of zinc, when imposed during the early postnatal period resulted in a substantial reduction in immunological responsiveness, particularly T cell-mediated immunity (Beach *et al.*, 1979, 1980c,d) (Table VII). These studies serve to underscore the importance of two critical aspects of any study of zinc deprivation: (1) the timing of the deprivation with respect to the life cycle of the animal and (2) the magnitude of the deprivation. Differences in methodology could account for the supposedly varied effects of zinc deficiency on such immunological parameters as natural killer cell activity and antibody-dependent cell-mediated cytotoxicity (Chandra *et al.*, 1980; Fernandes *et al.*, 1979).

Nonspecifically activated aspects of immunity are also affected by zinc status (Weston *et al.*, 1977) (Table VIII, Fig. 8). Reasonably extensive information now exists concerning the effect of zinc on activated macrophages. Overall, zinc ions in concentrations as low as 20 μM exert a markedly inhibitory effect on macrophages that have been activated; cells in the resting stage are not affected by zinc (Chvapil, 1976). When such activated macrophages are exposed to zinc *in vitro*, O_2 consumption via the hexose monophosphate shunt, phagocytosis of yeast cell particles, and intracellular killing of *E. coli* are inhibited (Chvapil *et al.*, 1977a). *In vitro* inhibition of PMN leukocytes and neutrophils was also observed (Chvapil *et al.*, 1977c). When animals received supplementary zinc *in vivo*, decreased mobility of peritoneal inflammatory cells (e.g., depressed chemotactic response of PMN leukocytes) was observed (Chvapil *et al.*, 1979). The high zinc content of prostatic fluid has been shown to immobilize cells such as PMN leukocytes effectively (Chvapil *et al.*, 1977b). The actions of zinc depend on its concentration. Physiological concentrations of zinc generally are inhibitory; other trace elements cannot effectively replace it (Chvapil *et al.*, 1976). It would appear that the influence of zinc ions on these cells is mediated at the plasma membrane level, since metal-complexing agents such as 8-hydroxyquinolone and 3-ethoxy-2-oxobutyraldehyde bis(thiosemicarbazone, KTS), which are also effective anticancer drugs, mediate this metal–cell interac-

Table VII

Relative Organ Weights as a Percentage of Total Body Weight at 4 Weeks of Age[a,b]

Diet[c]	Heart[d]	Kidney[d]	Liver[d]	Spleen[d]	Thymus[d]
100 ppm zinc Ad libitum-fed controls	0.46 ± 0.19^1	0.66 ± 0.01^1	$5.65 \pm 0.1g^1$	0.39 ± 0.04^1	0.39 ± 0.04^1
100 ppm zinc Inanition controls	0.49 ± 0.01^1	0.71 ± 0.02^1	5.97 ± 0.17^1	0.30 ± 0.01^2	0.44 ± 0.02^2
9.0 ppm zinc Marginal deficiency	0.60 ± 0.01^2	0.86 ± 0.02^2	4.82 ± 0.17^2	0.29 ± 0.02^2	0.18 ± 0.01^3
5.0 ppm zinc Moderate deficiency	0.62 ± 0.02^2	0.83 ± 0.03^2	3.99 ± 0.14^3	0.16 ± 0.01^3	0.11 ± 0.003^4
2.5 ppm zinc Severe deficiency	0.67 ± 0.01^3	0.88 ± 0.02^2	4.27 ± 0.15^2	0.09 ± 0.003^3	0.02 ± 0.002^5

[a]Reproduced with permission from Beach et al. (1979).

[b]Mean ± SE.

[c]Each dietary group represents 15 pups from at least 5 litters.

[d]Superscripts indicate values that differ significantly; $p < .01$ two-way analysis of variance and Duncan's multiple range; i.e., 1 is significantly different from 2, 3, 4, or 5.

Table VIII

Monocyte Chemotaxis and Plasma Zinc Levels[a]

Patient[b]	Zinc deficient	Oral supplemental zinc
Patient 1		
Chemotactic	2.88	16.10
cells (%)	$p < .01$	$p = $ ns
Plasma zinc	10.00	72.00
(μg/dl)	$p < .001$	$p = $ ns
Patient 2		
Chemotactic	4.20	18.02
cells (%)	$p < .05$	$p = $ ns
Plasma zinc	47.00	80.00
(μg/dl)	$p < .001$	$p = $ ns
Patient 3		
Chemotactic	3.32	8.25
cells (%)	$p = .01$	$p = $ ns
Plasma zinc	30.00	135.00
(μg/dl)	$p < .001$	$p = $ ns

[a]Reproduced with permission from Weston et al. (1977).

[b]p values compare results in patients 1, 2, and 3 to mean of 30 normal controls that were plasma zinc, (mean ± SE) 88.3 ± 2.5, and monocyte chemotaxis, 11.6 ± 0.6.

tion and do not cross the plasma membrane (Chvapil et al., 1976; Petering et al., 1967).

Other nonspecific immune substances with which zinc has been shown to interact include complement and interferon. The complex series of serum proteins known as C (complement) require divalent cations (e.g., Mg^{2+} and Ca^{2+}) at many of the steps toward immune lysis (Amivaian et al., 1974). In the presence of optimum Ca^{2+} and Mg^{2+} concentrations, low concentrations of zinc reduced the lytic activity of guinea pig complement (Amiraian et al., 1974). It was proposed that ionic zinc blocked formation of the active terminal complex through inhibition of C9 binding (Yamamoto and Takahashi, 1975). However, at higher concentrations, many of which were within a physiological range, zinc inhibited hemolysis of rabbit erythrocytes by aerolysin, a toxic, hemolytic bacterial product (Avigad and Bernheimer, 1976), as well as complement-mediated lysis of antibody-sensitized sheep erythrocytes in vitro (Montgomery et al., 1979). Such inhibitory activity was postulated to occur by preventing coalescence of an

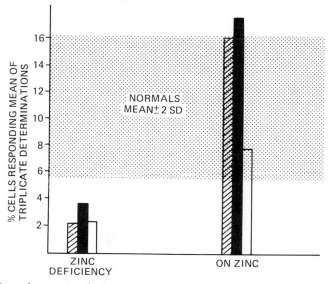

Fig. 8. Mean chemotaxis of monocytes during two phases: (1) zinc deficiency with mild symptoms of acrodermatitis enteropathica (AE) and (2) after symptoms and AE were corrected and plasma zinc levels returned to normal. ⊿, A; ■, B; □, C. A, B, and C, refer to patients 1, 2, and 3. (Reproduced with permission from Weston *et al.,* 1977.)

active complement–antibody–red blood cell complex (Montgomery *et al.,* 1979). When individual complement components were examined under such conditions, C2, C3, and C6 were inhibited most notably, while C7 and C8 were affected to a much smaller extent (Montgomery *et al.,* 1979). In contrast, C1, C4, and C9 were not affected by zinc concentration, and C5 activity was strongly enhanced (Montgomery *et al.,* 1979). If any of these complement components were already bound to the cell plasma membrane where they were exposed to the physiological zinc concentration, the zinc ions no longer had very much effect (Montgomery *et al.,* 1979). Zinc ions must be present as tertiary reactants during the binding-activation stage of complement-mediated immune lysis. Physiological zinc concentrations may play a central role in the mechanisms designed to regulate complement activation and function.

Relatively little is known regarding further interactions between zinc and other aspects of immune function. Mast cells have one of the highest local concentrations of zinc found in humans or animals (Angyal and Archer, 1968), a role ascribed to zinc is the binding of histamine, through a chelating action, within mast cells (Kazimierczak and Maslinski, 1974). Mast cells may be affected by zinc in an inhibitory fashion similar to that observed with macrophages, PMN leukocytes, and platelets (Chvapil, 1976; Chvapil *et*

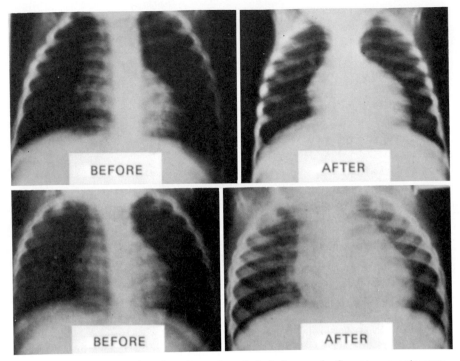

Fig. 9. Chest radiographs of patients 1 and 2 before and after zinc supplementation. (Reproduced with permission from Golden *et al.,* 1977.)

al., 1977a,c). Zinc may also affect the polymerization of IgM molecules (Anissimova, 1939). A single study on the interaction of zinc and interferon production and activity failed to determine its nature (Gainer, 1977). Much more work is needed regarding the effect of zinc on both interferon and interferon inducers such as Poly I : Poly C (Dion *et al.,* 1974). *In vitro* incubation of B lymphocytes with $ZnCl_2$ results in a significant restriction in the mobility of B-cell surface markers (Maro and Bornens, 1979). Such incubation with zinc results in delayed formation of lymphocyte caps and support the hypothesis that there is an interaction between the cellular membrane, the cytoskeleton, and the zinc content of the immediate environment.

Finally, in addition to the host's immunological response to a variety of pathogens, the effect of the local zinc environment must be considered. While zinc affects the viability and replication of bacteria and parasites (Failla, 1977), most is known regarding the effect of zinc on viruses. The viruses studied include herpes simplex *(*Fridlender *et al.,* 1978; 154), vaccinia virus, sindbis virus (Bracha and Schlesinger, 1976), human rhinovirus

1A (Butterworth and Korant, 1974), polio virus (Butterworth and Korant, 1974), encephalomyocarditis virus (Butterworth and Korant, 1974), and foot-and-mouth disease virus (Firpo and Palma, 1979). The effects of altering the local zinc environment include changes in thymidine kinase activity, DNA polymerase activity (Fridlender *et al.,* 1978), and reverse transcriptase activity (Auld *et al.,* 1974), all of which have been shown to be zinc-dependent enzymes or metalloenzymes. This results in aberrations such as accumulation of high molecular weight polypeptide precursors (Bracha and Schlesinger, 1976), inhibition of viral RNA synthesis and virus production (Firpo and Palma, 1979), posttranslational cleavage (Butterworth and Korant, 1974), and an overall reduction in the synthesis of virus-induced polypeptides; with each virus, the susceptibility to different concentrations of zinc varies considerably. Many of these viral systems have provided important insights into the role of zinc in the structure and function of higher animals. The important point here is to consider the direct effect of the internal milieu on any type of invasive organism.

The mechanism by which zinc acts on immune responsiveness remains obscure. One important theory emphasizes the role of increased adrenal weights and elevated levels of corticosteroids and their role as immunosuppressive agents (DePasquale-Jardieu and Fraker, 1979, 1980; Quarterman and Humphries, 1979). While such increases in steroid hormone levels can partially account for the observed immunodeficiency syndrome (DePasquale-Jardieu and Fraker, 1979), they cannot completely account for all of the observed defects (DePasquale-Jardieu and Fraker, 1980). Direct effects of zinc on the effector cells of the immune response may also account for a significant share of the role that zinc plays in intact immunocompetence. The notable effects of zinc ions on the response of T and B lymphocytes to mitogens *in vitro* (Alford, 1970; Chesters, 1972; Phillips, 1976; Phillips and Azaki, 1974; Rao *et al.,* 1979) and the remarkable effect of a dietary deficiency of zinc on mitogen responsiveness (Beach *et al.,* 1979) both argue for a direct influence of zinc on cells of the immune response, such as lymphocytes. Specific populations of lymphocytes may be particularly sensitive to lack of zinc, such as helper T cells (Fraker *et al.,* 1978). In addition, zinc seems to have a direct effect on the nonspecifically activated cells of the immune response, such as macrophages and PMN leukocytes (Chvapil, 1976; Chvapil *et al.,* 1976, 1977a,b,c; 1976). Zinc repletion has the potential to increase the thymic mass. (Fig. 9).

At what level do trace metals act on such cells? Sound evidence exists that zinc acts at the plasma membrane (Chvapil *et al.,* 1976), but it may also act on the nuclear membrane or on the histones or chromosomes directly, affecting the expression of various cellular products and thereby possibly modulating immunocompetence (Andrews, 1979; Andvonikashvili *et al.,*

1974; Falchuk, 1977). The role of zinc in numerous enzymes involved in the metabolism of basic cellular components may also affect immunological function (Dreosti and Duncan 1975; Dreosti and Hurley, 1975; Swenerton *et al.,* 1969; Vallee, 1976). Enzymes such as terminal deoxynucleotidyl transferase, which is present almost exclusively in thymus and which has been demonstrated to be a zinc metalloenzyme, may be of particular importance in the interaction between zinc and immunity (Chang and Bollum, 1970). Most likely, the observed dysimmunity in zinc deprivation (Beach, *et al.,* 1979; Beach *et al.,* 1980d; Chandra *et al.,* 1980; Fernandes *et al.,* 1979; Fraker *et al.,* 1977) is the result of numerous alterations in host functions, including some direct influences on the cells responsible for intact immunocompetence. Long-term studies in rhesus monkeys are currently underway to address these and similar issues (Golub *et al.,* 1982, 1984a,b,c; Leek *et al.,* 1984).

COPPER

The small amount of copper present in the human body participates in a large number of critical metabolic functions (Underwood, 1977). Like other essential trace metals, copper acts largely in conjunction with various enzyme systems, either in metalloenzymes (Mason, 1979), or as a more loosely attached cofactor (Mason, 1979). In some instances, deficiency symptoms can be correlated directly with altered activity of key enzymes (Underwood, 1977).

The mammalian cuproproteins are enzymes that contain copper as an integral part of their structure and have a defined ratio of protein subunits and copper atoms. These copper-containing metalloenzymes include ceruloplasmin (also called *ferroxidase*), which is involved with copper transport in the blood, mobilization of plasma iron, and biogenic amine regulation (Osaki *et al.,* 1966); SOD, which scavenges potentially damaging free radical intermediates of oxygen reduction (McCord and Fridovich, 1969); cytochrome C oxidase, the terminal enzyme of oxidative phosphorylation (Beinert, 1966); lysyl oxidase, which catalyzes oxidative deamination of ε-amino groups of hydroxylysine or peptidyllysine, critical for cross-linking of collagen (Harris and O'Dell, 1974; Siegel *et al.,* 1970); tyrosinase, involved in the conversion of tyrosine to melanin (Brown and Ward, 1959); dopamine hydroxylase, which catalyzes the formation of norepinephrine from dopamine (Friedman and Kaufman, 1965); and metallothionein, which is not actually an enzyme but which functions in the storage and transport of plasma and tissue copper (Porter *et al.,* 1964). Additional copper metalloenzymes include monoamine oxidases (McEwen, 1965), diamine oxidases (Yamada *et al.,* 1967), albocupreins (Fushimi *et al.,* 1971), uricase (Mahler, 1963), tryptophan-2,3-dioxygenase (Brady *et al.,* 1972), pink copper protein (Reed *et al.,* 1970), ascorbate oxidase (Dawson *et al.,* 1975), and mitochondrial monoamine oxidase (Nostrand and Glantz, 1973). This elaboration of enzymes known to contain copper as an integral structural feature serves to point out the widespread importance of copper in mammalian metabolism.

Perhaps more than with any other trace element, manifestations of copper deficiency vary greatly with species, sex, and age. One expression of copper deficiency is defective iron metabolism and consequent anemia (Lahey *et al.,* 1952; Van Wyk *et al.,* 1953); however, the precise nature of the anemia is variable, ranging from a hypochromic, microcytic anemia in pigs (Lahey *et al.,* 1952) to a normochromic, normocytic anemia in dogs (Bettger *et al.,* 1980). The principal defect is reported to involve ceruloplasmin and oxidation of ferrous iron (Osaki *et al.,* 1966). However, recent findings suggest that high ferroxidase activity is necessary for iron mobilization only under conditions of rapid hemoglobin synthesis, such as for growth, or when dietary iron is low (Cohen *et al.,* 1984). Another common feature of severe copper deficiency in most species is skeletal abnormalities, including deformities and susceptibility to fractures (Rucker *et al.,* 1969). The biochemical lesion responsible for these skeletal anomalies is a decreased activity of the cuproenzymes lysyl and amine oxidases, resulting in diminished cross-linking of bone collagen (Lahey *et al.,* 1952; Rucker *et al.,* 1969; Van Wyk *et al.,* 1953). Impaired disulfide cross-linking is also responsible for impeded keratinization in copper-deficient animals (Suttle *et al.,* 1970); this may be one of the principal defects in Menkes' disease, a heritable disorder of copper metabolism resulting in manifestations of copper deficiency (Danks *et al.,* 1972).

Cardiovascular disorders have also been observed in many species under conditions of severely limited copper availability (Goodman *et al.,* 1970; Shields *et al.,* 1962; Weissman *et al.,* 1963). Specifically, the pathogenesis involves the appearance of large areas of a dense, collagenous, fibrotic tissue replacing the degenerated myocardium. In addition, the elastin content of the aorta is markedly decreased in a number of species, leading to aortic aneurysms (Weissman *et al.,* 1963). Copper-deficient lambs experience enzootic neonatal ataxia associated with notable myelin aplasia and a significant reduction in ovine brain copper content and cytochrome oxidase activity (Mills and Williams, 1962). The decreased cytochrome oxidase activity is the result of depressed synthesis of the essential prosthetic group heme in a process strictly dependent on copper availability (Gallagher *et al.,* 1956). A breakdown in the conversion of tyrosine to melanin is responsible for the achromotrichia, or altered pigmentation, observed in the fur and skin of many species (Smith and Ellis, 1947). In female rodents, a profound influence of copper deprivation on reproduction was observed, with a significantly increased incidence of fetal death and resorption (Hall and Howell, 1969). Metabolic antagonisms with molybdenum in cattle resulted in diarrhea (Davis, 1950). Finally, disordered phospholipid synthesis and altered C_{16} and C_{18} fatty acid metabolism have been observed in copper deficiency (Fell et al., 1975).

The importance of copper for an effective response to a wide variety of pathogenic challenges has gained some attention (Newberne and Gebhardt, 1973; Newberne et al., 1968; Omole and Onawunmi, 1979; Wedgewood et al., 1975). In addition, animals supplemented with dietary copper show a significant reduction in pathological damage caused by the invading organism (Omole and Onawunmi, 1979). Suggestions on the precise nature of the lesion range from a blockade of the reticuloendothelial system (Newberne et al., 1968) to a defect in the IgM-to-IgG switching mechanism for the secondary antibody response (Sullivan and Ochs, 1978). It has also been proposed that patients with Menkes' disease (Danks et al., 1972; Menkes et al., 1962) may suffer from a basic T-lymphocyte defect, as reflected by their increased susceptibility to T cell–mediated infections (Pedroni et al., 1975). Numerous divalent cations have been shown to be intimately involved with cellular function, and the importance of copper in the function of a wide range of cell types including antibody-forming cells (Bazhora et al., 1974), PMN leukocytes (Rigas et al., 1979), T lymphocytes (Roberts and Aldous, 1951), and macrophages (Chvapil, 1976; Rabinovitch and Destefano, 1973) has been adequately demonstrated. $CuSO_4$ in conjunction with D-penicillamine, when administered to rheumatoid arthritis patients, almost completely inhibits the in vitro response of human T cells to mitogens; the same synergistic combination of agents has no significant impact on B cells and their immunoglobulin-secreting capacity (Lipsky and Ziff, 1980; Room et al., 1979). Helper T cells are particularly affected by $CuSO_4$ administration, and such interaction between $CuSO_4$ and D-penicillamine may help to explain their therapeutic efficacy in rheumatoid arthritis patients and their ability to reduce antiglobulin titers (Lipsky and Ziff, 1980).

Copper may also be closely involved with the function of complement, since copper ions inhibit the complement-mediated hemolysis of antibody-sensitized SRBC in vitro, seemingly by preventing the formation of an active red cell–antibody–complement complex (Montgomery et al., 1974). In addition, copper ions prevent the formation of the active terminal complement complex by inhibiting the binding of C9 (Yamamoto and Takahashi, 1975). Both dietary excess and deficiency of copper involve a notable decrease in phagocytic cell number and activity (Kolmitseva et al., 1969). Copper also seems to be involved in the inflammatory process, at certain times potentiating and at other times inhibiting it (Milanino et al., 1979). A severely copper-deficient diet leads to a pro-inflammatory effect. This may, in part, explain why serum copper and ceruloplasmin levels are elevated in rheumatoid arthritis patients (Grennan *et al.,* 1980) and why copper complexes, especially copper salicylate, are used widely in the treatment of rheumatoid arthritis and other degenerative diseases (Sorenson and Handgarter, 1977).

The mechanism by which copper alters immune responses may involve an interaction at the level of the plasma membrane, since copper has been shown to ameliorate the toxic effects of diethyldithiocarbamate on both T cells and PMN leukocytes, an interaction that must occur at the cell membrane (Rigas *et al.,* 1979). In addition, the interaction may involve enzymes such as copper-SOD which is important for the maintenance of cellular integrity. Additionally, copper is intimately involved in the three-dimensional structure of immunoglobulin molecules (Baker and Hultquist, 1978; Schrohenloher, 1978). Copper takes part in the catalysis of the thermal aggregation of human γ globulin as well, which is a key feature in the pathogenesis of rheumatoid arthritis (Kazuna *et al.,* 1979). Blocking this process may provide a new avenue of treatment for this condition.

Serum copper and ceruloplasmin levels increase in a variety of acute infectious disorders (Beisel, 1976) as opposed to the decrease in other trace metals such as zinc and iron. LEM seems to act as a key regulatory factor, influencing host–pathogen interaction and its effect on the metabolism of copper and other trace elements (Pekarek *et al.,* 1972). While many aspects of the role of copper in the host defense against a wide variety of pathogens remain to be investigated, many of the preliminary results indicate the potential for a significant interaction.

OTHER MINERALS

Interest in the interaction between selenium and immune function originated with the demonstration of this element as an anti-inflammatory agent in veterinary practice (Boyne and Arthur, 1979). Subsequent studies have indicated that selenium supplementation, within a limited range, results in significant enhancement of humoral immunity (Sheffy *et al.,* 1979; Mulhern *et al.,* 1981). Such potentiation of humoral immune responsiveness is substantiated by a heightened response to a variety of pathogens, including typhoid, canine distemper, and malaria (Desowitz *et al.,* 1980). Selenium deficiency is associated with a depression of humoral immune responsiveness, with a delay in its appearance and lower eventual titers of antibody.

Animals deprived of dietary magnesium develop reduced immune responses (McCoy *et al.,* 1975; Elin, 1975; Alcock *et al.,* 1974; McCreary *et al.,* 1973; Haas *et al.,* 1980; Haas *et al.,* 1978; Kraeuter *et al.,* 1980; Bois,

1963; Battifora *et al.,* 1968; McCreary *et al.,* 1967; McCreary *et al.,* 1966; Hungerford *et al.,* 1960). In contrast to many other nutrient deficiencies, magnesium deficiency is accompanied by marked thymic hyperplasia (Haas *et al.,* 1980); nonetheless, magnesium-deficient experimental rats and mice are characterized by impaired humoral and cell-mediated immunological responsiveness (McCoy *et al.,* 1975; Elin, 1975; Alcock *et al.,* 1974). Serum immunoglobulin profiles in magnesium-deficient animals may be altered significantly, with depressed levels of IgG_1, IgG_2, and IgA; however, not all such circumstances lead to changes in immunoglobulin levels. Magnesium-deficient animals immunized with sheep erythrocytes show only a minmal plaque-forming cell response; antibody titers are also markedly reduced. The appearance of malignant lymphoma in an increased proportion of magnesium-deficient rats has also been reported (Haas *et al.,* 1978). As with zinc, magnesium intake by elderly humans has been reported to be far below recommended daily allowance levels (Sempos *et al.,* 1982).

The potentially negative effects of iron deficiency on the immune system have been studied in humans and animals (Tables IX-XI). Blastogenic responses are reduced in humans and experimental animals suffering from iron deficiency (Lipschitz *et al.,* 1979). The number of circulating T Cells has also been reported to be reduced with iron deficiency (Joynson *et al.,* 1972; Fletcher *et al.,* 1975; Sawitsky *et al.,* 1976). Some improvement in immune dysfunction in iron deficiency with dietary iron supplementation has been reported in animals (Kuvibidila *et al.,* 1983) and humans (Bhaskaram *et al.,* 1977). However, other investigators have not found a consistent impairment of the immune system with iron deficiency in humans (Kulapongs *et al.,* 1974; Gross *et al.,* 1975), and have been unable to find an association between iron deficiency and an increased risk of infection (Gross *et al.,* 1975; Burman 1972). Detailed studies on the effects of iron deficiency on immunocompetence, including relationships with trace elements, have not been done.

MINERAL INTERACTIONS

A major consideration in the study of any aspect of trace element metabolism is the interactions between different essential and nonessential metals. and other nutrients (Baly *et al.,* 1984). In considering the effects of an excess or deficiency of any ingested trace mineral, direct actions of the metal on the organism must be distinguished from the effects of that metal on the metabolism of other metals and consequently on the whole organism. Copper, manganese, and zinc are all known to interact with each other and with many other trace elements such as cadmium, molybdenum,

Table IX

Serum Immunoglobulin and Complement C3 Levels (Means and Standard Deviations Are Presented)[a]

Group	Number of children	IgG (mg/dl)	IgA (mg/dl)	IgM (mg/dl)	Complement C3 (mg/dl)	Number showing C3 conversion products
Healthy	50	1080 ± 192	110 ± 29	88 ± 21	136 ± 31	0
Iron deficient						
Without infection	16	1163 ± 215	98 ± 36	80 ± 29	121 ± 42	0
With infection	4	1870 ± 203	148 ± 27	131 ± 39	92 ± 27	2

[a]Reproduced with permission from Chandra and Saraya (1975).

Table X

Opsonic Activity of Plasma and PMN Functions (Means and Ranges of Values Are Given)[a]

Group	Opsonic activity of plasma tested on control PMNs[b]	Phagocytosis in presence of control plasma[b]	Bactericidal capacity[c]	Reduction of nitroblue tetrazolium[d]
Healthy	484	484	9	0.27
	(431–576)	(431–576)	(2–27)	(0.16–0.39)
Iron deficient				
Before treatment	507	459	42	0.08
	(410–624)	(375–560)	(11–112)	(0.01–0.21)
After treatment	—	—	18	0.21
			(3–41)	(0.14–0.35)

[a]Reproduced with permission from Chandra and Saraya (1975).
[b]Expressed as number of yeast particles ingested by 100 PMN's in 30 min.
[c]Expressed as percentage of the number viable intracellular bacteria at the end of 2 hr of culture divided by the number at 20 min of culture.
[d]Expressed as the difference in optical density of cell extract of cultures containing latex particles for phagocytosis and of resting cultures without latex.

iron, silver, mercury, selenium, arsenic and chromium. In general, metals with the same electron valence structures may compete in membrane penetration and for the binding sites on certain enzymes. In human physiology, interactions between the trace elements zinc, copper, iron, molybdenum, and cadmium are most likely to have a significant impact on the whole organism.

One of the most widely studied interactions is that between copper and zinc. An excess of either was correlated with a decrease in serum and hepatic levels of the other. This was thought to be due to competition between these metals in membrane transport processes, and for binding sites on enzymes and on a class of metalloproteins called *metallothioneins*, which are present chiefly in liver, spleen, kidney, pancreas, and mucosa of

Table XI

Cutaneous Delayed Hypersensitivity[a]

Group	Number of children	Number with positive reaction				
		Candida	Trichophyton	Sk-St	Mumps	PPD
Healthy	20	18	16	17	12	6
Iron deficient	20	12	11	10	5	5

[a]Reproduced with permission from Chandra and Saraya (1975).

the small intestine and which are particularly important in copper homeostasis. In experimental animals, high levels of zinc in the diet were associated with anemia involving decreased hemoglobin levels, which was overcome by increasing the copper level of the diet. The best example of this interaction in humans occurred in patients with sickle-cell disease who were receiving high doses of zinc as treatment and consequently developed copper deficiency. Subsequent administration of appropriate levels of copper rapidly alleviated the deficiency syndrome. Further speculation on the importance of copper–zinc interactions involves the effects of a high zinc : copper ratio on associated hypercholesterolemia and a subsequently increased risk of ischemic heart disease. Experiments in animals have indicated that the risks of a high dietary intake of copper can be reduced by increasing the zinc intake, and the deleterious effects of a high zinc intake can be ameliorated by increasing the intake of copper.

Cadmium is also related to the metabolism of copper and zinc; generally, there is an antagonism between zinc and cadmium, which affects copper metabolism. Addition of zinc to the diet of cadmium-treated animals markedly reduces the toxic effects attributed to cadmium. Cadmium is also related to copper in that there is an increased mortality if animals are simultaneously copper deficient.

Metabolism of manganese is also related to the metabolism of these other essential and nonessential minerals. Elevated levels of manganese in the diet of experimental animals result in decreased hemoglobin synthesis and reduced iron stores. This alteration of iron metabolism due to high manganese levels can be overcome by the addition of extra iron to the diet. There are also interactions between copper, silver, and mercury. Silver causes reduced hemoglobin synthesis and elastin content in copper-deficient chicks but not in copper-supplemented controls, indicating an antagonistic relationship between these two trace elements in chickens. In contrast, mercury inhibits growth and increases mortality in copper-supplemented animals. Molybdenum is also closely associated with the metabolism of iron and copper in that it is a cofactor of xanthine oxidase, an enzyme responsible for the reduction of cellular ferric to ferrous ferritin. Furthermore, interactions between these essential trace metals and other elements such as arsenic, tin, tellurium, vanadium, and chromium have been described. Clearly, our understanding of these interactions is extremely limited at present.

9

Vitamins

INTRODUCTION

Vitamins represent an exceptionally heterogeneous group of compounds that are related to each other only in that they are each essential only in minute amounts for normal physiological function. Beyond this, they are chemically diverse and have different biochemical functions. For many of the vitamins, a great deal remains to be elucidated regarding their cellular basis of action and their comparative requirements in various species. The latter is particularly true with respect to the role of vitamins in the development and maintenance of intact immunocompetence and in the maintenance of host defense against a wide range of pathogens.

It is nonetheless interesting to note that vitamin A, for example, was found to modulate host defense against infection over 50 years ago (Green and Melanby, 1930). It has also long been known that children suffering from PEM with superimposed vitamin A deficiency have a much poorer prognosis than do children with uncomplicated PEM. These observations are being applied to the use of *retinoids,* as the various forms of vitamin A have come to be known collectively, in protecting against the pathological sequelae of invasive microorganisms. Yet we have only the most rudimentary clues as to how this essential fat-soluble factor exercises its influence. Such information is of particular interest in the case of vitamins because, in addition to their possible role in normal immunological function, they may have potential in clinical medicine if administered in pharmacological rather than physiological doses. This chapter will cover both fat-soluble and water-soluble vitamins.

VITAMIN A

As noted above, the discovery that vitamin A might play an important role in immune processes was made over 50 years ago. Indeed, one of the first functional properties ascribed to vitamin A was that of an anti-infective agent (Green and Melanby, 1930). Animals fed a diet devoid of vitamin A developed multiple septic foci and had a very high mortality rate. In contrast, rats fed adequate levels of β-carotene, a precursor form of vitamin A obtained from plants, grew normally and gained complete immunity to spontaneous infection. Additional studies have confirmed these early findings (Boynton and Bradford, 1931; Bang *et al.,* 1975). Vitamin A, in addition to its possible effect on cells directly responsible for mediating immunological function, is essential in the maintenance of normal epithelial tissues (Hays, 1971). Thus, vitamin A deficiency may allow the entry of basic pathogens that might ordinarily be excluded from intact mucosal surfaces. Indeed, vitamin A deficiency in chicks infected with Newcastle disease virus (NDV) had a synergistically negative impact on the host (Bang *et al.,* 1975). Moreover, the combined impact of NDV infection and dietary vitamin A deficiency results in a marked depletion of lymphoid cells from bone marrow, as well as the depletion of lymphoid cells localized to the nasal region and paranasal glands. Therefore, when the influence of vitamin A on the response of the host organism to disease is investigated, it is important to note that any alteration in resistance to infectious challenge might be attributed to either changes in host mechanical barriers to infection and/or alterations of host immunocompetence.

While vitamin A deficiency results in an increased susceptibility to infectious disease, excess vitamin A has a protective effect. For example, vitamin A palmitate produces a significant decrease in mortality if given before challenge with either *Pseudomonas, Listeria monocytogenes,* or *Candida albicans* (Fig. 1) (Cohen and Elin, 1974). This effect can be noted for up to 5 hr postchallenge; vitamin A–treated mice continue to exhibit sterile blood, while control animals experience persistent bacteremia. The mechanism responsible for this protection has been postulated to be an enhancement of the nonspecific defense mechanisms of the reticuloendothelial system.

Vitamin A deficiency has been investigated in several species. In all studies, it resulted in marked leukocytosis with a concurrent increase in the number of PMN leukocytes and a decrease in the number of lymphocytes in peripheral blood (Turner and Loew, 1931). Complement levels were also lower in serum obtained from vitamin A–deficient animals. Recent studies have confirmed these classic observations. The effects of vitamin A deficiency on lymphoid tissues has also been investigated. In rats subjected to vitamin A deficiency, there was a decrease in the size of both primary and secondary lymphoid organs (Table I) (Krishnan *et al.,* 1974). Histological examination revealed a near-total atrophy of the thymic cortex and a marked involution of the germinal centers (Fig. 2). Although the lobular integrity of the thymic medulla was maintained, the total size of the thymus

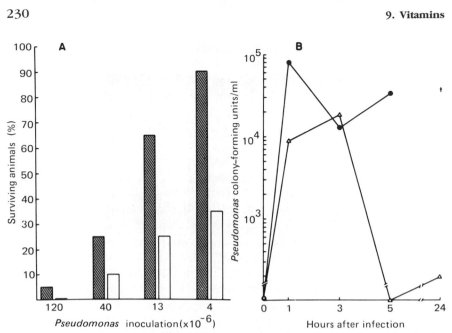

Fig. 1. (A) Percentage of mice treated with vitamin A or with saline that survived 72 hr after infection with *Pseudomonas aeruginosa.* Each bar represents the 25 mice from three separate experiments. (B) Clearance of *P. aeruginosa* from blood of mice treated with either vitamin A or saline, and then injected ip with 10^7 organisms. Groups of four mice were bled periodically by aseptic technique from the retrobulbar sinus, and the mean number of colony forming units/ml was determined at each interval by quantitative culturing. † = all control animals dead. (A) ▨, vitamin A treated; □, controls. (B) ●, control; △, vitamin A treated. (Reproduced with permission from Cohen and Elin, 1974.)

Table I

Effect of Vitamin A and Protein-Calorie Deficiency
on the Size of Thymus and Spleen[a,b]

	Thymus (mg per 100 g body weight)	Spleen (mg per 100 g body weight)
Control	398 ± 63 (6)[c]	400 ± 20 (6)
Vitamin A *cum* protein-calorie deficiency	214 ± 61 (6)	188 ± 12 (6)
Pair-fed	355 ± 71 (6)	262 ± 74 (6)

[a]Reproduced with permission from Krishnan *et al.* (1974).
[b]Average values ± SD of the mean.
[c]Figures in parentheses denote the number of animals studied in each group.

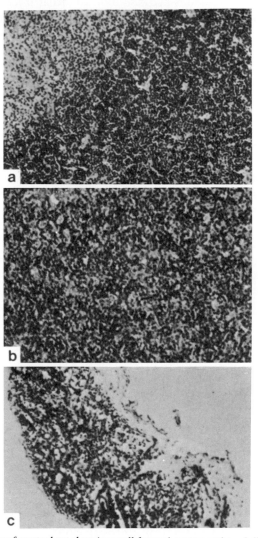

Fig. 2. (a) Thymus of control rat showing well-formed cortex and medulla. (hematoxylin & eosin, × 122.) (b) Thymus of pair-fed rat showing mostly medullary tissue. The epithelial cells are intermingled with a fair number of lymphoid cells. The cortex is not well defined. (Hematoxylin & eosin, × 122.) (c) Thymus of vitamin A-deficient rat. The cortex is completely depleted of lymphocytes and is not seen as a separate entity. (hematoxylin & eosin, × 122.) (Reproduced with permission from Krishnan *et al.*, 1974.)

was reduced. Other studies on the influence of supplemental levels of vitamin A on lymphoid tissues likewise indicated that injection of vitamin A resulted in a decreased cellularity of peripheral lymph nodes (Taub *et al.,* 1970). More recent studies have emphasized possible divergent results depending on the analog of vitamin A employed. In mice fed supplemental retinal acetate (250-mg/kg diet for 3 weeks), an enlargement of peripheral lymph nodes in the thymus was observed. However, elevated levels of retinoic acid (up to 1000 mg/mouse/day for 7 days) were found to result in a decrease in lymphoid organ size, with a concomitant decrease in the cellularity of the spleen and thymus (Dennert and Lotan, 1978). In contrast, no such effect was noted in the cellularity of bone marrow. Consequently, it is concluded that vitamin A excess and deficiency can both result in notable changes in lymphoid organ size and histological architecture. Moreover, specific retinoids may differ in the form and magnitude of the effect observed.

Many of the earlier studies of vitamin A and immunological phenomena focused on the levels of antibody titers in response to challenge with a variety of antigens. Administration of excess retinoic acid, whether orally or by intramuscular injection, had no significant impact on bacterial clearance or antibody titers (Uhr *et al.,* 1963). In contrast, vitamin A–deficient chicks displayed significantly lower bursal weights and a significant decrease in antibody titer following challenge when compared with *ad libitum*-fed controls (Panda and Combs, 1963). In contrast, no such changes were noted in the weights of the spleen, thymus, or adrenal glands. Similar results were found in pigs raised on a vitamin A–free diet (Harmon *et al.,* 1963). After a period of 6–7 weeks of dietary vitamin A repletion, antibody levels returned to control values.

Vitamin A, given as a single injection of retinol, could act as an adjuvant when administered simultaneously with bovine γ globulin (Dresser, 1968). Such administration of vitamin A prevents tolerance. Retinol suspended in incomplete Freund's adjuvant resulted in the highest titer of antibodies to bovine serum albumin of several other adjuvants examined. With increasing concentrations of adjuvant, there was a concurrent increase in the antibody titer to a plateau level (Spitznagal and Allison, 1970). Further studies indicated that five daily injections of 200 IU/g body weight/day (or approximately 40% of the LD_{50} of vitamin A palmitate) resulted in a substantial increase in the titer of hemagglutinating antibodies in response to sheep erythrocyte immunization. Mice given large doses of vitamin A for 4 days showed enhanced responsiveness to heterologous erythrocyte immunization. With administration of less than 1000 IU/day for 4 consecutive days, there was no observed effect on antibody production; maximum responsiveness was noted in a dose of 3000 IU/day (Jurin and Tannock, 1972;

Cohen and Cohen, 1973). Finally, simultaneous administration of vitamin A counteracted the immunosuppressive action of corticosteroids. In addition, retinol was shown to be capable of acting as an adjuvant for the production of IgE to either ovalbumin or ovalbumin absorbed to aluminum hydroxide on secondary challenge (Figs. 3, 4) (Bryant and Barnett, 1979). Thus, vitamin A is capable of acting as an adjuvant in the production of IgE antibodies as well as other classes. Finally, while previous studies have demonstrated that retinol acetate and retinol palmitate both stimulate the humoral immune response to heterologous erythrocytes, retinoic acid did not result in an enhancement of responsiveness to SRBC (Dennert and Lotan, 1978).

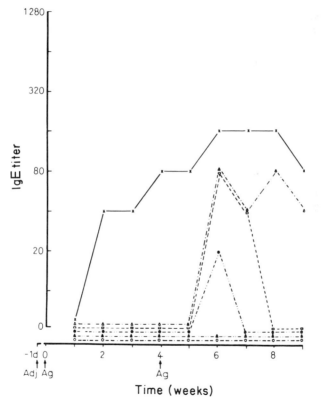

Fig. 3. The adjuvant effects of retinol pretreatment on the IgE response to OA in BALB/c mice. Treatment on day −1 with either 1000 (●), 3000 (□), 5000 (△), 9000 IU (▲) of retinol : Tween 80 or saline · Tween 80 (○) intraperitoneally. On days 0 and 30, all experimental groups (except one) received an intraperitoneal injection of OA : saline. One group (X) received saline only on day −1 and OA : Al(OH)₃ on days 0 and 30. IgE titers were determined by the 48-hr PCA reaction. −Id, −Iday; Adj, adjuvant; Ag, antigen. (Reproduced with permission from Bryant and Barnett, 1979.)

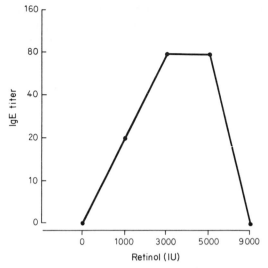

Fig. 4. Dose response of retinol pretreatment on IgE production to OA : saline at 6 weeks after primary immunization. (Reproduced with permission from Bryant and Barnett, 1979.)

In contrast to administration of supplemental levels of vitamin A, feeding a diet deficient in vitamin A resulted in a response to SRBC immunization that was depressed by approximately 50%, as measured by the hemagglutination titer (Krishnan *et al.,* 1974). In another study, rats fed a vitamin A–deficient diet produced only $17.5 \pm 4.8 \times 10^3$ plaques per spleen compared with $56.4 \pm 9.0 \times 10^3$ plaques per spleen in pair-fed control animals ($p < .01$) (spleens were not significantly different in size, so plaques per spleen was a valid reflection of immunocompetence) (Tables II, III) (Chandra and Au, 1981). There was a fundamental difference in these observations, since no differences between vitamin A–deficient animals and pair-

Table II

Plaque-Forming Cell (PFC) Response[a]

| | | Direct PFC per spleen ($\times 10^{-6}$) | |
Group	Number of rats	Background	5th day postimmunization
Vitamin A deficient	6	0.39 ± 0.08	17.5 ± 4.8
Pair-fed control	6	0.24 ± 0.09	56.4 ± 9.0
p		.05	.01

[a]Reproduced with permission from Chandra and Au (1981).

Table III
Organ Weights[a]

Group	Number of animals	Thymus weight (mg)	Spleen weight (mg)
Vitamin A deficient	6	181 ± 39	317 ± 41
Pair-fed control	6	208 ± 28	339 ± 47
Ad libitum-fed control	6	281 ± 40	387 ± 59

[a]Reproduced with permission from Chandra and Au (1981).

fed controls were noted in direct plaque-forming cell responsiveness. Krishnan et al. (1974) did note such a difference. However, they did indicate that responses to diphtheria and tetanus toxoids were markedly reduced in vitamin A–deficient animals, whether compared with ad libitum-fed or pair-fed controls. It would therefore appear that vitamin A is essential for normal antibody production in response to a specific antigen, and under many circumstances may act to enhance antibody production if supplemented at higher than normal levels.

The administration of excess retinoic acid resulted in a notable suppression of delayed-type hypersensitivity responses to diphtheria toxoid in complete Freund's adjuvant (Uhr et al., 1963). In addition, Arthus reactivity and the generalized inflammatory response to diphtheria toxoid administration were also suppressed by supplementation with retinoic acid. Five daily injections of 200 IU/g body weight/day of vitamin A palmitate resulted in a significant augmentation of skin graft rejection (Jurin and Tannock, 1972). This reaction, utilizing minor differences in histocompatibility, was noted whether the injections of vitamin A were initiated 5 days prior to the graft transplant or up to 6 days after grafting (Table IV). In addition, C3H mice treated with weekly doses of either 100 or 200 mg retinoic acid per kilogram of body weight rejected CBA/H skin homografts more rapidly than did controls, i.e., in only 20 days as opposed to over 40 days in the ad libitum-fed control animals (Floersheim and Bollag, 1972). In contrast, auto- and isografts were not affected by the administration of similar doses of retinoic acid. Higher doses of retinoic acid did affect the latter two types of grafts, but it was suggested that such graft breakdown was mediated by a toxic effect on wound-healing processes rather than by an immunological mechanism. More recent studies have shown that the median survival time of skin allografts was reduced by the administration of retinal acetate from 27.5 to 16.5 days (Medawar and Hunt, 1981). Furthermore, concomitant administration of antilymphocyte serum was demonstrated to reduce the action of vitamin A.

Table IV

Influence of Vitamin A on Rejection of C57BL/6 Male Skin by Isologous Females[a]

Group	Vitamin A injected on days[b]	Number of mice	Mean time to total rejection ($\pm$ SE)	Mean time from onset to completion of rejection ($\pm$ SE)
1	$-5--1$	12	24.3 $\pm$ 0.2	5.0 $\pm$ 0.3
2	0–4	12	23.8 $\pm$ 0.3	3.5 $\pm$ 0.3
3	6–10	18	23.1 $\pm$ 0.2	5.9 $\pm$ 0.3
4	Controls (saline injected on days 0–4)	18	33.3 $\pm$ 0.9	12.8 $\pm$ 0.6

[a]Reproduced with permission from Jurin and Tannock (1972).
[b]Skin grafts were done on day 0.

Mitogen responsiveness has also been utilized to investigate the influence of vitamin A levels on immune responsiveness. An impaired level of mitogen responsiveness was noted in animals deprived of vitamin A. For example, rats fed a vitamin A–deficient diet showed only approximately one-third the response to mitogens of either pair-fed or *ad libitum*-fed control animals (Nauss *et al.,* 1979). The response to concanavalin A (Con A) was only 24,767 $\pm$ 4209 cpm in vitamin A–deficient rats compared to 56,535 $\pm$ 11,250 cpm and 76,438 $\pm$ 12,848 cpm in *ad libitum*-fed and pair-fed controls; a similar marked reduction in the level of response to the T-cell mitogen phytohemagglutinin (PHA) was also noted (Table V) (Chandra and Au, 1981). The response to the B-cell mitogen LPS was also markedly reduced in the vitamin A–deficient rats. Repletion with 500 μg retinal acetate resulted in restoration of mitogen responsiveness to normal levels in the vitamin A–deficient animal.

Retinoic acid added to cultures of human lymphocytes resulted in enhanced DNA synthesis in response to the T-cell mitogen PHA and to rabbit anti-human thymocyte globulin (ATG) (Abb and Deinhardt, 1980). In contrast, responses to Con A and pokeweed mitogen were not altered by *in vitro* addition of retinoic acid.

Studies of vitamin A and the immune response have obviously become increasingly sophisticated. One facet of immunocompetence that seems to be particularly affected by vitamin A levels is cell-mediated cytotoxicity. By manipulating the level of retinoic acid administration (25–300 μg retinoic acid) and the dosage of allogeneic tumor (myeloma) cells (3 $\times$ 10^6 cells), it was possible to obtain a 10-fold increase in the level of cell-mediated cytotoxicity (Dennert and Lotan, 1978). This potentiation of cell-mediated

Table V

Mitogen Stimulation Response[a]

Group	Number of rats	PHA-induced stimulation index		
		0.2 μg[b]	0.5 μg	2.0 μg
Vitamin A deficient	6	20.7 ± 8.8	37.5 ± 19.0	38.7 ± 31.9
Pair-fed control	6	87.8 ± 39.5	104.8 ± 36.4	121.8 ± 57.5
p		<.05	<.01	<.01

[a]Reproduced with permission from Chandra and Au (1981).
[b]Amount of PHA in each well of microtiter plate.

cytotoxicity was noted whether the assays were performed *in vivo* or *in vitro*. At higher concentrations of retinoic acid, instead of an increase there was suppression of cell-mediated cytotoxicity. Thus, it would appear that the ability of retinoic acid to modulate immune responsiveness, at least as measured by cell-mediated cytotoxicity, is also dose dependent and is most effective within a specific range. Moreover, retinoic acid was found to act specifically on cytotoxic T lymphocytes rather than acting as a general adjuvant or as a T-cell mitogen. This demonstrated that retinoic acid did not cause an enhancement of the response of mixed lymphocyte culture proliferation or to the T-cell mitogens Con A and PHA. Delayed-type hypersensitivity responsiveness to SRBC and the induction of cooperating T-cell types was not appreciably stimulated by retinoic acid administration (Dennert and Lotan, 1978).

Repeated intraperitoneal administration of retinoic acid for as little as 6 days or as long as 3 months resulted in the potent stimulation of T-cell-mediated cytotoxicity (Dennert *et al.,* 1979). This was true of both an allogeneic system and a syngeneic system utilizing an *in vitro* challenge with tumor cells. The enhanced cell-mediated cytotoxicity was antigen dependent and antigen specific; in the allogeneic system it was specific for H-2 antigen, and in the syngeneic system it was specific for the tumor antigens. Therefore, vitamin A in the form of retinoic acid does not act as a polyclonal activator. The precise locus of the enhancement effect may be the cytotoxic T cell; the activity was abolished by pretreatment with anti-θ serum plus complement.

Perhaps the most clear and convincing investigation of the potential influence of vitamin A on immunological function was published most recently (Malkovsky *et al.,* 1983). When 6- to 9-week-old inbred mice were fed a diet supplemented with vitamin A acetate, 0.5 g/kg diet, they were found to respond to a suboptimal dose of semiallogeneic cells (10^5 cells) in a positive host-versus-graft reaction (HVGR). Control mice fed the conventional diet but without additional vitamin A showed no evidence of an HVGR. Moreover, these investigators were able to modulate the immunocompetence of the mice fed the conventional diet by utilizing cell transfer experiments. By injecting lymphoid cells obtained from the vitamin A— fed mice into control recipients, they enhanced the HVGR ability of control mice. The dose of lymphoid cells needed to observe this transfer of enhanced immunological reactivity was relatively low, indicating that the function of the responsible cell type was most likely that of a helper or inducer rather than an effector. By applying a positive selection technique utilizing a panel of monoclonal antibodies against a variety of T-cell determinants, the authors demonstrated that the cell most likely responsible for this immunopotentiation is the Lyt-1+,2− T cell or helper cell. This effect was quite specific, since analysis by fluorescence-activated cell sorter (FACS) indicated that a higher proportion of cells of the Lyt-1.1+ cells were present in lymph nodes of mice fed vitamin A than in control counterparts. In contrast, the proportion of Lyt-2.1+ cells was not significantly altered. These results suggest confirmation of recent studies indicating involvement of Lyt-1+ cells in response to both H-2 and non−H-2 alloantigens and underscore the potential use of nutritional manipulations to investigate basic immunological phenomena. The authors also suggest that these results help support the hypothesis that the anticancer action of retinoids is mediated by immunological processes and may act through an increase in the activity of the helper/inducer Lyt-1+2− phenotype T-cell subpopulation.

In addition, retinoic acid has been shown to enhance the activity of NK cells for humans and mice (Goldfarb and Herberman, 1981). Such enhancement could be partially reversed by simultaneous addition of the tumor promoter phorbol-12-myristate-13-acetate (PMA), which, when added alone, was shown to result in a decrease of NK cell activity. A combined treatment of NK cells with both retinoic acid and interferon, which had also been shown to enhance NK cell activity, resulted in less augmentation of NK cell activity than did similar treatment with either agent alone. These results are of biological significance since they show that the addition of the tumor promoter PMA inhibits NK cell activity, whereas addition of retinoic acid, an agent associated with prevention of tumors, augments this activity. These results may help to emphasize the importance of NK cell activity and host defense against oncogenic challenge. It may also help to explain the antineoplastic influences of various retinoids.

Vitamin A also affects interferon production and action. For example, it can inhibit the antiviral activity of interferon. The biochemical basis for this inhibition was found to be due to a direct action on the interferon molecule (Blalock and Gifford, 1975). Subsequent studies also indicated that retinoic acid suppressed interferon production (Blalock and Gifford, 1976). Other groups have studied the structural requirements of vitamin A with regard to inhibition of interferon production as well as interferon activity. In terms of antiviral activity, retinol was most potent, with retinoic acid slightly less so, and β-carotene possessing slightly less than one-half of the suppressor function of retinol and retinoic acid. Other retinoid analogs were markedly less effective in suppressing interferon antiviral activity. In contrast, with regard to its effect on interferon production, far less difference was noted between the various vitamins, with retinoic acid and retinal displaying the highest levels of suppressive activity (Table VI). Thus, inhibition of interferon antiviral activity is most affected by the configuration of the molecule's side chains. Retinoic acid also induces repressor protein synthesis, which blocks interferon production at the level of transcription (Table VII) (Blalock and Gifford, 1977). Thus, vitamin A exerts its influence on gene expression, probably at the level of transcription. These results have been recently confirmed. Production of both γ- and α-interferon by human peripheral blood lymphocytes in response to stimulation by synthetic polynucleotides, viruses, mitogens, bacterial products, and tumor cell lines *in vitro* was suppressed by concurrent addition of retinoic acid (Abb *et al.,* 1982). Interferon production by human lymphoblastoid cell lines was likewise reduced by addition of retinoic acid. The observed effects were dose dependent, with increasing inhibition as the level of retinoic acid was increased.

VITAMIN D

Vitamin D functions in the absorption and utilization of calcium. In the absence of vitamin D, calcium metabolism is altered and skeletal maturation cannot occur. There are many genetic disorders of vitamin D metabolism, e.g., vitamin D–dependent rickets. Patients with these syndromes have growth failure, rickets, and occasionally hypophosphatemia. Excessive amounts of vitamin D are detrimental and result in impairment of osteogenesis and the development of pathogenic fractures. Moreover, vitamin D is necessary for the development of mammary glands and/or normal lactation. Pregnant rats treated with vitamin D showed fatty degeneration of the liver and elevated levels of esterified fatty acids.

Vitamin D–deficient rickets is often accompanied by infections. It is unclear whether the infections are due to accompanying diseases or to increased exposure to infectious agents. For example, rickets occurs frequently in families of lower socioeconomic status, in whom there is an increased possibility of infectious diseases. In contrast, there is some evidence that rickets may also cause an increased incidence of infections. This

Table VI

Comparison of the Suppression of Interferon Production and Inhibition
of Its Action by Vitamin A and Related Compounds[a]

| | Percentage of suppression of interferon | | | | | |
| | Antiviral activity | | | Production | | |
Compound tested[b]	Replicate experiments[c]	Mean ±SD	P	Replicate experiments	Mean ±SD	P
Retinoic acid	60, 64, 65, 65	63 ± 3	<.001	75, 67, 61	68 ± 7	<.001
Retinol	57, 100	79 ± 21	<.01	67, 47	57 ± 14	<.01
Retinal	24, 17	21 ± 5	NS[d]	75, 68	72 ± 5	<.001

Structures of Retinoic acid, Retinol, and Retinal.

240

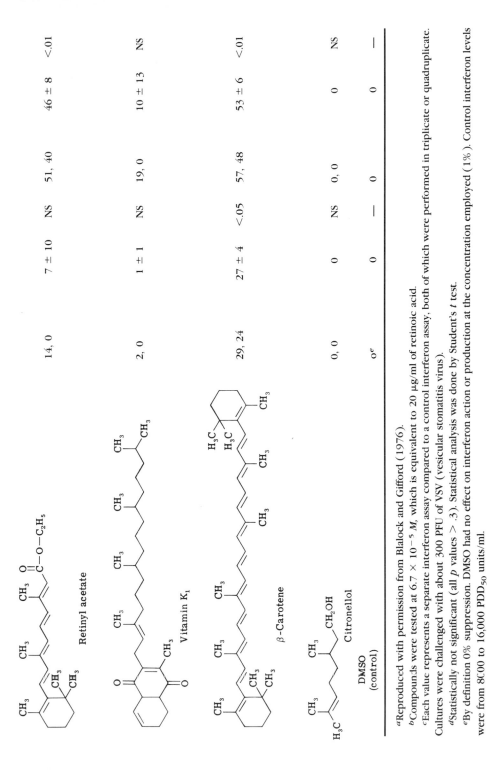

Retinyl acetate

Vitamin K₁

β-Carotene

Citronellol

DMSO (control)

14, 0	7 ± 10	NS	51, 40	46 ± 8	<.01		Retinyl acetate
2, 0	1 ± 1	NS	19, 0	10 ± 13	NS		Vitamin K₁
29, 24	27 ± 4	<.05	57, 48	53 ± 6	<.01		β-Carotene
0, 0	0	NS	0, 0	0	NS		Citronellol
0[e]	0	—	0	0	—		DMSO (control)

[a]Reproduced with permission from Blalock and Gifford (1976).

[b]Compounds were tested at 6.7×10^{-5} M, which is equivalent to 20 μg/ml of retinoic acid.

[c]Each value represents a separate interferon assay compared to a control interferon assay, both of which were performed in triplicate or quadruplicate. Cultures were challenged with about 300 PFU of VSV (vesicular stomatitis virus).

[d]Statistically not significant (all p values > .3). Statistical analysis was done by Student's t test.

[e]By definition 0% suppression. DMSO had no effect on interferon action or production at the concentration employed (1%). Control interferon levels were from 8000 to 16,000 PDD₅₀ units/ml.

241

Table VII

Effect of Retinoic Acid on NDV, SFV, and Poly I·Poly C Induction of Interferon[a]

Interferon inducer	Retinoic acid (20 μg/ml)	Interferon yield, PDD$_{50}$/ml	Inhibition of interferon yield (%)	Virus yield,[b] PFU × 10^6
NDV[c]	+	2,600	74	
	−	10,000		
SFV[d]	+	260	71	1.70 ± 0.45
	−	900		1.65 ± 0.40
Poly I·Poly C	+	100	86	—
	−	700		

[a]Reproduced with permission from Blalock and Gifford (1977).
[b]PFU, plaque-forming units.
[c]NDV (Newcastle disease virus) abortively infects L-929 cells and therefore no virus is produced.
[d]Sandfly fever virus.

possibility is supported by the observation of decreased cellular and humoral immunity in young rats with experimentally induced rickets. In one study, examinations of phagocytosis, bacteriotoxicity, and complement levels were performed in infants with rickets. *Escherichia coli* was used in all experiments because children are usually exposed to this bacterium early in life and subsequently produce antibodies against it (Stroder and Kasal, 1970).

Children with rickets were shown to have normal bactericidal capacity of leukocytes to *E. coli*, but all had impaired phagocytosis. These findings provide a possible explanation for the observations of increased infections in rickets (Table VIII, Fig. 5).

Table VIII

Phagocytosis of *E. coli* in Normal Serum
and Serum in Rickets by Normal
and Rickets Leukocytes[a]

Source of serum	Source of leukocytes	
	Normal	Rickets
Normal	60%[b]	63%
Rickets	42%	46%

[a]Reproduced with permission from Stroder and Kasal (1970).
[b]% *E. coli* phagocytized.

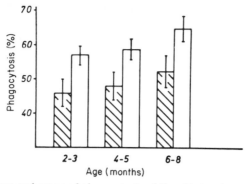

Fig. 5. Average values and range of phagocytosis of *E. coli* at various ages. Children with rickets in striped columns, controls in white columns. (Reproduced with permission from Stroder and Kasal, 1970.)

VITAMIN E

The tocopherols, known collectively as vitamin E, have been investigated less intensively than the retinoids. One of the factors hampering investigative efforts is the fact that the metabolic function of vitamin E and the basis for its essentiality as a nutrient remain to be clearly established. There is considerable controversy regarding the possible role of vitamin E in altering aging and retarding the progression of or preventing a number of chronic degenerative diseases. The level of vitamin E that might become harmful to humans also remains unclear. In addition, the metabolism of vitamin E is closely related to that of a number of other essential nutrients, most notably selenium and the polyunsaturated fatty acids; these nutrient interactions vary substantially among species. Consequently, the information regarding the role(s) of vitamin E and immunological function is a bit fragmentary. Nonetheless, it is evident that the potential exists for favorably manipulating various aspects of immunocompetence.

Most of the experimental investigation of vitamin E nutriture and immunological function has involved the administration of higher levels of vitamin E than those generally considered to be required. In animals deprived of vitamin E, there was a significant decrease in PFC responsiveness to heterologous erythrocytes and the production of very low levels of IgG hemagglutination titers. However, because vitamin E deficiency is considered to occur only rarely in human populations, little more has been done to discover what influence vitamin E deficiency might have on the development and maintenance of immunocompetence. Recent studies indicate that premature infants may routinely suffer from vitamin E deficiency, but it is not known if the immunological development of these infants is impaired. Consequently, additional studies of vitamin E deficiency, particularly during critical periods of development, are necessary.

In contrast to the relative lack of data regarding vitamin E deficiency, numerous studies have been conducted concerning supplemental vitamin E and immunological function. In experiments with mice, it was found that when vitamin E was supplemented as DL-α-tocopherol acetate at higher levels than those suggested as being required by mice, there was a significant increase in the humoral immune response, as reflected by the number of PFC per spleen in response to sheep erythrocyte immunization and in the hemagglutination titers in response to immunization with either SRBC or tetanus toxoid. There was also significantly enhanced resistance to infectious challenge. When hens were fed a diet supplemented with vitamin E, chicks hatched from their eggs showed a significant enhancement of antibody production, as reflected by the direct PFC responsiveness to heterologous erythrocytes, as well as by hemagglutination inhibition testing (Tables IX, X) (Nockels, 1979). Vitamin E excess prior to immunization with *Brucella abortus* also increased the level of passive immunity.

Guinea pigs supplemented with vitamin E and then challenged with live attenuated Venezuelan equine encephalitis virus showed an increase in the immune response, as reflected by elevated antibody titers. It was found,

Table IX

Effect of Feeding Vitamin E to the Hen
on Passively
Acquired Immunity of the Chick[a,b]

Maternal vitamin E added (IU/kg)	2 days old		7 days old	
	Number of chicks	Agglutinin[c] titer $\log_2$	Number of chicks	Agglutinin titer $\log_2$
0	26	2.68A[d]	50	2.16A
90	31	2.94ABC	62	2.18A
150	22	3.18BC	38	2.65B
300	20	2.59A	40	2.12A
450	21	3.34C	40	2.62B
900	14	2.79A	31	2.19A

[a]Reproduced with permission from Nockels (1979).

[b]Hens were immunized intramuscularly with *Brucella abortus* 4 weeks prior to incubating the egg.

[c]All 2- and 7-day titers within a treatment were different ($p < .01$).

[d]Means followed by different capital letters differ significantly ($p < .01$).

Table X

Effect of Feeding Vitamin E to Nonimmunized Hens
on Primary Immune Response of Chicks[a,b]

Maternal vitamin E added (IU/kg)	21 days old[c]		28 days old	
	Number of chicks	Agglutinin titer $\log_2$	Number of chicks	Agglutinin titer $\log_2$
0	49	3.96A[d]	44	5.72a
90	33	4.47AB	31	5.44a
150	48	4.07A	47	5.61a
300	34	3.85A	36	5.94a
450	33	4.91B	31	6.37b
900	46	4.13A	41	5.90a

[a]Reproduced with permission from Nockels (1979).

[b]Chicks were immunized intramuscularly with *Brucella abortus* at 14 days of age.

[c]Chicks were 21 and 28 days old when blood taken for hemagglutination titer.

[d]Means followed by different capital letters differ significantly ($p < .01$) and by different small letters differ ($p < .05$).

however, that the chemical form of the vitamin E and the route of administration were critical in determining this enhancement. For example, the feeding of DL-α-tocopherol acetate to these guinea pigs did not enhance antibody production; this form of vitamin E did not appear to be absorbed effectively from the intestinal lumen. Although DL-α-tocopherol can be injected and does result in a significant elevation of antibody titers in response to Venezuelan equine encephalitis immunization, the injection results in a severe tissue reaction at the injection site.

Finally, to investigate the protective influence of vitamin E on resistance to infectious disease, chicks and turkeys were fed supplemental vitamin E and were subsequently infected with *E. coli* (a slow lactose-fermenting strain) (Heinzerling *et al.,* 1974). The authors observed a decreased rate of mortality and increased weight gain following infection in the chicks supplemented with vitamin E (Table XI). The enhanced resistance to *E. coli* infection was most likely due to an enhanced humoral immune response, as reflected by elevated hemagglutination and inhibition titers to *E. coli* (Heinzerling *et al.,* 1974). Similarly, sheep fed elevated levels of DL-α-tocopherol acetate and subsequently challenged with chlamydia experienced increased weight gain, with no chlamydia detected on examination in the supplemented animals. In contrast to these observations, no notable differences in resistance to infection with *L. monocytogenes* were found in mice fed a diet high in vitamin E (a 20-fold increase over normal levels) for 4 weeks.

Table XI

Effect of Vitamin E on Growth and Survival of *E. coli*–Infected and Noninfected Chicks[a,b]

Dietary vitamin E added (mg/kg)	*E. coli* infected	Trial 1				Trial 2			
		Number of chicks	Number of deaths	Mortality (%)	2–4 weeks average weight gain (g)	Number of chicks	Number of deaths	Mortality (%)	2–4 weeks average weight gain (g)
0	+	36	9	25.0 B	284 B ±21	42	13	31.0 B	395 A ±43
	−	36	0	0.0 A	348 A ±34	40	0	0.0 A	411 A ±33
150	+	34	3	9.3 A	313 A ±27	40	2	4.9 A	367 A ±51
	−	36	0	0.0 A	332 A ±28	40	0	0.0 A	396 A ±40
300	+	37	2	5.4 A	330 A ±39	40	0	0.0 A	387 A ±35
	−	36	0	0.0 A	340 A ±32	40	0	0.0 A	408 A ±32

[a]Reproduced with permission from Heinzerling *et al.* (1974).
[b]Weight gains represent the average gain of survivors. Means followed by different capital letter indicate significant differences ($p < .01$).

A number of studies have attempted to elucidate the site of action of vitamin E. Mice fed various levels of this vitamin (i.e., 0, 20, or 200 mg/kg food) were immunized 50 days after initiation of the diet with hamster red blood cells (HRBC) and secondarily immunized with an HRBC-trinitrophenol (TNP) conjugate. Vitamin E supplementation resulted in an increased hemagglutination inhibition titer to HRBC and TNP. In addition, when mice were primed with HRBC, there was a beneficial influence of vitamin E supplementation on hapten-specific responses. This indicates that vitamin E acted specifically at the level of the helper T cell. That the helper T cell was the locus of the vitamin E influence was further established by experiments indicating that it facilitated the shift of production of IgM-class antibodies to IgG-class antibodies.

Mice consuming a diet containing approximately 20 times the vitamin E found in control diets experienced a significant increase in antibody-dependent cellular cytotoxicity (ADCC) within 7 days of initiation of the diet. Mice that began to consume the high vitamin E diet at 3 weeks of age showed a much earlier attainment of adult levels of ADCC than did control counterparts, indicating an accelerated maturation of ADCC. However, when such high vitamin E diets were consumed for a prolonged period of time, an actual decrease in ADCC was noted in mice. There were no such changes observed in [^{3}H]thymidine incorporation by lymphocytes stimulated by PHA (Lim *et al.,* 1981). The mechanism of these changes in immune function may involve alterations in the level of corticosteroids, which were also noted to decrease in mice consuming high vitamin E diets.

Dietary supplementation of mice with 180 mg DL-α-tocopherol acetate resulted in a fourfold increase in the phagocytosis of *Streptococcus pneumoniae* type I (Heinzerling *et al.,* 1974). Administration of vitamin E to humans for 2–3 weeks resulted in an increase in PMN leukocyte function.

Because earlier studies have shown that vitamin E was capable of stimulating Con A and PHA responses when adherent cell populations had been removed, Corwin and coworkers investigated the possibility that Ia$^+$ cells are required as direct targets for vitamin E (Corwin and Schloss, 1980; Corwin and Gordon, 1982). It was found that even in the presence of anti-Ia^k serum, vitamin E stimulated responsiveness to low levels of Con A by threefold. Removal of Ia$^+$-adherent cells did not alter the ability of vitamin E to enhance the responsiveness to the remaining Ia-nonadherent cell populations. Through experiments that required washing of the spleen cells, it was found that a splenic suppressor factor that must undergo oxidation to an active form inhibited the responsiveness of spleen cells, and this influence was reversible with the addition of vitamin E. The washing of spleen cell populations results in an increase in their mitogenic responsiveness to a degree that cannot be further enhanced by the addition of vitamin E. Thus, the stimulation of mitogen responsiveness by vitamin E was found to be dependent on the very presence of such splenic inhibitory factors. The tocopherols were also shown to enhance markedly the mixed lymphocyte reaction (MLR), which depends on the response of Ia⁻ cells to Ia⁺ stimulator cells (Corwin and Gordon, 1982). Nonetheless, it must be emphasized that the significance of these observations remains to be established.

The effect of vitamin E on mitogenesis by polyclonal activators was studied, and the vitamin was found to be stimulatory but selective in its action. Vitamin E itself is a mitogen for murine spleen cells. At suboptimal concentrations, it was capable of stimulating the response to low levels of the thymus-dependent lymphocyte (T-cell) mitogen, Con A, but not when Con A was itself at optimal levels. When vitamin E was added to the diet at normal levels, it was not as effective in stimulating mitogenesis as it was at much higher levels. The effect of the vitamin on T-cell mitogenesis could be modified by the degree of unsaturation of the dietary fat; it was more effective when dietary polyunsaturated fatty acids were low. Under several conditions, it was shown that vitamin E can increase the PHA/Con A response ratio, which may suggest an effect of the vitamin on the maturation of T cells. In normal mice, vitamin E also stimulated the response to LPS, a "bursa-equivalent" lymphocyte (B-cell) mitogen, but it was unable to do so when spleen cells from athymic, nude mice were used. This suggests a requirement for thymic factors in order for vitamin E to stimulate the mitogenesis of B cells (Corwin and Schloss, 1980).

B COMPLEX VITAMINS

Some of the greatest advances in clinical medicine resulted from observations that animals with deficiencies of water-soluble vitamins were particularly susceptible to bacterial infection. Although the mechanism was unclear, it was known that multiple vitamins were involved. This led to the elucidation of specific relationships between the lack of water-soluble vitamins and the total number of peripheral blood leukocytes. Such observations were critical in further understanding diseases such as pernicious anemia and folic acid deficiency. Specific sequential changes in the metabolism of water-soluble vitamins occur early in the course of chronic diseases. Thus, it was appreciated that while the body has significant stores of fat-soluble vitamins, it is considerably easier to produce deficiencies of non-stored, water-soluble vitamins.

Some of the earliest studies of water-soluble vitamins in relation to immune function were performed in pyridoxine-deficient animals. Pyridoxine (vitamin B_6) deficiency significantly reduces the immune response. This has been shown in a variety of animals, including mice, hamsters, and guinea pigs. The immunosuppression seen with vitamin B_6 deficiency can also be induced by administration of isoniazid (INH) in patients with tuberculosis; therefore, pyridoxine is given during INH treatment. Animal studies showed specific suppression of antibody responses to bacteria including *Salmonella.* These observations, while first noted with vitamin B_6, were also seen with pantothenic acid and riboflavin. The effects on immune function could be seen as early as 2 weeks following discontinuation of these B vitamins. Moreover, they were all reversible following repletion of the vitamins.

Similar studies have been carried out on the effects of B complex water-soluble vitamins on delayed hypersensitivity. For example, vitamin B_6–deficient guinea pigs have depressed reactions to skin sensitization with BCG. Moreover, such animals also have a reduced lymphocyte blastogenesis response to PHA and Con A. Similarly, vitamin B_6 deficiency reduces the ability of T cells to reject allografts. These effects do not appear to be selective to T-cell subpopulations, but seem to reduce all aspects of cell-mediated responses.

The mechanism by which vitamin B_6 deficiency affects immune function is related to its influence on cell transformation and multiplication. Vitamin B_6 deficiency reduces nucleic acid and protein biosynthesis (Felice and Kirksey, 1981). Similar effects are seen in riboflavin- and panthothenic acid-deficient animals, but not to the same extent with respect to reduction of the immune response. This is probably due to the relatively easy depletion of vitamin B_6 and its greater effects on both nucleic acid and protein biosynthesis (Fig. 6).

Thoracic duct lymphocytes TDL from vitamin B_6–deficient rats were found to have a reduced capacity to respond to foreign lymphoid cells in the MLR, to produce normal lymphocyte transfer reactions, and to incorporate [^{3}H]uridine *in vitro*. These findings indicate that specific nutritional deficiencies may impair cellular immunity and that this impairment can be monitored by the MLR. It is suggested that the reduction in MLR activity and in uridine uptake by TDL cells reflects either a shift in the proportions of T and B cells in the TDL and/or an impairment in the capacity of such cells to function in the MLR and in the *in vitro* test for [^{3}H]uridine incorporation (Robson and Schwarz, 1975).

The influence of dietary pyridoxine on passive antibody transfer from dams to pups and on active humoral antibody formation by the pups was studied. Rats were fed diets containing 20.0, 0.6, 0.45, or 0.3 mg pyridoxine·HCl/kg during gestation and 20.0, 0.4, 0.3, or 0.2 mg/kg during lactation (diets A, B, C, and D). Diets B, C, and D contained 100, 75, and 50% of the requirement for pyridoxine during gestation and lactation. After pups in groups B, C, and D developed signs of pyridoxine deficiency, all dams were fed diet A on days 9–21 of lactation. On day 9, vitamin B_6 levels were lower

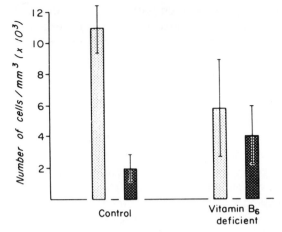

Fig. 6. Concentrations of lymphocytes and neutrophils in the peripheral blood of adult rats fed either a control diet or a 2-week vitamin B_6–deficient diet. Narrow bars represent the range. ▢, lymphocytes; ▓, neutrophils. (Reproduced with permission from Robson and Schwarz, 1975.)

in pup spleens and thymuses and in the milk of groups B, C, and D than in the others. However, IgG in the sera of dams and pups, and in milk, indicated that passive antibody transfer was similar for all groups. After weaning, pups in groups A, B, C, and D were fed diets containing 20.0, 0.4, 0.2, and 0 mg vitamin B_6/kg, respectively. On day 35, vitamin B_6 levels were lower in spleens and thymuses of pups fed inadequate amounts of pyridoxine (groups B, C, and D). These pups had fewer spleen cells and splenic antibody-forming cells (AFC) and lower levels of humoral antibody than pups of dams fed adequate amounts of vitamin B_6. The reduction in spleen cells and splenic AFC resulted in part from lower food intake but was intensified by pyridoxine deprivation (Debes and Kirksey, 1979; Groziak *et al.,* 1984).

FOLATE AND VITAMIN B_{12}

Folic acid and vitamin B_{12} deficiency have been extensively studied both in clinical conditions and in experimental manipulation of humans. Both substances are essential for protein and nucleic acid biosynthesis. Thus, deficiencies of either of these water-soluble vitamins produces a depression in immune competence. This can be shown in both humans and mice in cell-mediated immunity and humoral immunity. Moreover, the changes tend to parallel changes seen in the bone marrow with respect to hematopoiesis.

Table XII

Mortality Following Oral Challenge with 10^9 *Shigella flexneri* 2a[a]

Time of death following challenge	Diet		
	Folic acid-deficient (18)[b]	Folic acid-supplemented (18)	Optimal (16)
< 24 hr	9	0	0
24–48 hr	3	1	0
48–72 hr	2	0	0
16–31 days	2	2	0
Deaths not associated with *Shigella* infection	0	3	0

[a]Reproduced with permission from Haltalin *et al.* (1970).
[b]Numbers in parentheses are the numbers of animals in each group.

Ninety-five guinea pigs, aged 2–4 days, were fed three different diets: (1) a folic acid–deficient diet, (2) a folic acid–deficient diet supplemented with folic acid, and (3) an optimal diet. Animals were sham-infected or challenged with 10^9 *Shigella flexneri* 2a administered intragastrically 2 weeks later. Eighty-nine percent of the animals fed the deficient diet died following challenge with *Shigella;* 50% succumbed within the first 24 hr. Seventeen percent of the animals given the deficient diet supplemented with folic acid died because of *Shigella* infection, but none did so within the first 24 hr (Table XII). None of the animals fed the optimal diet showed adverse effects consequent to challenge with *Shigella.* The presence of bacteremia correlated strongly with a fatal outcome. Effects of challenge with *Shigella* were also evaluated with respect to physical growth (Fig. 7), hematologic changes, patterns of excretion of *Shigella,* recovery of organisms at postmortem, and serial hemagglutinin responses. The data indicate that folate acid deficiency was one factor responsible for inducing susceptibility to fatal *Shigella* infection. The folate-deficient state was confirmed by low levels of serum folate and megaloblastic changes in the bone marrow (Haltalin *et al.,* 1970). However, the difference between the folic acid supplemented diet and the "optimal" diet was not explained.

Wistar-Lewis rats were fed either a control (folate-supplemented) or a folate-free diet from weaning. After 4 weeks of the respective diets, they were sensitized with skin grafts from Brown Norway (BN) rats. Following initial sensitization, all animals received weekly ip injections of 3×10^7 BN thymocytes. When compared with controls at age 3 months, the folate-

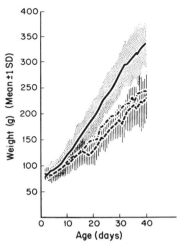

Fig. 7. Comparison of growth curves observed in sham-infected animals on the 3 different diets. ▬▬, optimal diet ($n = 14$); - - - -, folic acid–deficient diet ($n = 15$); ——·——·——, folic acid–supplemented diet ($n=14$). (Reproduced with permission from Haltalin *et al.,* 1970.)

deficient rats had mild megaloblastic changes in the bone marrow and small intestine, a mild decrease in cellularity in both the thymus and the thymic-independent areas of the spleen, decreased folate serum levels, and decreased overall body weight. Hematocrit levels and weights of the spleen and thymus did not differ significantly from those of controls. However, the cytotoxic activity of splenic lymphocytes of folate-deficient animals exposed to BN thymocytes *in vitro* decreased significantly, as did the sensitivity to stimulation by the T-cell mitogen phytohemagglutinin (Table XIII). The number of T cells in the spleen and peripheral blood of folate-deficient rats was significantly lower than in controls; the number of T cells in the thymus of deficient rats was also lower than in the control group, but not significantly so (Williams *et al.,* 1975).

Lymphocyte transformation responses to the mitogen phytohemagglutinin were measured in 20 patients with proven pernicious anemia (PA) and 20 matched controls using [³H]thymidine label. The patients with PA showed significant depression of lymphocyte transformation to the three doses of PHA employed, as judged by β counting (Figure 8); however, radioautographic examination of PHA-stimulated cells indicated that the results were due to a failure of intranuclear incorporation of [³H]thymidine by PA lymphocytes, rather than a failure of PHA to induce blastogenesis. The percentages and numbers of T and B lymphocytes in peripheral blood were measured in 30 patients and controls by rosette and immunofluorescence techniques, respectively. There was no significant difference in the B-cell

Table XIII

[^{3}-H]Thymidine Uptake by PHA-Stimulated Spleen Cells[a]

	Control (cpm)	Folate-deficient (cpm)	Significance
PHA stimulation			
No PHA	1315 ± 312	1405 ± 102	
	(877–1701)	(910–1966)	
+PHA	19,398 ± 1014	4263 ± 579	
	(14,501–23,412)	(1789–8248)	
Stimulation			
Index	14.8	3.0	$p < .005$
	$n = 8$	$n = 10$	

[a]Reproduced with permission from Williams *et al.* (1975).

subpopulations between patients and controls; the T-cell subpopulation was slightly lower in the PA patients (mean, 62.4%) than in the controls (mean, 65.5%), but the difference was not statistically significant. The depressed uptake of [^{3}H]thymidine by stimulated lymphocytes in PA would seem to reflect a chemical defect rather than an inherent immunologic abnormality (MacCuish *et al.,* 1974).

Morphological and quantitative neutrophil abnormalities are common in

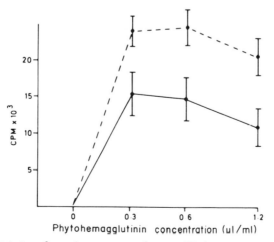

Fig. 8. Lymphocyte transformation responses (mean ±SEM) in 20 patients with PA (●——●) and 20 matched controls (●- - -●), at three concentrations of PHA. The mean response in the patients is significantly lower ($p < .01$) than in the controls at all concentrations. (Reproduced with permission from MacCuish *et al.,* 1974.)

the megaloblastic anemias of vitamin B_{12} and folic acid deficiency. Little is known, however, about the role of these vitamins in normal leukocyte function. Seven patients with megaloblastic bone marrow, four with vitamin B_{12} deficiency, and three with folic acid deficiency were studied to determine the effect, if any, of these deficiencies on leukocyte function. Phagocytosis of staphylococci, hexose monophosphate shunt activation with phagocytosis, and microbicidal capacity against *Staphylococcus aureus* were determined prior to the institution of therapy. In two instances, these studies were repeated following treatment. There was no impairment of phagocytosis per se, and the resting metabolism was not significantly decreased. With phagocytosis, however, metabolic activation was decreased to 35–36% of control values in the leukocytes of patients with vitamin B_{12} deficiency, but not in those of patients with folic acid deficiency. Bacterial killing was slightly decreased in vitamin B_{12} but not in folic acid deficiency. These abnormalities of function were reversed after therapy. These findings suggested a role for vitamin B_{12} in the production of intermediates necessary for normal cell function (Kaplan and Basford, 1976).

VITAMIN C

Somewhat more controversial than the effects of the vitamin B complex is the effect of vitamin C on the immune response. Much of the interest in vitamin C and immunity has been derived from the controversial book *Vitamin C and the Common Cold* by Linus Pauling. Although many clinical anecdotes have been published, there are no convincing data that an excess of vitamin C improves the immune response. The validity of the thesis that high levels of vitamin C augment the immune response and prevent colds has not been proven, and carefully controlled double-blind studies have not provided evidence in favor of this hypothesis. Indeed, it appears that large doses of vitamin C are rapidly excreted and do not change either the immune response or the course of infectious illnesses. Nonetheless, it is certain that a *deficiency* of ascorbic acid is significantly immunosuppressive. For example, ascorbic acid is required for both neutrophils and monocyte chemotaxis. Vitamin C also increases the immune response *in vitro* to Con A and PHA-P. Thus, animals or humans fed ascorbic acid–deficient diets are more susceptible to infectious diseases than controls fed adequate vitamin C, and have reduced levels of both humoral and cell-mediated responses. This has been shown in mice and guinea pigs and in clinical observations of humans. For example, in one study, guinea pigs were divided into three dietary groups, including ascorbic acid–deficient, pair-fed, and *ad libitum*-fed groups. In vitamin C deficiency, the antibody responses were reduced, as were the responses to Con A and PHA-P. Similarly, ascorbic acid–deficient guinea pigs had reduced macrophage phagocytosis.

Because ascorbate potentiates the chemotactic activity of normal leukocytes, the effect of vitamin C on PMN leukocytes from normal patients and from a patient with the Chediak-Higashi syndrome have been studied. The exposure of human granulocytes to ascorbic acid *in vitro* results in stimulation of the hexose monophosphate shunt, augmentation of random migration and chemotaxis, and inhibition of aldehyde formation and iodination of protein; however, neither the bactericidal nor the phagocytic capacity of these cells is altered. Pauling has suggested that the prophylactic ingestion of massive doses of L-ascorbic acid may prevent viral infections in humans. The possible consequences of such doses on granulocyte function are of considerable interest. Accordingly, Smith studied these potential effects by measuring the influence of varying concentrations of L-ascorbic acid on neutrophil function (Table XIV, Fig. 9) (Smith *et al.*, 1975).

Scorbutic guinea pig neutrophils (PMN), as well as control PMN, produce H_2O_2 and kill *Staph. aureus*, suggesting that scorbate does not contribute significantly to phagocyte H_2O_2 production or bacterial killing. Total and

Table XIV

Stimulation of the Hexose Monophosphate
Shunt in Human Granulocytes[a]

	Increase in ^{34}C-1-glucose oxidation (%)
10 mM LAA (9)[b,c]	64.4
20 mM LAA (10)	232.3
50 mM LAA (10)	296.7
100 mM LAA (6)	453.0
200 mM LAA (6)	305.6
Polystyrene beads (7)	599.6
Bread yeast (9)	974.3
S. aureus (11)	1276.2

[a]Reproduced with permission from Smith *et al.* (1975).

[b]The figures in parentheses indicate the number of experiments. The ratio of phagocytic particles to white blood cells was 400:1 for polystyrene beads, 1:1 for bread yeast, and 100:1 for *Staphylococcus aureus*. L-Ascorbic acid was not added to flasks stimulated with phagocytic particles.

[c]L-ascorbic acid (LAA).

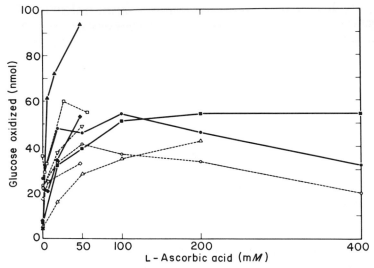

Fig. 9. Effect of L-ascorbic acid on the hexose monophosphate shunt in resting human granulocytes. Leukocytes (5×10^6) were incubated at $37°C$ in 10% AB serum-HBSS with $1[^{14}C]$glucose (7.6 nmol and 0.5 µCi glucose) and L-ascorbic acid. After 1 hr, the quantity of $^{14}CO_2$ generated was determined. The open and closed geometric figures represent individual experiments. The results are expressed as nanomoles of glucose oxidized/hr/5×10^6 granulocytes. (Reproduced with permission from Smith *et al.,* 1975.)

reduced ascorbate contents of human PMN were observed to fall on phagocytosis, whereas dehydroascorbate increased to a lesser extent. These observations are consistent with the view that ascorbate constitutes a functional part of the PMN's redox-active components, and may thus function to protect cell constituents from denaturation by the oxidants produced during phagocytosis (Stankova *et al.,* 1975).

It is well known that glycolytic and hexose monophosphate shunt activities of leukocytes increase during phagocytosis. The relevance of these metabolic changes to particle uptake and destruction is also well established. In one study, the metabolic activities were studied to assess the phagocytic function of leukocytes isolated from ascorbic acid–deficient guinea pigs. Glycolytic activity, which provides the necessary energy for particle uptake, was found to be decreased in both resting and phagocytizing leukocytes of ascorbic acid–deficient guinea pigs. The direct oxidation of glucose through the hexose monophosphate shunt was stimulated to a significantly lesser extent during phagocytosis in ascorbic acid–deficient leukocytes. There was a progressive decline in phagocytosis-induced shunt activity of leukocytes as the deficiency of ascorbic acid progressed. These findings show that particle uptake (as indicated by glycolytic activity), as well as particle destruction (as indicated by hexose monophosphate shunt activity) by leukocytes, is impaired in ascorbic acid deficiency. The bactericidal capacity of leukocytes against *E. coli* was also found to be low in ascorbic acid–deficient guinea pigs compared to those of the pair-fed control group (Shilotri, 1977).

PANTOTHENIC ACID

Six volunteer subjects (three pairs of men) were studied to determine whether the immunologic responses of men deficient in pantothenic acid were different from those of men given adequate diets. Two men received a balanced formula, two were given a formula deficient in pantothenic acid, and the other two were fed the deficient formula containing an antagonist of the vitamin omega methyl pantothenic acid.

Antibody responses to typhoid, Asian influenza, and tetanus vaccines were identical for typhoid and indeterminate for Asian influenza. However, volunteers who were deficient in pantothenic acid had fewer antibodies to tetanus. Similarly, heterologous skin grafts were accepted poorly by deficient subjects and were rejected at least as rapidly as they were in the control subjects. The rejection may have been hastened by secondary infections in these four subjects. The length of time required for healing was the same in all groups. These data are very limited but more recent studies likewise suggest the need for more definitive studies using pantothenic acid (Bendich *et al.,* 1983).

Similar observations have been made in animals. Rats fed a diet deficient in pantothenic acid failed to develop primary serum hemolytic titers following SRBC immunoglobulin comparable to those of control rats. In order to determine a possible basis for this defect, the localized hemolysis in gel assay was utilized to assess AFC production. The AFC response at varying times after intravenous injection of sheep erythrocytes was decreased in spleens of pantothenic acid–deficient rats. The defect was alleviated by administration of pantothenic acid 9 days prior to injection of antigen. Injection of large doses of sheep erythrocytes did not improve the response of deficient rats. Catabolism and phagocytosis of labeled sheep erythrocytes by the reticuloendothelial system were not critically affected by pantothenic acid deficiency (Lederer *et al.,* 1975).

BIOTIN

Three siblings presented in early childhood with central nervous system dysfunction, *Candida* dermatitis, keratoconjunctivitis, and alopecia. Two were studied immunologically and had absent delayed hypersensitivity skin test responses and absent *in vitro* lymphocyte responses to *Candida* antigen. One of them had selective IgA deficiency and no antibody response to pneumococcal polysaccharide immunization, and the other had a subnormal percentage of T lymphocytes in peripheral blood. The first two siblings died with progressive central nervous system deterioration and overwhelming infection. The third child, who presented with a perioral *Candida* dermatitis, alopecia, keratoconjunctivitis, and intermittent ataxia at 18 months of age, had intermittent lactic acidosis and elevated excretion of α-hydroxypropionate, methylcitrate, α-methylcrotonylglycine, and α-hydroxyisovalerate in urine. After 4 days of oral biotin, 10 mg/day, the metabolites in her urine were significantly reduced, suggesting a biotin-responsive multiple carboxylase deficiency. These findings, together with previous reports of immune defects in patients with disorders of branched chain amino acid catabolism, suggest a new biochemical basis for primary immunodeficiency disease.

10

Lipids

INTRODUCTION

The relationship of lipids to the immune response is multifactorial, and its study involves several disciplines (Gurr, 1983). For example, in addition to the interaction of lipids and immune function at the nutritional level, one must consider biochemical initiations at the cellular level, since lymphocytes contain a large number of essential and nonessential fatty acids. In addition, many of the events involved in lymphocyte activation and function are related to arachidonic acid metabolism. Unfortunately, lipids as components of lymphocyte membranes have often been neglected by immunologists in favor of the protein components. The reasons for this have been discussed by Meade *et al.* (1978) and include the difficulty of preparing antisera against lipids. Moreover, few immunologists are expert in lipid biochemistry.

Dietary manipulation of fatty acids has been used with several animal species, including mice, rats, and guinea pigs, to study both excess and deficiency of fatty acids and the degree of lipid saturation. Further, subcutaneous injection of lipids has been used to alter the levels of specific lipids within lymphoid tissue. The dietary levels and the relative balance of different lipids are particularly important to the tissue concentrations of polyunsaturated fats. Polyunsaturated fats, including linoleic acid, cannot be synthesized in the body. Recent recommendations to reduce the level of saturated fats and increase the level of unsaturated fats in the diet may produce effects on the immune system. Indeed, alterations of dietary lipids have been shown to influence a variety of diseases in animal models, including carcinogen-induced tumors, experimental allergic encephalomyelitis, and the immune response to both thymic-dependent and thymic-independent antigens (Meade and Mertin, 1978).

In general, animals fed higher levels of polyunsaturated fatty acids have reduced immune competence. This is manifested in several ways and will be discussed in depth in the balance of this chapter. First, in studies of mice and guinea pigs, there was a decrease in the total number of B cells as well as a reduction in serum immunoglobulins. Second, the immune response to thymic-dependent antigens was reduced. The effect of polyunsaturated fatty acids increases with the number of double bonds in the chain. Thus, polyunsaturated fatty acids with a higher number of double bonds have a more suppressive effect. Deficiencies of polyunsaturated fatty acids also reduce B-cell function and depress responses to thymic-independent antigens. However, a reduction in polyunsaturated fatty acids appears to improve cell-mediated immunity. This results, for example, in enhanced lymphocyte blastogenesis to concanavalin A and phytohemagglutinin. In addition, mice have an increased ability to reject skin allografts when levels of polyunsaturated fats are reduced (Meade and Mertin, 1978).

Many experiments have investigated the influence of a deficiency of essential fatty acids. Generally, the results, at least in mice, suggest that diets deficient in essential fatty acids produce a significant reduction in humoral responses. Such reductions were seen within a few weeks of initiation of the diet and appeared much earlier than the effects of fatty acid deficiencies on other aspects of animal health, including growth and general appearance. The deficient antibody responses occurred with both thymic-independent and thymic-dependent antigens and were shown to affect both IgM and IgG responses. All of these effects were reversible; that is, when diets deficient in essential fatty acids were changed to normal diets, the immune response recovered.

The effects of diets containing polyunsaturated fat depend a great deal on the fat levels chosen. It is clear that feeding both mice and rats diets containing high levels of polyunsaturated fats inhibits conconavalin A–induced blastogenesis of splenic lymphocytes. Moreover, the sera of mice and rats fed high levels of polyunsaturated fats are capable, via transfer, of suppressing the lymphocyte response of normal rats. The inhibition factor in the serum includes at least one lipoprotein, and probably other serum factors as well (Curtiss et al., 1980).

DIET AND CELL MEMBRANES

We will not discuss the lipid components of cell membranes in depth, since this subject is far beyond the scope of this volume. Nonetheless, one should note that the cell membranes surrounding mononuclear cells are similar to those of other cells and are composed of phospholipids and proteins. The distribution of proteins within the cell membrane is relatively random, and the interactions that occur at the cell membrane level depend a great deal on the communication and cooperation between antigens and membrane receptors (Resch and Ferber, 1974; Ferber and Resch, 1976) (Tables I, II). These involve both protein and lipid components. Some critical changes occur in membrane phospholipids during lymphocyte blastogenesis. These changes can be induced by the reaction of lymphoid cells with either allogeneic cells or plant lectins. The most dramatic changes are reflected by increases in arachidonic acid levels and increases in fatty acid turnover. Stimulation of lymphoid cells with concanavalin A and analysis of phospholipid fatty acids in cell membranes leads to some characteristic changes. Compared with liver cells, phosphatidylcholine of unstimulated lymphocytes contains relatively high amounts of palmitic acid in position 2 and oleic acid in position 1. After stimulation, the content of polyunsaturated fatty acids (linoleic and arachidonic acids) increases and the ratio of polyenoic acids ($18 : 2 + 20 : 4$) to saturated fatty acids doubles when compared to control cells. Similar results can be obtained after *in vivo* stimulation with *Bacille Calmette Guerin* (BCG) (Ferber *et al.,* 1974) (Table II).

These changes appear to be important for lymphocyte activation; alterations in membrane phospholipids are important for triggering lymphocytes. Lymphoid and other cells methylate phospholipids using membrane-associated methyltransferase enzymes. With successive methylation of phospholipids, the active sites are translocated from the inside to the outside of the membrane. When lectins, immunoglobulins, or chemotactic peptides bind to the cell surface, they stimulate the methyltransferase enzymes and reduce membrane viscosity. This methylation of phospholipids releases arachidonic acid, lysophosphatidylcholine, and prostaglandins. This facili-

Table I

Alterations in Fatty Acid Content of Phosphatidyl Choline from Rabbit Thymus Cells Following Stimulation by Con A[a,b]

	Moles (%)						Polyunsaturated/ saturated fatty acids
	16:0	18:0	18:1	18:2	20:4	22:6	
Position 1							
Control	50.6	17.9	22.5	4.9	—	—	0.072
Con A	58.1	16.0	20.7	5.2	—	—	0.070
Position 2							
Control	47.4	3.2	20.0	19.4	7.8	—	0.538
Con A	39.0	1.6	21.7	20.3	17.2	—	0.924

[a]Reproduced with permission from Ferber and Resch (1976).
[b]The cells were cultured for 4 hr in Eagle's medium with 5 μg concanavalin A/ml.

Table II
Fatty Acid Composition of Phosphatidylcholine and Phosphatidylethanolamine
from Rat Liver and from Lymphocytes of Different Species[a–c]

	16:0	16:1	18:0	18:1	18:2	20:4	22:6
Phosphatidylcholine							
Rat liver	28.5	2.3	25.4	9.7	11.7	18.9	1.9
Pig lymphocytes	38.6	3.7	16.6	19.3	9.2	12.4	—
Rabbit lymphocytes	42.4	1.9	9.6	17.9	18.1	8.0	—
Rabbit thymus	47.9	5.8	6.9	17.2	14.4	5.1	—
Calf thymus	34.6	3.2	8.0	29.4	20.2	2.3	—
Phosphatidylethanolamine							
Rat liver	27.8	2.5	25.0	5.6	4.1	21.4	12.0
Pig lymphocytes	18.7	2.5	28.1	14.4	4.8	31.3	—
Rabbit lymphocytes	12.9	2.4	27.0	14.6	9.9	27.9	0.4
Rabbit thymus	16.8	3.4	24.8	14.2	9.5	26.1	—
Calf thymus	16.1	0.5	25.1	25.4	12.8	19.3	—

[a]Reproduced with permission from Ferber *et al.* (1974).
[b]Phosphatidylethanolamine: including alk-1-enylacyl ethers from plasmalogen.
[c]The results are expressed as mol %.

tates transmission of signals through membranes. It can result in the generation of adenosine 3′,5′-monophosphate in virtually all immune cells, including release of histamine in mast cells and basophils, mitogenesis in lymphocytes, and chemotaxis in neutrophils (Table III) (Hirata and Axelrod, 1980).

The increased turnover of cell membrane phospholipids that occurs during blastogenesis involves the increased synthesis of phospholipids as well as the transfer and incorporation of new fatty acids. Lymphocytes are ideal cells for studying such interactions because they are relatively rich in the enzymes required for changes in phospholipid activity during blastogenesis. These changes have been studied both *in vitro* and *in vivo* and appear to be consistent, whether peripheral lymphocytes, lymph node, or spleen are studied. Moreover, the alterations in phospholipids that occur on stimulation have been shown in a variety of animals.

It has also been hypothesized that the formation of free fatty acids during lymphocyte stimulation may be important to the cytotoxic action of lymphocyte subpopulations (Pelus and Strausser, 1977). Dietary levels of fatty acids and changes in fatty acid saturation can alter cell membrane biochemical profiles. For example, SJL/J mice were fed two nutritionally adequate, purified diets that differed only in polyunsaturated versus saturated fatty acid content. The fatty acid composition of membranes from spleen and thymus cells was determined after the diet was initiated. Dietary fat significantly altered the fatty acid composition of lymphocyte membrane

Table III

Phospholipid Methylation, Arachidonic Acid Release, and Signal Transduction
in a Variety of Cell Types[a]

Cell type	Stimulus	Phospholipid methylation	Arachidonic acid release	Biological effect
Rat reticulocyte	β-Adrenergic agonists	+	?	Cyclic AMP
C$_6$ glioma astrocytoma	β-Adrenergic agonists	+	+[b]	Cyclic AMP
	Benzodiazepine agonists	+	?	?
HeLa cells	β-Adrenergic agonists	+	+[b]	Cyclic AMP
Mast cells	Con A IgE receptor	+	+	CA^{2+} influx, histamine release
Leukemic basophils	IgE specific antigens	+	+	Histamine release
Lymphocytes	Con A	+	+	Ca^{2+} influx, mitogenesis
Neutrophils	Chemotactic peptides	−	+	Chemotaxis
Fibroblasts	Bradykinin	+	+	Cyclic AMP
Platelets	Thrombin, epinephrine	No effect	No effect	Aggregation

[a]Reproduced with permission from Hirata and Axelrod (1980).
[b]After long-term stimulation.

phosphatidylcholine and phosphatidylethanolamine (Cinader *et al.,* 1983).

The role of arachidonic acid and its metabolites has been a particularly fertile area for research because of evidence that prostaglandin derivatives may be important as immunoregulatory substances. These agents interact with a variety of receptors, including hormone receptors. In addition, it appears that one mechanism of action of corticosteroids is mediated by a direct interaction with the release of phospholipids, the metabolite of arachidonic acid, and the production of free fatty acids within cells. Although the majority of these observations involve lymphocytes, similar data are also available for macrophages and PMN leukocytes.

The metabolites of arachidonic acid, namely, the mediators produced either through the cyclooxygenase or the lipoxygenase system, have profound effects on the immune system. These effects can be shown primarily *in vitro* but have been also shown *in vivo.* For example, prostaglandins of the E series reduce the ability of PHA-P and Con A to stimulate T lymphocytes. The effects of prostaglandins on T lymphocytes appear to be highly dose dependent and to have different actions depending on the species. Generally, PGE reduce the ability of PHA-P and Con A to stimulate T lymphocytes. Because PGE are readily produced during the activation of lymphocytes, it is postulated that they are important in both feedback stimulation and inhibition of the immune system (Kelly and Parker, 1979).

It is not surprising, therefore, that a great deal of attention has been paid to the role of dietary fats in the modulation of immune responsiveness.

Although there are several human lipid disorders, generally characterized by excesses of one or more lipid components, most attention has been directed to animal systems in which either specific lipid deficiencies or excessive polyunsaturated/saturated fatty acids have been fed. Therefore, in this chapter, we deal with the influence of both arachidonic acid and its metabolites and specific lipid disorders and their relationship to dietary manipulation.

IN VITRO STUDIES

Fatty acids are essential components of cell membranes. A variety of experiments have been used to investigate the role of dietary fat in the modulation of the immune function. This has been reviewed by Meade and Mertin (1978). Nonetheless, the results of many experiments are difficult to interpret because they failed to include pair-fed control groups. In addition, some laboratories have simply altered the percentage of fat in the diet, whereas others have varied both the percentage and the type of fat. There are major differences between the effects of dietary polyunsaturated and saturated fats. Finally, we should note that fatty acids and their esters are water insoluble. Therefore, all experiments, whether *in vitro* or *in vivo*, must take into account the way in which the fatty acid is presented to the cell or to the gastrointestinal system for digestion. This problem has led to many artifactual complications, including the influence(s) of the vehicle, in some cases alcohol, in which the fatty acids have been dissolved. Fatty acids have also been studied as dissolved salts, often with vehicles, or bound to albumin (Mertin and Hughes, 1975; Weyman *et al.,* 1977). Obviously, the latter can be a problem because of the chemical relationship with and association between fatty acids and albumin (Tonkin and Brostoff, 1978).

More effort has been directed to the role of fatty acids in *in vitro* than *in vivo* function, including observations of human, mice, rat, and guinea pig cells. Linoleic acid as well as arachidonic acid, when added *in vitro,* suppresses both PHA-P and Con A induced lymphocyte transformation. These results have been reported by numerous groups (Mertin *et al.,* 1974; Mertin and Hughes, 1975) and are often quite impressive. In contrast, other fatty acids, particularly stearic and oleic acids, do not appear to have such activity. This suggests that the degree of polyunsaturation is important in determining which fatty acids are involved, since oleic and arachidonic acids are polyunsaturated, while stearic and oleic acids are saturated. Therefore, experiments to investigate the role of polyunsaturated versus saturated fatty acids *in vitro,* as well as to determine the mechanism of action of arachidonic acid, have been performed by many groups. The results have shown that the activity of arachidonic acid is highly dose dependent; it can either stimulate or suppress blastogenesis. Second, it is clear that the suppressor role of arachidonic acid is not due to cell death (Mihas *et al.,* 1975; Offner and Clausen, 1974) (Fig. 1). However, studies by other laboratories suggest that the degree of polyunsaturated versus saturated acids is not the sole factor in suppression of T-cell mitogenesis. In particular, Weyman *et al.* (1977) found that the saturated fatty acids, stearic acid and heptadecanoic acid, as well as the model unsaturated acid, oleic acid, were also suppressive. Considerable attention is still being directed to these observations, particularly to the mechanism by which saturated fatty acids inhibit the interaction of lymphocytes and plant lectins. As reported by Robak *et al.* (1975), certain saturated fatty acids can inhibit the conversion of arachidonic acid to PGE_2. These observations are important because PGE_2 can be shown to inhibit directly the incorporation of [^{3}H]thymidine and the lym-

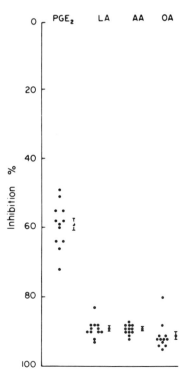

Fig. 1. Inhibitory effect of 16, (16) prostaglandin E_2 (PGE_2), linoleic acid (LA), arachidonic acid (AA), and oleic acid (OA) on PHA-induced lymphocyte transformation from 12 normal subjects. (Reproduced with permission from Mihas *et al.,* 1975.)

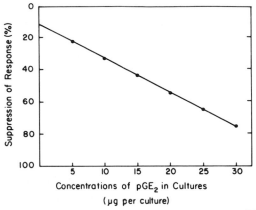

Fig. 2. Relation of PGE$_2$ concentration to its suppressive activity on PHA-induced lymphocyte transformation. (Reproduced with permission from Mihas *et al.*, 1975.)

phocyte transformation reaction in response to phytohemagglutinin (Figs. 1, 2) (Mihas *et al.*, 1975).

The work cited above concerning the role of fatty acids in immune function has been criticized because many of the studies, including that of Mertin and Hughes (1975), added fatty acids to the cultures in a solution of ethyl alcohol. Free fatty acids are bound to serum albumin *in vivo* (Tonkin and Brostoff, 1978; Spector, 1968). Thus, the addition of fatty acids in alcohol is inappropriate and unphysiological. Furthermore, the results appear to differ depending on the source of sera for the lymphocyte transformation test. Accordingly, Tonkin and Brostoff (1978) added free fatty acids bound to bovine serum albumin in their lymphocyte transformation assays. They found much less suppression of PHA transformation than did Mertin and Hughes. Nonetheless, when lymphocytes were cultured in human AB serum instead of fetal calf serum, an entirely different result was obtained. In that case, neither inhibition nor stimulation was seen. The authors argue that since human AB serum is more physiological, the results of others using *in vitro* cultures are likely to be artifacts since they would be unlikely to occur *in vivo*.

More recent studies have also been concerned with the effect of fatty acids on the mitogen response of peripheral blood lymphocytes. These studies have added an additional dimension to the observations: When a sufficient range of concentration is used, linoleic acid, as well as oleate, or phosphatidyl inositol, can either stimulate or suppress lymphocyte transformation (Arai *et al.*, 1977). Kelly and Parker (1979) studied a wide range of concentrations of arachidonic acid and other unsaturated fatty acids on PHA induced stimulation of human peripheral blood lymphocytes (Table IV). Arachidonic acid was found to produce significant enhancement of DNA synthesis, as manifested by increased thymidine incorporation. Several

Table IV

Effect of Fatty Acids on E-PHA-Induced [^{3}H]thymidine Uptake
in Medium Containing 10% Fetal Calf Serum[a,b]

Fatty acid (μm/ml)		E-PHA (1 μg/ml)[b] cpm $\pm$ SEM	SR[c]
		41,524 $\pm$ 4,101	
+ Arachidonic acid	1.0	71,942 $\pm$ 10,653	1.75 $\pm$ 0.3
	0.5	57,457 $\pm$ 7,261	1.4 $\pm$ 0.2
	0.1	34,762 $\pm$ 4,271	0.8 $\pm$ 0.1
+ Linoleic acid	1.0	54,037 $\pm$ 5,827	1.3 $\pm$ 0.1
	0.5	44,034 $\pm$ 4,162	1.0 $\pm$ 0.1
	0.1	62,128 $\pm$ 2,329	1.5 $\pm$ 0.2
+ Oleic acid	1.0	47,755 $\pm$ 10,259	1.1 $\pm$ 0.2
	0.5	40,268 $\pm$ 9,048	0.9 $\pm$ 0.2
	0.1	41,214 $\pm$ 11,248	0.9 $\pm$ 0.2
+ Linolenic acid	1.0	60,891 $\pm$ 2,412	1.4 $\pm$ 0.1
	0.5	58,293 $\pm$ 719	1.3 $\pm$ 0.1
	0.1	46,841 $\pm$ 8,767	1.0 $\pm$ 0.2
+ Dihomo-γ linolenic	1.0	56,151 $\pm$ 1,980	1.3 $\pm$ 0.1
	0.5	36,741 $\pm$ 6,040	0.8 $\pm$ 0.2
	0.1	38,077 $\pm$ 5,595	0.8 $\pm$ 0.2
+ Arachidic acid	1.0	44,192 $\pm$ 4,252	1.0 $\pm$ 0.1
	0.5		
	0.1	39,399 $\pm$ 4,883	0.9 $\pm$ 0.1

[a]Reproduced with permission from Kelly and Parker, 1979.

[b]The cells were cultured for 72 hr at 37°C, with 1 μCi of [^{3}H]methyl thymidine present during the final 5 hr. The basal (unstimulated) [^{3}H]thymidine uptake was 292 ($\pm$35 SEM).

[c]Stimulation ratio (SR) = $\dfrac{\text{cpm experimental (PHA + fatty acid)} - \text{cpm basal}}{\text{cpm PHA alone} - \text{basal}}$

other unsaturated fatty acids were also stimulatory but were not as significant as arachidonic acid. Most importantly, this stimulation was shown in a variety of media, including media supplemented with 10% fetal calf serum. The alterations were also seen when uridine incorporation, total cell number, and blast transformation were quantitated, suggesting to the authors that the effects of arachidonic acid were not due to thymidine transport or pool size (Kelly and Parker, 1979). Finally, arachidonic acid did not interact with PHA binding on cells. Nonetheless, at higher concentrations, fatty acids were inhibitory. This observation is important because unsaturated fatty acids have been reported to enhance the formation of human E rosettes (Offner and Clausen, 1978). Furthermore, the addition of fatty acids has been shown to increase the number of avid T lymphocytes that bind more than 10 SRBC; thus, increased fatty acids might change the lipid of the plasma membrane and stimulate T-cell immunity. Although these observations appear reproducible, many groups would argue that the data are unphysiological because of the nature of the presentation of fatty acids *in vitro* (Offner and Clausen, 1978).

There also appear to be significant differences in the effects of saturated versus unsaturated fatty acids on phagocytosis. It has long been known (DiLuzio and Blickens, 1966) that intravenous fats alter phagocytosis. Intravenous administration of methyl palmitate produces a marked depression of the phagocytic activity of the reticuloendothelial system. Histological evidence indicates that the effect of methyl palmitate is due to suppression of Kupffer cell phagocytosis (Di Luzio and Wooles, 1964). Hawley and Gordon (1976) isolated human neutrophils and performed *in vitro* function tests including phagocytosis, bactericidal activity, and chemotaxis after incubation with long chain fatty acids. Unsaturated fatty acids (oleic acid) caused no changes in bactericidal activity and only moderate decreases in phagocytosis and chemotaxis at very high concentrations. Saturated fatty acid (palmitic acid) at high concentrations produced virtually complete inhibition of chemotaxis and moderate depression of phagocytosis and bactericidal ability. Lower concentrations of saturated free fatty acids, within a physiologic range in humans, caused a marked inhibition of chemotaxis. The functional changes observed were associated with ultrastructural alterations. The neutrophils contained numerous cytoplasmic neutral lipid droplets (Hawley and Gordon, 1976).

Many similar studies have been performed in humans who have received lipid injections to demonstrate the interactions of fat pigment and fat droplets in phagocytic cells. Others studies have focused on the effect of lipid on the morphology and function of peritoneal macrophages. Guinea pig macrophages were exposed to lipids for up to 48 hr *in vitro*. The macrophages ingested the lipids over 48 hr, as confirmed by transmission electron microscopy and by oil red 0 staining. Moreover, the lipid uptake was associated with a decreased ability of the cells to spread, decreased complexity of membrane ruffles, a reduction of latex bead phagocytosis, and lastly, a reduced capacity to adhere to and ingest sheep erythrocytes coated with IgG. Clearly, compromised reticuloendothelial cell function could compromise the host defense against infectious agents (Table V) (Strunk *et al.,* 1979).

The mechanism of these effects has been studied in several ways. In particular, methods were developed to measure the incorporation of exogenous fatty acids into membrane lipids. Schroit and Gallily (1979) prepared chromatograms of macrophages grown in the presence of exogenous

Table V

Effect of Intralipid (IL) on the Capacity of Guinea Pig Peritoneal Macrophages to Associate with Opsonized Latex Particles (5.7 μm Diameter)[a]

Time (hr)	IL (mg/dl)	Number of experiments	Macrophages associated with latex (%)[b]	p	Ave. No. latex beads/ macrophage[c]	p
0	—	12	72.6 ± 11.1	—	2.50 ± 0.35[c]	—
4	.0	17	70.3 ± 15.7	—	2.41 ± 0.36	—
	37.5	17	70.2 ± 13.2	—	2.54 ± 0.36	—
24	0	35	80.4 ± 15.7	—	3.13 ± 0.44	—
	37.5	32	46.9 ± 24.4	<.001[d]	2.24 ± 0.60	<.001[d]
48	0	4	89.4 ± 0.08	—	3.60 ± 0.08	—
	37.5	4	51.7 ± 12.7	<.001[e]	2.37 ± 0.51	<.01[e]

[a]Reproduced with permission from Strunk *et al.* (1979).
[b]Mean ± SD.
[c]Mean ± SD. Only macrophages associated with at least one latex bead were used in this calculation.
[d]p value for two-tailed Student *t* test comparing value with that obtained at 24 hr without IL.
[e]p value for two-tailed Student *t* test comparing value with that obtained at 48 hr without IL.

unsaturated fatty acids (palmitoleic, oleic, elaidic, linoleic, linolenic, and arachidonic acids). These fatty acids were incorporated into the cells and selectively altered the fatty acyl composition of phospholipids. Up to 38% of the total cellular phospholipids were found to be derived from the exogenous fatty acid supplements. More importantly, the incorporation of the different fatty acids into cellular phospholipids had striking effects on cellular phagocytic activity. The effects on phagocytosis were found to correlate with the degree of unsaturation and with the *cis-* or *trans-*double bond configuration. Thus, macrophage phagocytic ingestion rates of ^{125}I-labeled *Shigella flexneri* were found to be altered by more than twofold after the cells were cultivated in the presence of cis-unsaturated fatty acids (Schroit and Gallily, 1979).

In explaining these effects, the biophysical alterations produced by dietary fats continue to be the major focus of attention. Adams *et al.* (1983) examined isolated plasma membranes of splenic lymphoid subpopulations as a function of diet. Fluorescence polarization of 1,6-diphenyl-1,3,5-hexatriene (DPH) decreased in lymphocyte populations from mice fed a diet containing 8% or 20% polyunsaturated fats. Moreover, fluorescence polarization measurements in T and B splenic cells and their purified plasmalemma implied differential alteration of physical properties in whole cells and membranes as a function of diet. High-resolution nuclear magnetic resonance (NMR) scanning indicated a shift in the distribution of phosphatidylcholine in the membrane bilayer from the outer to the inner leaflet in lymphocytes of mice fed high polyunsaturated fat diets. Spectral changes observed by NMR indicated alterations in the motional properties of phospholipid headgroups *in situ* on the membrane surface as a function of dietary manipulation, with the phospholipid headgroups moving more rapidly in the presence of high polyunsaturated fat diets. Dietary lipids may therefore modulate the level of immune responsiveness by differential effects on plasma membrane lipid structure in lymphocyte subpopulations (Adams *et al.,* 1983).

Fatty acid biosynthesis and the attendant synthesis of structural lipids of appropriate fatty acid composition play a prominent role in the generation of cytotoxic lymphocytes (CTL) (Table VI) (Kung *et al.,* 1979). This has been shown by determining the role of fetal calf serum (FCS) in generating CTL. Dialyzed fetal calf serum (dFCS) is a poor source of serum supplement for *in vitro* CTL generation. Serum dialysate or biotin fully restores dialyzed

Table VI

Inhibition of CTL Generation by Avidin
and Restoration with Biotin[a]

Experiment	Serum supplement	Avidin[b] (μ/ml)	Biotin (ng/ml)	Lysis (%)
I	2% FCS	—	—	69
	5% FCS	—	—	84
	10% FCS	—	—	91
	2% FCS	—	200	74
	5% FCS	—	200	82
	10% FCS	—	200	90
	2% FCS	15	—	0
	5% FCS	15	—	2
	10% FCS	15	—	32
	2% FCS	15	200	74
	5% FCS	15	200	84
	10% FCS	15	200	89
	10% FCS[c]	—	—	2
II	5% FCS	—	—	75
	5% dFCS	—	—	31
	5% dFCS	10	—	6
	5% dFCS	10	150	62
	5% FCS[c]	—	—	0

[a]Reproduced with permission from Kung *et al.* (1979).
[b]Avidin and biotin additions were made at initiation of cultures.
[c]All cultures received 2×10^6 C57BL/6 spleen cells and 5×10^4 DBA/2 peritoneal cells except these negative controls that received 2×10^6 C57BL/6 spleen cells alone.

FCS to activity levels comparable to FCS. The active principle in serum dialysate is biotin; further dialysis is prevented by addition of avidin, a biotin-binding protein. Avidin inhibits CTL generation only when added during the early stages of mixed lymphocyte cultures, whereas biotin can restore activity even if added at a later time. When FCS enriched in a fatty acid mixture, or in palmitic acid alone, is used as the serum supplement, avidin-mediated inhibition of CTL generation is markedly reduced. Avidin also inhibits CTL generation in cultures containing killed macrophages as the stimulating cell and supplemented with concanavalin A–induced spleen cell supernatant, a source of helper factor(s) (Kung *et al.,* 1979).

IN VIVO EFFECTS OF FATTY ACIDS

The interaction of diet, lipids, and the immune system has been studied *in vivo* by numerous investigators (Meade *et al.,* 1978; Tsang *et al.,* 1976). Other groups have studied the influence of fatty acid injection on immune responsiveness (Ring *et al.,* 1974). We prefer, and will focus most of our attention in this chapter on, dietary manipulation because of its implications for nutrition. Moreover, subcutaneous administration of fatty acids is unreliable; slow absorption makes it difficult to quantitate the changes of fatty acids in the host.

Dietary fat modulates several aspects of immune responsiveness (Figs. 3–5). In mice subjected to prenatal and postnatal dietary manipulation, the weights of the spleen, thymus, and liver were significantly more influenced by dietary fat saturation and concentration than were those of other organs. Serum immunoglobulins IgG_1 and IgG_2, but not IgM or IgA, were higher in mice fed a polyunsaturated fat diet than in mice fed a staurated fat diet (Erickson *et al.,* 1980) (Table VII). While dietary manipulation generally did not influence the differential cell counts of peripheral blood, the percentage of immunoglobulin-positive splenic cells changed with dietary manipulation. Although the percentage of T cells was not influenced by the experimental diets, T-cell blastogenesis was affected by both the saturation and the concentration of dietary fat. Polyunsaturated fats, particularly at high levels, suppressed lymphocyte blastogenesis, whereas at low or deficient levels, they intensified mitogenic responses (Erickson *et al.,* 1980).

As noted above, early studies demonstrated that either subcutaneous or oral administration of linoleic acid, a polyunsaturated fatty acid, retarded the rejection of skin allografts (Figs. 4, 5). This delayed rejection was attributed to changes in T-cell immunity. In contrast, mice fed a diet deficient in polyunsaturated fatty acids rejected skin allografts more rapidly. Interestingly, the latter group of mice had a decreased rate of development

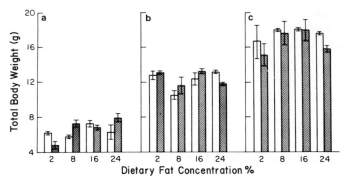

Fig. 3. Total body weights of (a) 2-, (b) 4-, and (c) 6-week-old C57BL/6 mice after dietary manipulation. Dams were fed a diet with either an unsaturated or saturated fat source at 2, 8, 16, and 24% concentration through pregnancy and lactation; then the offspring were weaned to the diets of the dam. Neither dietary fat concentration nor saturation influenced total body weight in any age mice. Brackets indicate SEM. □, safflower oil; ▨, coconut oil.   (Reproduced with permission from Erickson *et al.,* 1980.)

and a lower incidence of methylcholanthrene-induced tumors (Mertin and Hunt, 1976).

These observations led to similar studies attempting immunosuppression of polyunsatured fatty acids in patients undergoing renal transplantation. McHugh and colleagues (1977) carried out a double-blind control trial to assess the potential therapeutic value of feeding renal allograft recipients a diet containing polyunsatured fatty acids. Eighty-nine patients were studied for 6 months following transplantation. Approximately half of them consumed a diet rich in polyunsatured fatty acids; 45 received the placebo

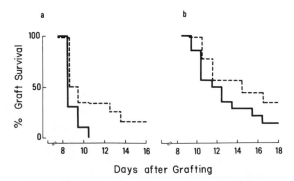

Fig. 4. Life tables of second set skin allograft survival times in (a) female and (b) male CBA mice grafted with C3H tail skin. The animals were C18:2 treated for 16 days only during the first set. ▬▬, control. - - -, C18:2. (a) Control, $n = 10$; C18:2 treated, $n = 12$. (b) Control, $n = 14$; C18:2 treated, $n = 9$.   (Reproduced with permission from Mertin and Hunt, 1976.)

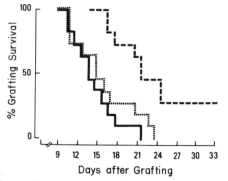

Fig. 5. Life table of skin graft survival in male CBA mice grafted with C3H tail skin. Untreated control and oleic acid (C18:1) or linoleic acid (C18:2) injected (sc) animals (11 per group). ▬▬, control; ·····, C18:1; - - -, C18:2. (Reproduced with permission from Mertin and Hunt, 1976.)

diet containing oleic acid. Initially, as suggested in the animal studies, graft survival was significantly better in the polyunsaturated fatty acid group than in the placebo group. However, after 3 months, and especially at the 6-month point of observation, there were no differences in the two groups. These results are perhaps not surprising, considering more recent data on the effect of polyunsaturated fatty acids on modulating T-cell response.

The changes in the lymphoid and reticuloendothelial systems produced by allografting could also be produced in ungrafted animals by polyunsaturated fatty acid treatment, including increased ^{125}IudR uptake by lymphoid

Table VII

Analysis of Variance of Quantitative Immunoglobulins[a]

Source of variation	df	Significance of F values							
		IgG$_1$			IgG$_2$			IgM	
		2w[c]	4w	6w	2w	4w	6w	4w	6w
Dietary fat concentration (F)	3	<.001	.01	>.10	.01	<.01	.04	>.50	>.40
Saturation (S)	1	<.001	>.50	.06	<.001	.001	>.50	>.40	>.50
Excess XS	3	.01	>.50	.06	.03	<.01	.05	>.50	>.30

[a]Reproduced with permission from Erickson *et al.* (1980).
[b]Significance as determined by a two-way analysis of variance.
[c]Age in weeks (w).

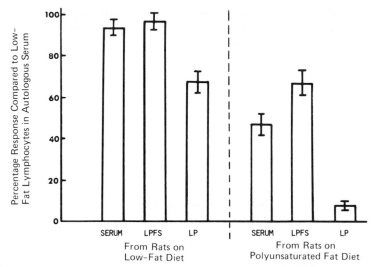

Fig. 6. Lymphocytes from rats on the low-fat diet were cultured in 2.5% autologous serum supplemented with 2.5% allogeneic serum, lipoprotein-free serum (LPFS) or the serum lipoprotein fraction (LP) taken from rats on the low-fat diet or the polyunsaturated-fat diet. Statistical comparisons were made with respect to the response of low-fat lymphocytes in autologous serum. The lipoprotein fraction from rats on the low-fat diet inhibited the blastogenic response ($p \leq .05$), whereas lipoprotein-free serum did not inhibit. Blastogenic response was inhibited by both lipoprotein-free serum ($p \leq .05$) and the lipoprotein fraction ($p \leq .001$) taken from rats on the polyunsaturated fat diet. Bars, SE. (Reproduced with permission from Kollmorgen *et al.,* 1979.)

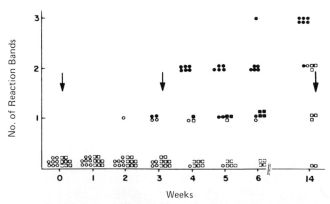

Fig. 7. Sequential development of precipitating antibodies against components of ovalbumin in control (circles) and hypercholesterolemic (squares) monkeys. The arrows indicate times of primary, booster, and skin test injections. High-titer ($> 1 : 8$) samples from each monkey are shown by solid symbols. The number of bands of precipitating reactions are shown on the ordinate. □, ○, negative or low titer; ■, ●, high titer. (Reproduced with permission from Fiser *et al.,* 1973.)

cells, increased spleen and lymph node weight, increased proportions of red pulp and granulocyte precursors in the spleen, and reticuloendothelial activation (Meade and Mertin, 1976). Interestingly, the combined effects of allografting and linoleic acid on peripheral lymph node weight were greater than the effects of either treatment alone, but fell short of the sum of both treatments. Prolonged treatment with linoleic acid led to destructive changes in the spleen. Nonetheless, immunoinhibition could be demonstrated even with only short treatments and before histological evidence of tissue destruction was apparent. These effects were reversible when linoleic acid treatment was discontinued (Meade and Mertin, 1976). Certain immunoinhibitory effects of the polyunsaturated fatty acid linoleic acid no longer occur after splenectomy of young adult CBA mice. This observation suggests that the spleen is a major intermediary in the action of linoleic acid on the immune system, implying that linoleic acid stimulates splenic suppressor cells or the synthesis of inhibitor prostaglandins by splenic macrophages (Mertin *et al.,* 1977).

Work by DeWille *et al.* (1981) demonstrated that *in vivo* antibody production was not reduced in mice fed a diet containing a high level of polyunsaturated fatty acids (50% corn oil). Indeed, reduced antibody responses were observed only in mice fed a diet deficient in essential fatty acids. The experiments, however, quantified only the number of B cell–secreting antibodies, using classic plaque systems. Because antibody production requires T helper cell function, the same group studied the effects of dietary fatty acids on delayed-type hypersensitivity in mice (DeWille *et al.,* 1981). Briefly, the effects of an essential fatty acid–deficient diet and a diet rich in polyunsaturated fatty acids were studied. Groups of animals were compared on the basis of the length of time they were fed the diet before alterations were seen in dinitrofluorobenzene (DNFB) delayed-type hypersensitivity. After 70 days, delayed-type hypersensitivity was reduced by nearly 30% in mice that were fed an essential fatty acid–deficient diet, whereas the response of mice fed the high polyunsatured fatty acid diet was equal to that of a control group. In contrast, the time required for the essential fatty acid–deficient diet to reduce delayed-type hypersensitivity was only 42 days. This reduction in T-cell immunity was rapidly corrected by feeding a control diet. Thus, although consumption of an essential fatty acid–deficient diet can reduce T-cell immunity, the reduction is transient and requires a significant period of time. In fact, those results were not as dramatic as those seen earlier, when the effects of essential fatty acid deficiency in different levels of dietary polyunsaturated fatty acids on humoral immunity in mice were studied.

A great deal of attention has focused on the role of fatty acid concentration and the relative influence of saturated versus unsaturated fatty acids on antibody responsiveness. The data from several laboratories are in reasonable agreement, provided that both of these features (level and saturation) are taken into account in data analysis. DeWille *et al.* (1979) conducted several experiments to investigate the influence of an essential fatty acid–deficient diet, including different levels of polyunsaturated fatty acids, on murine humoral immunity. Consumption of diets deficient in essential fatty acids (0% corn oil) significantly reduced the humoral response. This reduction was demonstrated even after only 28 days, a period far in advance of any ill effects of essential fatty acid deficiency on growth. The reduction in antibody response was seen in primary and secondary responses against both T cell–dependent and T cell–independent antigens. The influence of this diet on antibody production was readily reversible. After 56 days of feeding the deficient diet of 0% corn oil, mice were given a control diet of 13% corn oil for 1 week and they recovered from this humoral deficiency. In contrast, diets containing various levels of polyunsaturated fatty acids (2–70% of energy from corn oil) did not adversely affect antibody responses (DeWille *et al.,* 1979).

More impressive results have been provided by Carolomagno *et al.* (1983) on the effects of dietary fat, fed during the postweaning period, on immune ontogeny. Equal numbers of female rats, either prematurely weaned at 14 days of age or allowed to nurse for 21 days, were pair-fed a diet containing either vegetable oil- or cholesterol-enriched animal fat for 95 days. Thereafter, all animals received the animal fat diet until 11 months of age. Rats were then immunized with sheep erythrocytes, and the antibody response was quantified. There was no significant effect of early weaning or diet on the number of plaque-forming splenocytes or on serum hemolysins. A significant positive correlation between high-density lipid cholesterol and both plaque-forming cells and hemolysin titers was detected in the groups fed animal fat. Significant impairment in the splenocyte blastogenic response to phytohemagglutinin was observed in rats receiving animal fat prior to 95 days. Separate groups of rats were infected 5 days before death with *Listeria monocytogenes.* Splenocyte blastogenesis was impaired in the group fed animal fat. The degree of impairment was similar to that observed in uninfected rats fed the same diet, and there were increased numbers of bacteria recovered from the spleen and kidney of animals whose early diet contained animal fat. Thus, the fat content of the early postweaning diet has an impact on immune responses that persists into adulthood (Carolomagno *et al.,* 1983).

The route of antigen administration is also important for following the relative influence of dietary lipids on immune response. Weanling male Lewis rats and A/J mice were fed purified diets either adequate or deficient in essential fatty acids for 50–60 days. The animals were immunized with SRBC either iv or ip, and PFC responses were determined. When the antigen was injected iv, the essential fatty acid–deficient animals of both species showed an increased PFC response compared to controls, but when it was injected ip, there was no difference between the groups. It was also noted that the increase in PFC response in the mice immunized by the iv route correlated with a decreased synthesis of prostaglandin F (PGF) by the spleen (Boissonneault and Johnston, 1984).

Serum factors may be involved in the suppression of mitogens in rats fed a diet rich in polyunsaturated fats. Concanavalin A–induced blastogenesis of spleen lymphocytes was significantly inhibited when lymphocytes from rats fed a high polyunsaturated fat diet were compared to those from rats fed a low-fat diet. Responsiveness was dependent on the source of serum, since lymphocytes from rats fed a low-fat diet were suppressed by serum from rats fed a high-fat diet. Alternatively, lymphocytes from rats fed a high-fat diet were more responsive in autologous serum. One of the inhibiting factors in serum was the lipoprotein fraction; however, rats fed a high-fat diet probably had additional inhibitors in their serum (Kollmorgen *et al.,* 1979) (Fig. 6). Interestingly, the fatty acid profiles of the total lipid in plasma, spleen, and thymus can be altered without accompanying major changes in mitogen-induced blood lymphocyte transformation (Clifford *et al.,* 1983).

Other groups have similarly looked into the role of serum factors. A diet containing 20% by weight of fat rich in unsaturated fatty acids reduced the ability of guinea pigs to form antibody and reduced delayed hypersensitivity responses. Reduced responses *in vivo* were seen on primary immunization only; subsequent antigenic challenges showed responses similar to those of animals fed a normal diet. However, cells from animals fed large amounts of unsaturated fats, when cultured *in vitro* with antigen and sera of normal animals fed a low-fat diet, did not show reduced delayed hypersensitivity, as manifested by both macrophage migration inhibition and lymphocyte transformation. The serum of animals fed high-fat diets greatly inhibited the *in vitro* response to mitogens and antigens of lymphocytes from tuberculin-sensitized animals fed either low- or high-fat diets. Since serum from animals fed low-fat diets did not have this effect, the authors postulated that the inhibitory activity was due to a lipid or lipoprotein derivative of unsaturated fatty acids. Animals fed high-fat diets remained healthy (Friend *et al.,* 1980).

Triglycerides can also alter mitogen responsiveness. Weanling rats were fed casein-based diets containing purified and mixed triglycerides to evaluate the effect of these lipids on mitogen-induced lymphocyte transformation, lymphoid organ weights, and fatty acid profiles of the total lipid in plasma, spleen, and thymus. Test lipids were added at a level of 8 g/100 g diet. All diets contained 0.82 g/100 g safflower oil. The differences in mitogen-induced lymphocyte transformation in rats fed the various dietary lipids were unrelated to saturation of the lipid and correlated negatively with the total amount of lipid absorbed. Except for tripalmitin and tristearin, dietary lipids significantly altered the fatty acid profiles of the total lipids in plasma, spleen, and thymus.

The modulating effect of fat on the immune system clearly depends on the duration of feeding (Locniskar et al., 1983). Sprague-Dawley rats were fed either 5% mixed fat, 24% saturated fat, 24% polyunsaturated fat, or 24% partially saturated fat. After 2.5 months of dietary treatment, the high-fat groups showed evidence of splenic hyperplasia; however, no consistent morphologic changes were seen in the mesenteric lymph nodes. Splenocytes from rats fed the 24% polyunsaturated fat diet were cultured in fetal bovine serum and had a depressed lymphocyte transformation response, which persisted after 5 months of dietary treatment. Supplementing the culture medium with 10% rat serum altered the transformation response profile, but high-fat serum did not have an immunosuppressive effect.

Caution must be exercised in interpreting in vitro studies of lymphocyte transformation. When functions in cultured cells obtained from rats fed different dietary fats are studied, the dietary effect are found to be abrogated or modified by the use of fetal bovine serum in the medium (Loomis et al., 1983). Loomis et al. (1983) fed rats purified diets containing either 10% by weight corn oil or linseed oil for 8 weeks. Splenocytes from rats fed a control diet were cultured for 48 hr in media containing either fetal bovine serum or serum from rats fed stock diet, corn oil, or linseed oil. Cells were cultured with phytohemagglutinin, and the production of PGF_{2a} was determined. The serum from the corn oil–fed rats differed markedly in composition from that of the linseed oil–fed rats, and was notably higher in arachidonic acid and lower in timnodonic acid. These changes were reflected in the fatty acid composition of choline glycerophosphatide from the spleen. PGF_{2a} production was significantly depressed in the medium from linseed oil–fed rats compared to that of the corn oil–fed group. This effect was due to the competition of timnodonic acid for cyclooxygenase.

Similarly, there are differential responses of lymphoid subpopulations. Dietary lipids independently modulate the levels of T- and B-cell responsiveness (Adams et al., 1983). Lymphocyte transformation from dietarily manipulated mice in response to alloantigens was significantly greater in mice fed a diet containing minimal essential fatty acids (EFA) as the only fat source (EFA control) than in those fed an EFA-deficient dict. When the dietary fat concentration was increased, blastogenic responses decreased compared to the EFA control diet. High levels of dietary fat, particularly polyunsaturated fat, suppress lymphocyte functions when EFA requirements are met, whereas low levels (EFA control) intensify these responses. Clearly, there is a different susceptibility of T and B cells to these influences, but dose–response kinetics have not been well worked out.

There has been some concern that a diet rich in polyunsaturated fats may enhance tumorigenesis. In 1974, Dr. Bruce Mackie noted the development of malignant melanoma in five patients who had recently substituted polyunsaturated for saturated fats in the diet. Because of these findings and the frequent prescription of polyunsaturated fats for the treatment of hyperlipidemia, the problem has been investigated (Goldrick *et al.,* 1976).

Rats fed diets high in lipid and cholesterol have more dimethylhydrazine (DMH)-induced tumors than those fed diets low in lipid or lacking cholesterol. Rats were fed diets containing 20% safflower oil or coconut oil, with or without cholesterol (1%) and cholic acid (0.3%), for 35 weeks, during which time they were given DMH for tumorigenesis. Concurrently, the responses of T cells to PHA and natural killer cell activity (NKCA) of splenic lymphocytes were monitored. DMH injection did not result in any significant differences in either T-cell or NK-cell activity. T-cell mitogenesis, however, was profoundly affected by differences in diet. Nearly total suppression of PHA response was observed in the polyunsaturated fat diet groups, a 90% decrease compared to the saturated fat diet groups. Cholesterol in the diet was found to diminish T-cell activity (Krause *et al.,* 1980).

Of more importance, however, is the relationship between dietary lipid and macrophage function. The tumoricidal capabilities of macrophages can be reversibly inhibited by a lipoprotein of high molecular weight, and the inhibition appears to be reproduced by enrichment of macrophage plasma membranes with cholesterol (Chapman and Hibbs, 1977).

LIPIDS AND EXPERIMENTAL ALLERGIC ENCEPHALOMYELITIS

Linoleic acid and its polyenoic derivatives occur in relatively high proportional amounts in myelin ethanolamine, phosphatides and cerebrosides. These fatty acid derivatives are suggested to be of importance for the optimal stability of the myelin membrane. In support of this theory, rats bred and fed a diet deficient in polyunsaturated fatty acids have a higher susceptibility to allergic encephalomyelitis than rats fed a control diet. On the basis of this finding, it is suggested that a low content of linoleic acid derivatives in the brains of multiple sclerosis patients may be explained by a high intake during the newborn period and childhood of cow milk and its derivatives. The latter contains an amount of polyunsaturated fatty acids five times lower than that of mother's milk. Some groups believe that these observations correlate with geographic studies of the distribution of multiple sclerosis (Clausen and Moller, 1967).

There may also be a role for PGF synthesis in modulating the susceptibility of rats to experimental allergic encephalomyelitis (EAE) (Weston and Johnston, 1978). For example, a fat deficiency during development leads to increased susceptibility to EAE; a supplement of linoleic acid has a marked protective effect against this disease (Selivonchick and Johnston, 1975). Lewis rats were fed diets adequate or deficient in EFA. At 70–80 days of age, EAE was induced using adjuvants containing either *Mycobacterium butyricum* or *M. tuberculosis* H37Ra. When the former was used, the incidence of EAE was greater in the EFA-deficient rats than in the EFA-adequate controls. However, when the rats were challenged with *M. tuberculosis,* the incidence of the disease was the same in both dietary groups. Histochemical studies of brain from EFA-deficient rats showed marginally depressed levels of PGF compared to controls (Weston and Johnston, 1978).

On day 14 of gestation, Sprague-Dawley rats were assigned to a control diet, a fat-deficient diet, or a fat-deficient diet supplemented with ethyl linoleate. The same diets were continued during lactation. On weaning, the offspring were fed the same diets as their mothers. The rats were serially sacrificed, and the lipid compositions of the brain, brain myelin, and spinal cord myelin were determined. Experimental EAE was induced in animals from each group at 54 days of age. Development of body, brain, and brain myelin was slower in the fat-deficient and ethyl linoleate–supplemented rats during early life. At 68 days, the brain myelin from all groups reached mature composition, although the body and brain weights of fat-deficient and ethyl linoleate–supplemented rats remained lower than those of controls. The composition of spinal cord myelin from the two former groups was similar to that of control rats throughout the period of study. The greatest incidence and severity of EAE occurred in animals from the fat-deficient group, and the incidence of the disease in the ethyl linoleate–supplemented rats was similar to that in the controls. A reduction in total brain protein occurred in fat-deficient EAE rats and in control and fat-deficient EAE cerebrosides. Myelin from the brain and spinal cord of EAE rats did not differ appreciably in protein content or lipid composition from that of controls (Selivonchick and Johnston, 1975).

Because of these observations that experimental EAE was enhanced by EFA deficiency, a fat-free diet was studied in Lewis rats starting either in late gestation, at weaning, or in adult life. Contrary to previous reports, the diet did not influence the appearance of EAE. Retardation of growth, the typical dermatitis, increased water consumption, and testicular atrophy were seen in EFA-deficient rats. Control rats were fed either a complete diet or a fat-free diet supplemented with corn oil. EAE was induced in the EFA-deficient and control rats by conventional active sensitization with neural antigen and adjuvants or by passive transfer of living lymphoid cells from sensitized, nutritionally normal donors. Contrary to previous reports, EFA deficiency did not enhance EAE in any of seven experiments, and these results were supported by histological examination. In fact, inhibition of clinical signs, but not of histological lesions, occurred when EFA deficiency was moderately advanced. This was accompanied by (and probably related to) thymic atrophy, possibly due to nonspecific stress (Levine and Sowinski, 1980). Thus, the issue of the effect of dietary fat on EAE is far from resolved.

CHOLESTEROL

There is little information at present on the influence of cholesterol on immune function. The data that are available suggest that high levels of cholesterol in the diet produce a decrease in T-cell function, but have little effect on either antibody response or NKCA. In humans, high plasma levels of cholesterol are often associated with an increased incidence of infections. Moreover, the adjuvant effect of *Corynebacterium parvum* is reduced in animals fed high levels of cholesterol. Similarly, there is a decrease in the phagocytic activity of macrophages in animals fed diets high in cholesterol.

In an attempt to evaluate the role of blood leukocytes in the transport of lipids in circulation, the cholesterol content and ingested exogenous cholesterol-4-^{14}C were measured in leukocytes and plasma. Cellular lipids were fractionated chromatographically and measured spectrophotometrically. The leukocytes contained 1.8 and 0.6 mg/10^9 cells of free and esterified cholesterol, respectively. There was a predominance of free cholesterol in leukocytes (free ester ratio = 3 : 1), in contrast to a predominance of esterified cholesterol in plasma (1 : 2.5). Groups of 22 rabbits received intragastric administration of cholesterol-4-^{14}C and were serially sacrificed from 4 hr to 14 days later. In leukocytes, the free fraction of labeled cholesterol was highest after 7 days, but the esterified fraction remained low throughout the 14-day period. In plasma, the labeled cholesterol was also highest after 7 days, but the esterified fraction was higher than the free fraction throughout the experiment. The results indicate that blood leukocytes play a role in the transport of cholesterol in the circulation (Suzuki, 1968).

Similar studies have been carried out with rabbit macrophages. The composition and metabolism of lipid in peritoneal macrophages obtained from normally fed rabbits were compared with those of macrophages obtained from cholesterol-fed rabbits. Macrophages from cholesterol-fed rabbits had a higher cholesterol content and a markedly higher cholesterol ester content than did normal macrophages. The increase in cholesterol ester content was most marked for cholesterol oleate and cholesterol linoleate, with the cholesterol ester fatty acid composition of the cholesterol-fed macrophages resembling that of foam cells derived from aortic lesions of similarly cholesterol-fed rabbits. Metabolic differences were also demonstrated between the cells obtained from normal and cholesterol-fed rabbits (Table VIII). The incorporation of C-labeled acetate into cholesterol-fed rabbit macrophages was almost completely suppressed compared to macrophages from control rabbits. However, incubation *in vitro* of normal macrophages for up to 20 hr with hyperlipemic serum did not suppress cholesterol synthesis (Kar and Day, 1978).

Cholesterol is a constituent of all mammalian cells and a structural component of membranes. Thus, the above data are not surprising, since cholesterol–phospholipid interactions have been shown to influence the physical properties of cell membranes (Kroes and Ostwald, 1971; Steim, 1972; Poznansky *et al.,* 1973; Feo *et al.,* 1975). During phagocytosis, plasma membranes contribute to the constitution of lysosomes (Werb and Cohn, 1972). In phagocytosis, nearly all cellular cholesterol is located in plasma membranes and phagolysosomes (Cohn, 1972). A rise in plasma membrane free cholesterol is followed by inhibition of phagocytosis of latex particles or lipid droplets (Dianzani *et al.,* 1976).

These observations take on additional significance because cholesterol-fed rabbits were more susceptible to experimental infections than are control animals. Phagocytosis was unchanged in the cholesterol-fed animals. However, many functions of neutrophils and macrophages were significantly reduced. Three of five dehydrogenases and phosphatase were lower

Table VIII

Lipid Composition of Macrophages
from Normally Fed and Cholesterol-Fed Rabbits[a–c]

	Lipid composition (μg/mg of protein)		
	Normally fed	Cholesterol fed	P^d
Cholesterol (free)	24.6 ± 0.91	45.7 ± 3.80	<.001
Cholesterol (ester)	1.98 ± 0.36	79.8 ± 20.10	<.01
Triglyceride	11.68 ± 2.88	38.40 ± 3.7	<.01
Lipid P	6.98 ± 0.26	7.75 ± 0.79	NS

[a]Reproduced with permission from Kar and Day (1978).

[b]Mean ± SEM of five experiments.

[c]Normally fed rabbit macrophages contained 135 ± 6.7 μg of protein per 10^6 cells compared with 147 ± 16.0 μg of protein per 10^6 cells for cholesterol-fed macrophages.

[d]By Students t test.

in activity from cells obtained from cholesterol-fed rabbits than from controls.

These metabolic and functional alterations of cells from cholesterol-fed rabbits may explain the increased susceptibility to infection among these animals (Klurfeld *et al.,* 1979).

Humoral and cellular immune responses to several antigens were compared in control and hypercholesterolemic groups of monkeys (Fig. 7). When studied prior to infection, hypercholesterolemic monkeys exhibited impaired production of antibodies against ovalbumin, enhanced sensitivity to tuberculin antigen, and an increased rate of clearance of colloidal carbon from blood. During pneumococcal infection, the ability of neutrophils from hypercholesterolemic monkeys to reduce nitroblue tetrazolium dye was higher than in control monkeys (Fiser *et al.,* 1973).

Other experiments showed that hypercholesterolemia in mice causes an increase in susceptibility to coxsackievirus B, with a marked suppression of cellular infiltrates in infected tissues and increased mortality. Similarly, a hypercholesterolemic diet was associated with inhibition in host resistance, as measured by susceptibility to *L. monocytogenes* infection and the growth of two transplanted syngeneic murine tumors. Moreover, the ability of *C. parvum* to induce regression of a transplanted methylcholanthrene-induced fibrosarcoma was inhibited in hypercholesterolemic hosts, as was the histiocytic infiltration normally accompanying *C. parvum* inoculation. In contrast, the peritoneal macrophages from *C. parvum*–treated hypercholesterolemic mice were indistinguishable from similarly treated macrophages from normal mice with respect to their *in vitro* tumoricidal activity and the presence of a cell surface antigen associated with activated macrophages. Hypercholesterolemia was also associated with a decreased antibody response to sheep erythrocytes *in vivo,* but did not appear to exert a detrimental effect on B- or T-cell blastogenesis when tested *in vitro* (Kos *et al.,* 1979).

STUDIES IN HUMANS

There have been only a few studies on the effects of lipids on the immune response in humans. Many observations have depended on the study of lipid emulsions used in parenteral nutrition. This has been an important issue because of the increased incidence of infection in patients receiving TPN. In one study, 12 healthy humans were injected with lipid emulsions for 2 hr, and the influence of lipids on chemotaxis and lymphocyte migration was studied. During the infusion, there was a significant reduction in both chemotaxis and the random migration of leukocytes. These data correlated well with the increased incidence of infection in patients with high serum lipid levels. However, there has been little recent work on this subject, and a restudy would appear to be well justified (Nordenstrom *et al.,* 1979; Wagner and Silberman, 1983).

These observations should not be confused with those concerning the roles of some injected lipid preparations as nonspecific adjuvants. Studies have been conducted in several species that demonstrate enhanced responses to viral vaccines using the adjuvant activity of a metabolizable lipid emulsion. The lipid base consists of highly refined peanut oil emulsified in aqueous vaccines with glycerol and lecithin. Mice inoculated with lipid emulsion and Western or Venezuelan equine encephalitis vaccine were significantly more resistant than vaccinated controls to lethal homologous virus challenge. Similarly, sheep and rhesus monkeys given one dose of lipid emulsion plus Rift Valley fever vaccine developed significantly higher antibody titers than did control sheep. This lipid formulation has several advantages over other water-in-oil adjuvants for potential clinical use because they are metabolizable to normal host constituents, are readily emulsified with aqueous vaccines, and are nontoxic (Reynolds *et al.,* 1980).

11

Immunological Considerations of Breast Milk

INTRODUCTION

The composition of breast milk and its nutritional implications have been reviewed by Hurley (1981). For varying lengths of time, milk is virtually the only food of the human newborn. Even beyond the immediate neonatal period, milk remains a major source of nutrients. In order to review the potential impact of milk on immunity, it is necessary to examine its composition.

Milk is composed of water, fats, and nonfat solids. The fatty fraction consists of triglycerides and other fat-soluble compounds, including phospholipids, sterols, fat-soluble vitamins, and carotenoids. The nonfat solids include lactose and the nitrogenous materials casein, albumin, and globulin, proteoses and peptones, and certain enzymes. Milk also contains minerals, water-soluble vitamins, and nonprotein compounds. Casein is the major protein of milk in most species (but not in the human); albumin, also called *lactalbumin,* is the protein second highest in concentration. Milk can be distinguished by at least three materials that are unique to it: casein, lactose, and butterfat.

The composition of milk is species dependent and correlates with the growth rate of the offspring. Table I shows the relationship between growth rate and milk composition. The time required for the newborn animal to double its birth weight is shown for a number of species and is compared with the protein and ash concentrations of the milk. The amount of protein

Table I

Bunge's (1898) Original Table Showing the Relationship
between Growth and Milk Composition[a]

Species	Time in days for newborn animal to double its birth weight	100 parts of milk contain (parts)	
		Protein	Ash
Human	180	1.6	0.2
Horse	60	2.0	0.4
Ox	47	3.5	0.7
Goat	19	4.3	0.8
Pig	18	5.9	—
Sheep	10	6.5	0.9
Dog	8	7.1	1.3
Cat	7	9.5	—
Additional fast-growing species not included in Bunge's table			
Rabbit	6	14.0	2.2
Rat	6	12.0	2.0

[a]Reproduced with permission from Blaxter, as presented in Kon
and Civie (1961).

and ash varies inversely with the time necessary for the doubling of birth
weight. These variations may be related to differences in body surface area
per body weight rather than to body weight itself.

The natural food of human infants is human milk. Therefore, it is useful to
compare the composition of human milk with that of the commonly used
cow's milk. As can be seen in Table II, there are differences in the composition of milk as lactation proceeds. Colostrum is secreted by the mammary
gland within the first 3–5 days of lactation and has a composition different
from that of mature milk. The caloric value of colostrum, as well as its fat
and lactose concentrations, is lower than that of mature milk, while ash and
protein concentrations are almost twice those of mature milk. An important
component of colostrum is IgA; this provides valuable protection against
infection. During the course of lactation, even after the establishment of
mature milk, the composition of milk continues to change. Concentrations
of protein, ash, calcium, phosphorus, sodium, potassium, and zinc decrease
as lactation increases.

Most infant formulas are based on cow's milk. The water content and
caloric value of human and cow's milk are similar. However, there are also
some important differences. Cow's milk contains almost four times as much
protein, approximately three times as much calcium, and six times as much
phosphorus as human milk. Until recently, it was stated that breast milk

Table II

Mean Nutrient Content of Breast Milk Samples: 1–6 Months[a]

	Month					
	1	2	3	4	5	6
Energy (kcal/100 ml)	78.1 (10.0)[c]	75.3 (9.2)	73.6 (14.8)	78.7 (17.3)	74.7 (14.8)	74.8 (18.3)
Protein (g/100 ml)	1.44 (0.20)	1.33 (0.16)	1.32 (0.16)	1.30 (0.24)	1.25 (0.17)	1.27 (0.36)
Fat (g/100 ml)	4.92 (1.05)	4.58 (0.97)	4.58 (1.65)	4.62 (1.86)	4.36 (1.67)	4.30 (1.96)
Lactose (g/100 ml)	7.05 (0.56)	7.21 (0.62)	7.13 (0.79)	7.61 (0.40)	7.62 (0.33)	7.75 (0.27)[c]
Calcium (μg/ml)	261 (44)	275 (48)	270 (61)	255 (43)	248 (40)	256 (42)
Magnesium (μg/ml)	27.6 (4.7)	32.4 (4.1)[e]	33.6 (4.7)	35.1 (8.0)	33.8 (7.1)	33.9 (4.4)[c]
Iron (μg/ml)	0.31 (0.11)	0.22 (0.07)[f]	0.25 (0.11)	0.22 (0.09)	0.20 (0.08)	0.21 (0.10)
Zinc (μg/ml)	2.71 (0.36)	1.67 (0.68)[e]	1.35 (0.54)	0.89 (0.39)	0.57 (0.20)	0.64 (0.28)[c]
Copper (μg/ml)	0.36 (0.08)	0.28 (0.06)[e]	0.27 (0.07)	0.24 (0.05)	0.20 (0.09)	0.21 (0.07)[c]
Sodium (μg/ml)	227 (152)	264 (223)	184 (139)	175 (138)	166 (130)	134 (78)[d]
Potassium (μg/ml)	527 (70)	477 (79)	470 (81)	464 (89)	460 (85)	430 (63)[c]
(n)	(13)	(16)	(18)	(16)	(14)	(15)

[a]Reproduced with permission from Dewey and Lönnerdal (1983).
[b]Mean (SD).
[c]Paired t test of difference between 1 and 6 months significant: $p < .001$.
[d]$p < .01$.
[e]Paired t test of difference between 1 and 2 months significant: $p < .05$.
[f]$p < .01$.

contained 1.1–1.2% protein. Modern analysis has established the protein content to be 0.8–0.9%. Cow's milk also contains about five times as much riboflavin as human milk. Human milk, on the other hand, is one and a half times as high in carbohydrate value as cow's milk. In addition, lactose, vitamin D, vitamin E, and ascorbic acid concentrations are all higher in human than in cow's milk. There is considerable variation in the composition of human milk both within and between individuals. There are also differences between human and cow's milk in the composition of the proteins. Amino acid profiles are quite different, with higher levels of cystine and lower concentrations of tyrosine, phenylalanine, and tryptophan in human milk. In addition, human milk contains lactoferrin, an iron-binding protein, in considerable amount, and lysozyme, while cow's milk has only traces of these compounds. On the other hand, cow's milk contains a fairly large amount of β-lactoglobulin, which does not occur at all in human milk. The lipid components in human and cow's milk also differ. Cow's milk is higher in saturated fatty acids, while human milk is higher in unsaturated fatty acids.

In addition to these dissimilarities in chemical composition between human and cow's milk, there are important differences in other properties. The principal protein in cow's milk, casein, forms a relatively firm curd in the stomach even when it is pasteurized and homogenized. This hard curd is not easily digested by the infant's still immature digestive tract. Lactalbumin, the chief protein in human milk, forms a soft curd during digestion that a baby can easily digest and absorb. Another difference between the two types of milk is the high level of lactose in human milk, which is favorable to the absorption of calcium. The feeding of human milk also promotes the establishment of a gastrointestinal flora that is advantageous to the infant.

INFLUENCE OF NUTRITION ON LACTATION

Studies on the effects of dietary intake on the quantity and quality of lactation in women have been concerned mainly with the relationship of nutritional intake to the composition of milk. Lactation is remarkably efficient even under conditions of extreme malnutrition. For example, lactation occurred in some mothers subjected to the severe famine of the siege of Leningrad in World War II (Hurley, 1981). In the World War II internment camps of Japan, and even at the Belsen concentration camp in Germany, breast feeding took place, although there is some indication that it was not normal.

Both the quantity of milk produced and its composition in major nutrients were satisfactory even when the diet was inadequate. The caloric intake of mothers in India who had an extremely poor diet was only 70% of the recommended allowance of the Indian Council on Medical Research (Gopalan and Belavady, 1959). Their protein intake was 40% of the recommended amount, while their calcium intake was only about 22% and that of vitamin A 23%. Estimation of the quantity of milk produced by the women indicated that normal amounts were secreted, and in many of the women no weight loss occurred. In those who did lose weight, the amount lost was not very large and extended over nearly a year. The composition of the milk is summarized in Table III and compared with that from well-fed American women. It can be seen that the protein, mineral matter, and calcium content were unaffected by the poor dietary intake of the women. However, there were differences in the concentrations of potassium, magnesium, vitamin A, riboflavin, and vitamin C. There also seemed to be a depression in the fat concentration in the milk of the poorly nourished Indian women. Bantu and Chimbu women who did not receive an adequate diet during lactation also produced milk that was low in fat (Table III). Other studies have also shown a significant correlation between the fat content of a woman's diet and the concentration of fat in her milk.

The protein concentration of human milk is of importance and has received considerable attention because of the problem of protein-calorie

Table III

Composition of Human Milk in Relation to Dietary Adequacy[a]

		Diet		
			Inadequate	
Constituents	Adequate, U.S.	Indian	Bantu	Chimbu
Solids (%)	12.1	12.1	12.8	10.9
Fat (%)	3.4	3.4	3.9	2.4
Lactose (%)	7.5	7.5	7.1	7.3
Protein (%)	1.1	1.1	1.4	1.0
Minerals (%)	0.2	0.2	0.2	0.2
Calcium (mg/100 g)	34.4	34.2	28.7	
Phosphorus (mg/100 g)	14.1	11.9		
Potassium (mg/100 g)	51.2	34.7		
Sodium (mg/100g)	17.2	22.1		
Magnesium (mg/100 g)	3.5	2.6		
Vitamin A (μg/100 ml)	201	70		
Thiamin (μg/100 ml)	14.2	15.4		
Riboflavin (μg/100 ml)	37.3	17.2		
Vitamin C (mg/100 ml)	5.2	2.6		

[a]Reproduced with permission from Hurley (1980).

malnutrition. The protein content of human milk is relatively unchanged by malnutrition of the mother and therefore does not influence the development of protein-calorie malnutrition in children. The effect of protein supplementation on lactating women whose diets are low in protein content has also been studied. An increase in the protein intake from 61 to 99 g/day brought about an increase in the yield of milk. At the same time, the concentration of protein in the milk decreased somewhat, so that the overall milk protein produced in 24 hr was unchanged. In other studies, however, women who were existing on 15–20 g of protein per day during lactation did show an increased concentration of protein in milk when they were given a dietary protein supplement.

NUTRITIONAL REQUIREMENTS DURING LACTATION

Nutritional requirements in absolute terms are higher during lactation than at any other stage of the life cycle. In addition to the need for increased nutrients because of the amounts secreted in milk, nutrients are needed to make up for the energy used in the synthesis of the milk and its components. Furthermore, if the nutrient intake is insufficient, losses from the mother's tissues may occur.

The energy requirement for lactation is proportional to the quantity of milk produced. The caloric value of human milk is about 67–77 kcal/100 ml, and the efficiency of conversion of maternal calories to milk calories is about 80%. Thus, approximately 90 kcal are required for each 100 ml of milk. During pregnancy, body fat is stored and is later drawn on to supply part of the additional energy needed for lactation. According to the National Research Council, the recommended daily allowance for energy should be increased by 500 kcal/day during the first 3 months of lactation, with further additions beyond this time.

The RDA for protein during lactation is increased by 20 g/day above the maintenance amount recommended for a woman of a specific age and size. This is based on a consideration of 70% efficiency of protein utilization to synthesize the additional protein of the milk.

The RDA for vitamin A is also increased above that of the pregnant, as well as the nonpregnant, female in order to provide sufficient vitamin A for the milk. Similarly, for most of the other vitamins and minerals, requirements and RDAs are higher than at other stages of life.

The RDA for iron is not increased during lactation, since the iron concentration of milk is low. Furthermore, lactating women usually do not menstruate, so that loss of iron from the body is minimal.

NUTRITION OF THE INFANT

Information on the requirements of infants for specific nutrients is still limited. In addition, requirements often vary with age, size, rate of growth, and level of activity, as well as with the composition of the diet and the concentration of other nutrients. Thus, the amounts of specific nutrients that are recommended should not be interpreted too strictly.

The caloric requirements of the newborn are shown in Table IV. It is generally accepted that the basal metabolic need of newborn infants is approximately 48 kcal/kg/day. With additions for physical activity, fecal loss, specific dynamic action, and growth, the total requirement is 92 kcal/kg/day or 42 kcal/lb/day. For the premature newborn, 150 kcal/day is necessary.

The protein requirement during early infancy is highly correlated with both body size and rate of gain in body weight. Since caloric intake during *ad libitum* feeding is generally correlated with these variables, it is reasonable to express protein requirements in relation to caloric intake.

Estimates of infants' requirements for amino acids are shown in Table V and are compared with adult requirements. On a body weight basis, the infant has a much higher requirement than the adult for amino acids, and, because of metabolic differences, certain amino acids are dietary essentials for infants but not for adults.

Table IV

Approximate Caloric Requirements of Premature and Term Infants
After the First Week of Life[a]

	Daily caloric requirements per kilogram of body weight			
Individual factors	Premature infants		Term infants	
Basic metabolism	60		50	
Specific dynamic action and activity	10		20	
Total catabolism		70		70
Fecal loss	20		10	
Maintenance				80
Weight gain	30	90	20	
Total	120 (55/lb)		100 (45/lb)	

[a]Reproduced with permission from Nelson (1962).

Table V
Essential Amino Acid Requirements of Infants and Adults (Mg/Kg/Day)[a]

		Adult requirement		
Amino acid	Infant requirement	Men	Women	Average
Histidine	26	—	—	—
Isoleucine	66	10.4	5.2	7.8
Leucine	132	9.9	7.1	8.5
Lysine	101	8.8	3.3	6.1
Methionine	24	—	3.9	3.9
Phenylalanine	57	4.3	3.1	3.7
Cystine	23	—	—	—
Threonine	59	6.5	3.5	5.0
Tryptophan	16	2.9	2.1	2.5
Valine	83	8.8	9.2	9.0

[a]Reproduced with permission from Fomon (1974).

The RDAs for infants and children are summarized in Table VI. Infants also need other nutrients as well. They require EFA, and in the absence of adequate intake of linoleic acid, there has been clear evidence of abnormal symptoms. When linoleic acid intake provided less than 0.5–1.0% of the caloric consumption of otherwise normal infants, there were skin lesions typical of fatty acid deficiency (scaly skin) as well as growth impairment.

Other vitamins and minerals are also required by infants. These include vitamin K, folic acid, zinc, copper, manganese, iodine, and fluorine, although RDAs have not been developed for all of these factors.

It is recommended that the diet of the breast-fed infant be supplemented with iron-fortified infant cereals, iron-fortified formula, or medicinal iron at about the age of 4 months. Supplementation with vitamin D should begin within the first 2 weeks of life, and for the artificially fed infant, supplementation with vitamin C should occur soon after birth.

MODIFICATION OF COW'S MILK FOR INFANT FEEDING: FORMULAS

The basic principle of infant feeding, as of all dietary programs, is that the diet should be adequate but not excessive in calories and all essential nutrients, including water. There should be a reasonable distribution of calories from protein, fat, and carbohydrate. In addition, the diet must be easily digestible and free of harmful bacteria.

Table VI

Recommended Dietary Allowances for Infants and Children[a]

	Infants		Children		
	0.0–0.5	0.5–1.0	1–3	4–6	7–10
Weight (kg/lb)	6/14	9/20	13/28	20/44	30/66
Height (cm/in.)	60/24	71/28	86/34	110/44	135/54
Energy (kcal)	kg × 117	kg × 108	1300	1800	2400
Protein (g)	kg × 2.2	kg × 2.0	23	30	36
Vitamin A activity (IU)	1400	2000	2000	2500	3300
Vitamin D (IU)	400	400	400	400	400
Vitamin E (IU)	4	5	7	9	10
Ascorbic acid (mg)	35	35	40	40	40
Folacin (μg)	50	50	100	200	300
Niacin (mg)	5	8	9	12	16
Riboflavin (mg)	0.4	0.6	0.8	1.1	1.2
Thiamin (mg)	0.3	0.5	0.7	0.9	1.2
Vitamin B_6 (mg)	0.3	0.4	0.6	0.9	1.2
Vitamin B_{12} (μg)	0.3	0.3	1.0	1.5	2.0
Calcium (mg)	360	540	800	800	800
Phosphorus (mg)	240	400	800	800	800
Iodine (μg)	35	45	60	80	110
Iron (mg)	10	15	15	10	10
Magnesium (mg)	60	70	150	200	250
Zinc (mg)	3	5	10	10	10

[a]Reproduced with permission from Hurley (1980).

The differences between cow's milk and human milk necessitate the modification of cow's milk to make it suitable for the infant. Because of the difference in the type of curd formed by cow's milk compared to human milk, and because of the higher protein concentration of cow's milk, the milk is diluted with water. This procedure reduces the concentration of protein and at the same time decreases the problem of curd formation. Dilution of cow's milk, however, causes an equivalent reduction in the carbohydrate content, which reduces the caloric value. In order to return the calorie content to its original level, carbohydrate is added. Table VII shows the minimum vitamin and mineral levels that should be provided by an infant-feeding formula.

In studying the differences between human milk and cow's milk, the major focus of interest is the effects on the infant. During the past few decades, there has been a marked decline in many countries in the proportion of infants who are breast-fed. This change occurred very rapidly in

Table VII

Recommended Ranges of Nutrient Levels in Infant Formulas: AAP Committee on Nutrition, 1976 Recommendations with 1982 Modifications

Nutrient (per 100 kcal)	Lowest adequate		Not to exceed[a]	
Protein (g)	1.8[b]		4.5	
Fat (g)	3.3	(30% of Cal)	6	(54% of Cal)
Including				
Essential Fatty Acid (mg, linoleate)	300	(2.7% of Cal)		
Vitamins				
A (μg, retinol equivalents)[c]	75		225	
D (μg, cholecalciferol)[d]	1		2.5	
K (μg)	4		—	
E (mg, tocopherol equivalents)[e]	0.5		—	
C (ascorbic acid) (mg)	8		—	
B_1 (thiamine) (μg)	40		—	
B_2 (riboflavin) (μg)	60		—	
B_6 (pyridoxine) (μg)	20	μg/g protein	—	
B_{12} (μg)	0.15		—	
Niacin (μg)	250	(or 0.8 mg niacin equivalents)	—	
Folic acid (μg)	4		—	
Pantothenic acid (μg)	300		—	
Biotin (μg)	1.5[f]		—	
Choline (mg)	7[f]		—	
Inositol (mg)	4[f]		—	

Minerals[g]

Calcium (mg)	60[b]		—
Phosphorus (mg)	30[b]		—
Magnesium (mg)	6		—
Iron (mg)	0.15		2.5[i]
Iodine (µg)	5		25
Zinc (mg)	0.5		—
Copper (µg)	60		—
Manganese (µg)	5		100
Selenium (µg)	3		—
Sodium (mg)	20	(5.8 mEq/l)	60 (17.5 mEq/L)
Potassium (mg)	80	(13.7 mEq/l)	200 (34.3 mEq/L)
Chloride (mg)	55	(10.4 mEq/l)	150 (28.3 mEq/L)

[a] Where no upper limit is given, toxicity is not well defined. However, the Task Force is concerned that massive excesses may have adverse consequences.

[b] At least nutritionally equivalent to casein, quality recommended as outlined in "Statement: Commentary on Breast Feeding and Infant Formulas, including Proposed Standards for Formulas." *Pediatrics* **57**, 278–285, 1976.

[c] Retinol Equivalents: 1 RE = 1 µg retinol or 6 µg B-carotene (1 RE = 3.33 IU vitamin activity from retinol).

[d] Cholecalciferol 1 µg = 40 IU vitamin D.

[e] α, tocopherol equivalents: 1 mg of dl-α-tocopherol = 0.74 α – tocopherol equivalent (or 1.1 IU); 1 mg of d-α-tocopherol = 1α – tocopherol equivalent (or 1.49 IU); 1 mg of d-α-tocopherol acetate = 0.91α – tocopherol equivalent (or 1.36 IU); 1 mg of d-α-tocopherol succinate = 0.81α – tocopherol equivalent (or 1.21 IU). At least 0.5 mg per d-α-tocopherol per gram linoleic acid.

[f] Average present in milk-base formulas; should be included in this amount in other formulas.

[g] Formula should be manufactured with water low in fluoride and should contain less than 45 µg/100 kcal. (For explanation see "Statement: Fluoride Supplementation: Revised Dosage Schedule." *Pediatrics* **63**, 150–152, 1979.) It is not technically feasible at this time to reduce fluoride below this amount in certain formulas.

[h] Calcium to phosphorus ratio should be no less than 1.1 nor more than 2.

[i] Prudence indicates there should be an upper limit for iron. Formula labeled "infant formula with iron" should contain not less than 1 mg iron/100 kcal.

comparison with the million years during which human infants could only be breast-fed. In recent years, however, breast feeding has been increasing.

THE RELATIONSHIP BETWEEN MILK AND NEONATAL INFECTIONS

There are several important lines of evidence supporting the protective role of breast milk against infectious agents, particularly diarrheal diseases of the newborn. Discussion of these data must include a distinction between colostrum and later milk and the significance of secretory IgA.

Many studies have clearly demonstrated that both colostrum and milk contain cellular and soluble immunologic factors that mediate specific and nonspecific mechanisms of defense against infectious agents. The soluble substances observed in human colostrum and milk include predominantly secretory component, 11 S (secretory) IgA, 7 S (serum) IgA, and some IgM and IgG, as well as IgE and IgD, the complement system, lactoferrin, lactoperoxidase, lysozyme, chemotactic factors, lipid-associated staphylococcal resistance factors, monoglycerides containing antiviral activity, α-1-antitrypsin, and protease inhibitors. In addition, a variety of other factors including macrophage MIF, IgA-stimulating factors, interferon, and T-cell immunosuppressive substances have been found. A number of cellular components have also been found in the products of lactation. These include monocytic phagocytes, macrophages, T cells, B lymphocytes and plasma cells, PMN leukocytes, and epithelial cells (Ogra *et al.,* 1979). These often have significant antimicrobial immunity (Tables VIII–X).

Table VIII

Distribution of Immunoglobulins and Other Soluble Substances in the Colostrum and Milk Delivered to the Breast-Fed Infant during a 24-hr Period[a]

Soluble product	Concentration in mg/day weeks postpartum			
	<1	1–2	3–4	>4
Immunoglobulin				
IgG	50	25	25	10
IgA	5000	1000	1000	1000
IgM	70	30	15	10
Lysozyme	50	60	60	100
Lactoferrin	1500	2000	2000	1200

[a]Reproduced with permission from Ogra *et al.* (1979).

Table IX

Spectrum of Antimicrobial Activity in Human Colostrum and Milk[a]

Bacteria	Viruses	Fungi
Enterobacteriaceae	Enteroviruses	*Candida*
E. coli enterotoxin	Polio 1, 2, 3	
Clostridium tetani	Coxsackie A, B	
Diphtheria	Echo 6, 9	
Streptococcus pneumoniae	Rotavirus	
Salmonella	Herpes simplex	
Staphylococcus aureus	Influenza	
Vibrio cholerae	Arboviruses	
	Simliki Forest	
	Ross River	
	Japanese B	
	Dengue	
	Rubella	
	Respiratory syncytial	

[a]Reproduced with permission from Ogra *et al.* (1979).

There are many mononuclear cells present in colostrum. For example, in one study, colostrum and breast milk samples were obtained from 74 women. The mean total leukocyte count in colostrum was 3190 cells per millimeter. The proportions of macrophages, PMN leukocytes, and lymphocytes varied widely, but macrophages usually predominated. Serial sampling of some women showed (1) a small fall in total counts through delivery, (2) a

Table X

Cellular Components of Prepartum
and Early Postpartum Colostrum[a]

Cell type	No. per mm³		% of total cells
	Range	Mean	Mean (range)
Macrophage	350–7000	2140	66 (37–93)
Polymorphs	10–900	560	21 (2–41)
Lymphocytes	20–390	240	11 (2–30)
Epithelial cell	Rare	Rare	(1–2)
Total cells	1100–8000	3400	—

[a]Reproduced with permission from Ogra *et al.*(1979).

fall in total counts and in the proportion of neutrophils at the onset of lactation, and (3) after 1–2 weeks the appearance of cytoplasmic fragments and epithelial cells as the major cell type. The total number of leukocytes available to the neonate remained approximately constant during the first 2 weeks of lactation and fell thereafter. The macrophages in colostrum and breast milk resembled macrophages elsewhere (Ho *et al.,* 1979).

Newborn babies with hematogenous infections between the 4th and 10th day of life were compared with matched controls with respect to breast milk consumption. The patient group consumed significantly less milk than did the controls, suggesting that breast milk protected the newborn against early infections by enteric bacteria (Winberg and Wessner, 1971).

Colostrum and milk from malnourished populations were evaluated for antibodies against selected bacterial and viral pathogens. IgA levels were high in colostrum (333 mg/100 ml) as well as later in the protracted weaning period (242 mg/100 ml) (Table XI). IgM was detectable in colostrum (36 mg/100 ml) but not after 4 weeks of lactation. Antibody titers against bacterial and viral pathogens were detected in colostrum and, less frequently, in milk. A correlation was observed between the levels and frequency of antibody titers with the pathogens of the population (Wyatt *et al.,* 1973).

Although B cells found in human milk can synthesize IgG and IgM, only IgA production is generally seen. These observations have suggested that there may be a specific factor capable of stimulating differentiation of IgA-

Table XI

Statistical Analysis of IgA Concentrations
in Colostrum and Milk

Duration of lactation	n	Mean	SD
Colostra (3 days)	35	333.2[b]	71.3
Milk (weeks)			
1	20	195.7[b]	42.9
2	17	166.3	23.0
3	17	158.3	30.7
4	15	147.8	15.0
5–16	14	152.1	21.4
17–52	8	144.4	24.9
>52	7	241.7[b]	111.7

[a]Reproduced with permission from Wyatt *et al.* (1973).

Table XII

Cellular Content of Breast Milk

Cells	Cell count $\times$ 10[6]/ml milk		
	Day 1 ($N = 13$)	Day 3 ($N = 16$)	Day 5 ($N = 6$)
Lymphocytes	0.77 ± 0.72[b]	0.29 ± 0.51	0.27 ± 0.36
Macrophages	2.55 ± 3.21	1.30 ± 2.37	0.75 ± 0.71
Neutrophils	5.04 ± 5.99	1.48 ± 1.89	0.38 ± 0.76

[a]Reproduced with permission from Pittard (1979).
[b]Mean ± SD.

bearing B cells. To investigate this possibility, Pittard studied lymphocytes and macrophages from early (<5 days) and late (>8 days) milk (Table XII). These cells were incubated, and aliquots of their cell-free culture media were added to peripheral blood lymphocyte cultures. The release of IgA, IgG, and IgM by the blood lymphocytes in culture was quantitated using double-antibody (Ab) competitive radioimmunoassays (Table XIII). The cell-free media from early (colostral) milk cell cultures significantly stimulated IgA synthesis and had no effect on the production of IgG or IgM. There was no effect on immunoglobulin production when the milk cell supernatant came from cells isolated from mature milk. Therefore, the authors proposed that a soluble mediator(s) of immunologic regulation is released by human milk cells, and that this factor(s) is released in greater amounts by colostral cells than by cells in mature milk (Pittard, 1979; Pittard and Bill, 1979).

Bacterial counts in the stools of breast-fed infants were found to differ quantitatively and qualitatively from those of bottle-fed newborns. For ex-

Table XIII

Immunoglobulin Release in PBL Cultures with Early Milk
(≤5 Days) Cell Supernate[a,b]

	PBL alone (ng)	With cell supernate, 100 μl (ng)
IgA	200 (40–3000)	420 (60–3680)[c]
IgG	128 (40–1240)	120 (40–445)
IgM	140 (40–700)	142 (60–572)

[a]Reproduced with permission from Pittard and Bill (1979).
[b]$n = 40$. Values represent median, with range indicated in parentheses.
[c]$p < .0001$.

Table XIV

Bacterial Counts from Stools of Breast-Fed and Bottle-Fed Infants[a]

Bacteria	Number of bacteria/g of stool obtained from infants at various times after birth							
	1 day		2 days		3 days		4 days	
	Breast fed	Bottle fed	Breast fed	Bottle fed	Breast fed	Bottle fed	Breast fed	Bottle fed
Coliforms	1×10^7[b]	2×10^8	$<10^6$	4×10^9	$<10^6$	4×10^{10}	2×10^8	3×10^{10}
Lactobacilli	$<10^6$	$<10^6$	2×10^7	$<10^6$	3×10^8	$<10^6$	5×10^9	$<10^6$
Gram-positive cocci	4×10^6	2×10^6	3×10^7	5×10^7	4×10^8	5×10^8	6×10^8	3×10^8

[a]Reproduced with permission from Michael et al. (1971).
[b]Numbers given are averages from 20 infants in each group.

Table XV

Levels of Immunoglobulin in Colostrum
during the First 4 Days After Delivery[a]

Immunoglobulin	Immunoglobulin (mg/100 ml)			
	1 day	2 days	3 days	4 days
IgA	600[b]	260	200	80
IgG	80	45	30	16
IgM	125	65	58	30

[a]Reproduced with permission from Michael *et al.*
(1971).

[b]Numbers given are averages from 10 samples in each
group.

ample, during the first week of life, the coliform flora of the breast-fed infants was depressed, while the lactobacilli were more abundant (Table XIV). The levels of IgG, IgM, and IgA were highest in the mothers' colostrum immediately after delivery, and they rapidly declined during the first 4 days (Table XV). The colostrum contained substantial amounts of antibodies to *Escherichia coli.* Agglutinating and bactericidal activity against strains of *E. coli* was also detected in saline extracts of the stool of breast-fed infants (Table XVI). A direct correlation between the concentrations of immunoglobulins and the reduction of coliform bacteria in the stools of breast-fed newborns was observed (Michael *et al.,* 1971). These observations take on further significance because of more recent data. Enteric virus-specific IgA and IgG present in human sera and colostrums were compared. As expected, virus-specific IgA was present in colostrum, but virus-specific IgG was not present. Colostrum neutralized poliovirus and reovirus (Tables XVII, XVIII) (Palmer *et al.,* 1980).

Bacteriostatic activity of milk-sensitive and milk-resistant strains of *E. coli* were reduced when secretory IgA was removed from milk. Further lysozyme can be removed without loss of activity. The heat-labile, antigen-cliciting, bacteriostatic antibody for *E. coli* crossreacts with the antigen in other bacteria, e.g., *Proteus* and *Enterobacter* (Dolby and Honour, 1979).

Milk from 150 local mothers has been assayed for bacteriostatic activity for milk-sensitive and milk-resistant indicator strains of *E. coli.* Activity is greatest in colostrum. One week after delivery, milk is active against the milk-sensitive strain and becomes active against the milk-resistant strain in the presence of physiological amounts of bicarbonate and iron-binding protein. This activity decreases within 2–4 days when milk is kept unheated at

Table XVI

Agglutinating Activity of Colostral Antibodies
to Various Strains of *E. coli*[a]

E. coli	Reciprocal titers of agglutinating antibodies on postpartum day			
	1	2	3	4
0127	1024[b]	1024	256	64
055	2048	1024	512	64
0111	256	256	64	16
No. 1	2048	2048	256	32
No. 2	512	256	64	32
No. 3	128	128	32	4

[a]Reproduced with permission from Michael *et al.*
(1971).
[b]Numbers given are averages from eight samples
in each group.

Table XVII

Immune Response to Poliovirus[a]

Patient	ELISA antipoliovirus type 1 IgA or IgG in colostrum or serum			Poliovirus-neutralizing antibody in colostrum and serum	
	Colostrum IgA	Colostrum IgG	Serum IgG	Colostrum	Serum
1	8	—	32	8	32
2	—[b]	—	—	32	32
3	16	—	16	8	32
4	32	—	32	64	64
5	—	—	32	10	32
6	20	—	32	40	64
7	32	—	32	8	32
8	—	—	32	16	128
9	32	—	64	8	16
10	—	—	32	—	64
11	16	—	64	8	16
IgA pool				16	

[a]Reproduced with permission from Palmer *et al.* (1980).
[b]Denotes titer of <8.

Table XVIII

Immune Response to Reovirus[a]

	ELISA antireovirus type 1 IgA or IgG in colostrum or serum			Reovirus-neutralizing antibody in colostrum and serum	
Patient	Colostrum IgA	Colostrum IgG	Serum IgG	Colostrum	Serum
1	8	—	8	8	16
2	—[b]	—	16	4	8
3	8	—	16	4	8
4	16	—	64	4	8
5	10	—	128	—	16
6	20	—	32	—	4
7	8	—	8	4	4
8	8	—	64	—	4
9	32	—	64	—	16
10	—	QNS[c]	QNS	4	16
11	8	—	8	8	4
IgA pool	8				

[a]Reproduced with permission from Palmer et al. (1980).
[b]Denotes titer of <8.
[c]Quantity not sufficient.

4°C, but is preserved for at least 4 months and often up to 2 years in milk heated to 56°C and then stored at 4°C, or in milk frozen, unheated, at −28°C, provided it is not repeatedly thawed and frozen. Later-lactation milks are usually indistinguishable in activity from 1-week postpartum milk, but may be less stable on storage, particularly if frozen.

Human milk contains antibodies of the sIgA (secretory IgA) type against a variety of enteropathic viruses and food proteins. There seems to be a close link between the specific immune response in the mammary gland and the antigenic exposure in the intestine. As a consequence of this relationship, IgA provides protection against enteric microorganisms (Hanson et al., 1977). Similar data have been obtained in other studies. Breast milk samples from 74 women at different stages of lactation were analyzed for leukocyte concentration and bactericidal activity. The total leukocyte count in colostrum was 5000/mm, a concentration similar to that in circulation. As lactation became established, there was a decrease in leukocyte concentration to 2000/mm after 3 months. Neutrophils and macrophages constituted 90 95% of cells. The bactericidal activity of these cells was similar to that of circulating leukocytes. The total leukocyte concentration and the bactericidal capacity were similar in well-nourished and undernourished women. Thus, the protective factors of milk are not influenced by the nutritional status of the mother (Bhaskaram and Reddy, 1981).

Lactoferrin is often considered to be involved in the bacteriostatic effect of human milk on *E. coli.* In one study, milk from different individuals differed in its ability to produce bacteriostasis of three pathogenic serotypes of *E. coli.* The bacteriostatic effect was stable to heating at 60°C for 35 min. The bacterial iron-transporting compound, enterochelin, abolished the bacteriostatic effect of human milk. IgA was isolated from the milk samples in two forms that appeared to differ in molecular weight. When mixed with lactoferrin, some of these fractions induced bacteriostasis, which could be reversed by the Fc fragment. The authors concluded that the mechanism of bacteriostasis was identical in serum and milk (Rogers and Synge, 1978).

Bottle-fed infants do not gain weight as rapidly as breast-fed babies during the first week of life. This weight lag can be corrected by the addition of a small amount of alkali to the feed. The alkali corrects the acidity of cow's milk, which now assumes some of the properties of human breast milk. For example, it has a bacteriostatic effect on specific *E. coli in vitro,* and in infants it produces a stool with a preponderance of lactobacilli over *E. coli* organisms. When alkali is removed from the milk, there is a decrease in the infant's weight and the stools contain excessive numbers of *E. coli* bacteria. Alkali-corrected cow's milk is more physiological than unaltered cow's milk and may provide some protection against neonatal gastroenteritis. The bacteriostatic effect on specific *E. coli* may be of practical significance in feed preparations when terminal sterilization and refrigeration are not available (Harrison and Peat, 1972).

Finally, food allergy should be considered. Food antigens are taken up in immunologically considerable quantities, and antibody responses occur especially in patients with an atopic history. There are presumably elaborate control systems, but since they are poorly understood, their possible defects, which would be expected to contribute to food allergy, are even less clear. Some clinical observations, however, are providing certain indications; for example, there is growing evidence that feeding breast milk may delay the appearance of significant allergies.

12

Alcohol and Immune Function

INTRODUCTION

The effects of alcohol on immune responsiveness have been very difficult to define. Furthermore, experimental data are filled with inconsistencies. Although alcohol should be properly considered only as a pharmacological substance, it must also be viewed as an integral dietary constituent of many persons. In some individuals, particularly those suffering from chronic alcoholism, ethanol intake, with a value of 7 kcal/g, may represent the major form of caloric intake. This, of course, is a serious problem, not only in terms of the metabolic and psychological consequences in alcoholic patients but also because it reflects a substantial nutritional problem. Because alcoholic beverages contain few nutrients other than ethanol, the heavy drinker is forced to obtain all essential nutrients from the remainder of the diet. In addition, chronic ethanol intake has been implicated as a contributory factor in a variety of other physiological alterations including anorexia, malabsorption, and alterations in gastric and intestinal mobility. These latter factors reduce the availability of the already markedly limited nutrient supply of the alcoholic. The social and economic conditions that frequently accompany alcoholism are seldom conducive to the provision of a nutritionally adequate diet. These same parameters of socioeconomic status also generally result in poor overall health care; thus, the pathology and deficient nutriture accompanying alcoholism may go undetected for prolonged periods of time.

When considering the influence of alcohol on the immune response, it is important to distinguish between the direct toxic influences of ethanol and the effects of the nutritional deficiencies that may occur in the chronic alcoholic. Many of the studies of human alcoholics have not considered the nutritional status of the patients and therefore have failed to distinguish between these two factors. A further consideration is the influence of chronic alcoholism on the host's metabolic function. This is most apparent in the effects of ethanol on the liver and vice versa; nonetheless, other organs such as the stomach, small intestine, pancreas, and kidneys may also be damaged by chronic exposure to ethanol or by elevated levels of ethanol metabolic breakdown products such as acetaldehyde (Geokas *et al.,* 1972).

Alcoholic patients experience a wide variety of hepatic lesions ranging from fatty liver to hepatitis and cirrhosis. Immunological mechanisms have been frequently proposed as contributory factors in the pathological complications that occur secondary to chronic alcoholism. The compromised function of the liver has important implications not only for direct host immunocompetence but also for host nutriture, and thereby host immunological function.

ALCOHOL AND INFECTIOUS DISEASE

Nearly two centuries have passed since medical scientists began to postulate that there was a correlation between consumption of alcohol and increased susceptibility to a variety of infectious maladies, most notably respiratory ailments such as pneumonia and tuberculosis. Most early observations were anecdotal, but still served to establish firmly the connection between ethanol intake, especially when chronic, and infectious disease. Unfortunately, time has done little to alter the general situation with regard to studies of infectious complications of alcoholism. For example, many studies document a high proportion of alcoholics among patients suffering from tuberculosis, particularly in the general medical wards of public hospitals (Jones *et al.,* 1954). The latter, without any attempt to study control populations, have frequently been accepted as conclusive evidence that alcoholism alone predisposes to infectious disease. In addition, very little consideration has been given to controlling for other environmental factors that may also influence susceptibility to infection in chronic alcoholics, such as poor housing conditions, lack of medical care, inattention to medical problems even if such care is available, and concomitant use of illicit drugs and tobacco (Jones *et al.,* 1954). Nonetheless, there has been widespread acceptance of such an interaction, despite the fact that the statistical and epidemiological data to substantiate these clinical studies of alcohol and infectious disease have been, at best, weak and, at worst, totally lacking. Moreover, because of the widespread acceptance of this association despite the lack of reliable data, the necessary definitive clinical studies in this area have never been undertaken.

Studies on chronic alcohol intake and the epidemiology of infectious disease have been summarized and will not be covered in detail here (Tapper, 1980). The two diseases most frequently associated with long-term alcohol intake are bacterial penumonia and tuberculosis. While many of the early studies of these associations failed to characterize the specific pathogen associated with the lobar pneumonia frequently found in alcoholic patients, it is presumed that, in most cases, the etiologic agent responsible for disease was *Streptococcus pneumoniae*, a common pathogen found under such circumstances. Other organisms that have also been associated with pneumonia in alcoholics are *Haemophilus influenzae, Escherichia coli, Pseudomonas aeruginosa, Klebsiella pneumoniae. Bacteroides* spp, *Proteus* spp, *Achromobacter* spp., and some strains of anaerobic bacteria.

The other major disease entity that has been most strongly correlated with chronic intake of ethanol is tuberculosis. For instance, Jones *et al.* found the incidence of tuberculosis in skid-row alcoholics to be greater than 55 times that of normal residents of the same city during the same time period (Jones *et al.*, 1954). In addition, some studies have indicated not only that alcoholics are susceptible to a greater incidence of tuberculosis but also that its severity, especially among those with advanced pulmonary disease, may also be significantly greater (Holmdahl, 1967). Indeed, it has been suggested that such alcoholic populations tend to be major foci of harbored tuberculosis infections, thus continuing to infect the population at large (Fergus and Jackson, 1959). Chronic alcoholism has also been associated with both spontaneous bacteremia (Tisdale, 1961) and spontaneous bacterial peritonitis. However, in many of these cases, the disease process was complicated by trauma or surgical manipulations.

Acute pancreatitis and pancreatic abscess are both recognized as frequent sequelae of long-term, excessive intake of ethanol (Geokas *et al.*, 1972). A significant number of alcoholic patients may develop severe infectious complications when such pancreatic lesions fail to resolve spontaneously; substantial mortality may result (Warshaw, 1972). Finally, alcoholism has been noted as a predisposing factor in infectious endocarditis (Buchbinder and Roberts, 1973). In fact, a common tetrad in a subset of patients includes chronic alcoholism, pneumococcal endocarditis, pneumonitis, and meningitis. As noted above, the causative organism in most cases has proven to be *S. pneumoniae* (Buchbinder and Roberts, 1973).

One study has cast considerable doubt on the observation that chronic alcoholism per se predisposes to an increased incidence of infection (Bienia *et al.*, 1982). Alcoholic and nonalcoholic patients were compared to determine the incidence of infection, anemia, skin test anergy, total lymphocyte count, and mortality rate. This study was unable to detect any difference between these two populations with regard to any of these parameters (Bienia *et al.*, 1982). The lack of correlation held not only with regard to overall rates of infection but also specifically with respect to respiratory infections such as pneumonia and tuberculosis. However, the investigators did find that in either the alcoholic or the nonalcoholic population, malnutrition (as determined by alterations in at least two of the following parameters: serum albumin, serum transferrin, muscle circumference, or percent weight for height), was a critical factor in patient outcome (Bienia *et al.*, 1982). In both chronic alcoholics and their hospitalized control counterparts, malnutrition correlated closely with decreased total lymphocyte count, skin test anergy, an increased rate of infection, and, most importantly, an increased death rate (Bienia *et al.*, 1982).

STUDIES IN ANIMALS

A number of studies of experimental animals have involved challenge with a variety of pathogens after various periods and degrees of experimental alcoholization (Caren *et al.*, 1983). Alcoholized mice that inhaled a mist containing aerosolized bacteria such as *S. pyogenes, H. influenzae,* and *S. pneumoniae* experienced delayed clearance of bacteria, particularly pneumococci (Stillman, 1924). In addition, these alcoholized mice exhibited an increased frequency of infection, both locally (pneumonia) and systemically (bacteremia). In mice given ethanol, the bacteremia occurred much more rapidly and with greater frequency than in nonalcoholized controls (Stillman, 1924). More recent studies have shown that intake of ethanol apparently has a notable effect on certain strains of pathogenic organisms, while other strains are not affected. For instance, when cultures of mixed bacteria were inhaled by alcoholized mice, the clearance of *S. aureus* continued, although at a somewhat reduced rate, but the killing of *Proteus mirabilis* was almost completely inhibited (Green and Green, 1968). Thus, alcohol administration was capable of selectively inhibiting the clearance of specific bacterial pathogens, perhaps mediated by an influence on pulmonary alveolar macrophages, thus allowing bacterial proliferation. Similar mechanisms may be operative in the oropharynx of alcoholics, where selective inhibition of the removal of certain strains of pathogenic organisms may lead to the persistent carriage of gram-negative organisms, most notably various *Klebsiella* spp. (Mackowiak *et al.*, 1976). This condition may lead the oropharynx to act as a focus of infective organisms that continually seed, leading to subsequent infection in the tissues of the lower respiratory tract.

Some studies have elucidated the role of ethanol in altering susceptibility to a broader spectrum of organisms, including numerous viruses. In a study of acute alcoholization in mice, administration of ethanol resulted in an increased susceptibility to both influenza and encephalomyocarditis viruses, but only when the ethanol was administered after the inoculation of

Table I

Effects of Acute Alcoholization on EMC Virus Titers in Brains of Infected Mice[a]

		Virus titers (TCID 50/ml)				
		0.2 ml 40° GL ethanol[b]			0.5 ml 40° GL ethanol	
Days after infection	Control	30 min before infection	30 min after infection	Control	30 min before infection	30 min after infection
1	$<10^3$	$<10^3$	$<10^3$	$<10^3$	$<10^3$	$<10^3$
2	$<10^3$	$<10^3$	2.1×10^4	$<10^3$	$<10^3$	$<10^3$
3	2.9×10^6	$<10^3$	2.4×10^8	$<10^3$	$<10^3$	2.9×10^3
4	10^3	6.8×10^7	2.9×10^6	2.9×10^6	$<10^3$	2.9×10^6
5				2.1×10^5	3.7×10^8	4.2×10^7

[a]Reproduced with permission from Cotte *et al.,* 1982.
[b]Gay-Lussac (GL)-ethanol.

the virus (Cotte *et al.,* 1982) (Tables I–III). Mortality was substantially increased when ethanol was administered in this fashion; whereas 16.7% of the control animals died, 43.0% of the alcoholized mice died when ethanol was administered after virus inoculation (Cotte *et al.,* 1982) (Figs. 1, 2). However, no dose–response relationship was observed in this interaction. In contrast, alcohol administration after viral inoculation with herpes or vaccinia virus had no effect on the disease process. Moreover, administration of ethanol prior to viral inoculation had no significant impact on the pathogenesis of any of the viruses studied. This lack of effect of ethanol when administered before virus inoculation may have been due to alterations in virus dissemination in the alcoholized host. On the other hand, the enhanced viral proliferation with the administration of ethanol after inocu-

Table II

Effects of Acute Alcoholization on EMC Virus Titers in Spleen of Infected Mice[a]

		Virus titers (TCID 50/ml)				
		0.2 ml 40° GL ethanol		0.5 ml 40° GL ethanol	
Days after infection	Control	30 min before infection	30 min after infection	30 min before infection	30 min after infection
3	3.3×10^3	4.3×10^3	6.8×10^4	4.2×10^3	10^4
4	4.2×10^3	6.8×10^3	6.8×10^4	4.2×10^3	4.2×10^4
5	6.8×10^4	3.2×10^3	3.3×10^4	2.4×10^4	4.2×10^4

[a]Reproduced with permission from Cotte *et al.* (1982).

Table III

Effects of Acute Alcoholization on Mice Viremia after EMC Virus Infection[a]

Days after infection	Virus titers (TCID 50/ml)					
	0.2 ml 40° GL ethanol			0.5 ml 40° GL ethanol		
	Control	30 min before infection	30 min after infection	Control	30 min before infection	30 min after infection
2	$<10^2$	3×10^2	4.2×10^2			
3	2.4×10^4		2.1×10^4	3.3×10^3	3.3×10^4	1.5×10^4
4	$<10^2$	2.9×10^4	1.7×10^2	2.4×10^3	2.4×10^3	3.1×10^4
5				$<10^2$	1.7×10^3	3.2×10^4

[a]Reproduced with permission from Cotte *et al.* (1982).

lation with the virus may have been due to alterations in host immune responsiveness. In this study, the reticuloendothelial system was most markedly affected, whereas the impact on cell-mediated immunity was questionable. Indeed, as noted, there was no effect on herpes or vaccinia virus infections, which are primarily affected by cell-mediated host immune defenses. Alcoholization may also affect host susceptibility to viral infection by causing hypothermia, a factor known to result in enhanced viral growth (Carmichael and Barnes, 1969).

Ethical considerations preclude challenge of alcoholic patients with pathogenic organisms. However, some useful data have been generated in the study of the response of alcoholic and control patients to endotoxin. Patients with a history of chronic excessive ethanol intake, but without overt manifestations of alcoholic liver disease, were injected with endotoxin. Administration of endotoxin, using three doses of LPS purified from *Salmonella abortus,* resulted in a significant decrease in the incremental rise in the number of white blood cells appearing in peripheral blood as compared with the response of similar nonalcoholic controls (McFarland and Libre, 1963). Withdrawal of the ethanol from these patients resulted in a prompt improvement (i.e., within 20 days). The investigators in this latter study felt that a deficient granulocyte reserve was the basis of the ineffective response. This hypothesis was based on observation of bone marrow morphology, including decreased cellularity and an arrest of cellular maturation. A deficient granulocyte reserve in these patients may be easily exhausted in the face of infectious challenge, thereby contributing to the higher rates of morbidity in alcoholics (McFarland and Libre, 1963). Finally, it is important to consider the interactions of alcohol with other drugs (Watson *et al.,* 1983).

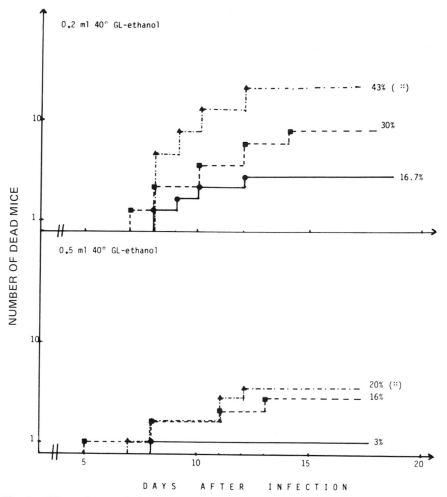

Fig. 1. Effects of acute alcohol intoxication on the mortality of mice infected with influenza virus. ●, control; ■, ethanol before infection; ▲, ethanol after infection; *, .02 < *p* < .05. (Reproduced with permission from Cotte *et al.*, 1982.)

ETHANOL AND HUMORAL IMMUNITY

Virtually no data exist regarding the influence of ethanol intake on B-cell function and humoral immune responses. Nonetheless, it has been suggested that alcohol has a substantial impact on humoral immune responses because of the hypergammaglobulinemia frequently found in alcoholic patients. This assumption is not valid, since it does not reflect responses to

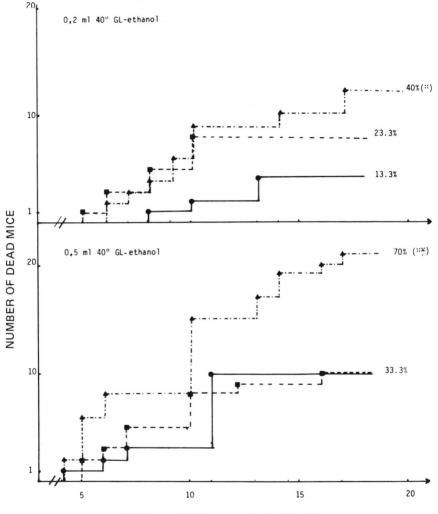

Fig. 2. Effects of actue alcohol intoxication on the mortality of mice infected with encephalomyocarditis virus. ●, control; ■, ethanol before infection; ▲, ethanol after infection; **, .01 < p < .02; *, .02 < p < .05. (Reproduced with permission from Cotte *et al.,* 1982.)

specific antigenic challenges. Hypergammaglobulinemia may merely reflect the increased antigenic encounters in the chronically alcoholic host or may reflect chronic liver disease. When specific antigenic challenges have been studied, the results have proven highly variable, with alcoholization resulting in the elevation of antibody titers in response to certain antigens (Havens *et al.,* 1954) and depression of the response to other antigens

(Gluckman *et al.,* 1977) (Table IV). There is clearly a need to study the influence of acute ethanol intake on the antibody response to specific antigenic challenge.

One study has considered the influence of longer-term alcoholization on humoral immunity in experimental animals. In rats treated with ethanol for 3 months, fatty liver but not cirrhosis was observed (Tennenbaum *et al.,* 1969). Such rats exhibited a delay in antibody formation in response to primary immunization with either *B. abortus* or typhoid H antigens. Such a delay in the appearance of normal antibody titers could alter the ability of the animal to respond to bacterial challenge, particularly if it occurs during the early periods of pathogen dissemination. Nonetheless, peak antibody titers were not significantly lower than those observed in nonalcoholic control animals. Likewise, there were no significant differences in the secondary responses to typhoid H antigens when a booster dose was administered at 28 days postprimary injection (Tennenbaum *et al.,* 1969). However, from these relatively preliminary observations, it is difficult to ascertain what effects ethanol might have on the host's response to actual pathogenic challenge, as mediated by alterations in host humoral immunity.

Most of the investigations on the influence of alcohol on humorally mediated immunity have been conducted among human populations in clinical settings. Thus, most studies were poorly controlled, and because of numerous intervening factors, e.g., nutritional or socioeconomic status, the results have frequently proven difficult to interpret. The major parameter that has confounded these studies has been the variable degree of liver disease in such patients. Only a few studies have been conducted in alcoholic patients without alcoholic liver disease. In alcoholic patients in whom liver disease was either mild or absent according to established clinical criteria (i.e., 71% of the patients had either one or no abnormal measurements of hepatic

Table IV

Keyhole Limpet Hemocyanin (KLH) Antibody Titer: Changes After Antigen Exposure[a]

Patient group (Number of patients)	Titer change	Comment
Controlled drinking alcoholics (5)	No change in three One-tube rise in two	Received KLH while drinking on CRC[b] maximum of one-tube titer rise
Controlled drinking alcoholic (1)	Three-tube rise	Received KLH 3 days after stopping drinking
Normal volunteers (9)	Three-tube rise in three Four-tube rise in six	No drinking

[a]Reproduced with permission from Gluckman *et al.* (1977).
[b]Clinical Research Center.

function) investigators found no change in the levels of circulating B cells (Lundy *et al.,* 1975). Other investigators found elevated levels of B cells in peripheral blood of alcoholics without complicating liver disease (Bernstein *et al.,* 1974). Moreover, the response of such B cells to pokeweed mitogen was within normal ranges. Serum levels of IgG, IgA, and IgM were all significantly elevated in such alcoholics (Lundy *et al.,* 1975). When treatment was instituted, there was some return of serum immunoglobulin levels toward normal values. In another study, in noncirrhotic alcoholics who were hospitalized in a controlled environment, the authors found a poor antibody response to immunization with keyhole limpet hemocyanin (Gluckman *et al.,* 1977). Thus, in patients with overt clinical symptoms of liver disease, it would appear that humoral immunity may be variably altered depending on which aspect of immunity is monitored. Beyond this, little is known regarding the impact of ethanol on humoral immune responsiveness when hepatic manifestations are absent. Further well-controlled studies will be required to establish the nature of such a relationship.

In patients with advanced alcoholic liver disease, one of the hallmarks of the disease process is hypergammaglobulinemia; such patients often present with a reversal of the albumin/globulin ratio (Triger and Wright, 1973). As demonstrated by experiments utilizing ^{131}I-labeled human γ globulin, such hypergammaglobulinemia is due largely to increased synthesis rather than decreased catabolism (Havens *et al.,* 1954). In these patients, changes in both lymph nodes and spleen have also been found, e.g., enlargement and increased numbers of AFC; these findings suggest elevated antibody production (Glagov *et al.,* 1959). Elevated titers of antibodies to a variety of infectious agents have also been documented (Triger and Wright, 1973); in addition, it is possible that the response to autoantigens may contribute to the hypergammaglobulinemia. Two possible basic mechanisms have been suggested: (1) the alcoholic host may be subjected to a hyperactive immune state, or (2) there may be an increased antigenic stimulation in the host. Because the alcoholic liver disease may involve considerable necrosis, an adjuvant effect may be produced by the breakdown products of liver cells. However, this cannot explain the hypergammaglobulinemia seen in chronic inactive alcoholic cirrhosis.

The anatomic position of the liver has been emphasized to play a central role in the hypergammaglobulinemia observed in alcoholic liver disease (Triger and Wright, 1973). A large variety of antigens arrive in the liver after absorption from the gastrointestinal tract and subsequent passage via the portal system. Because of its central position, the liver regulates the quantity of antigen that reaches the systemic circulation. This has major implications. For example, it has been shown that prior feeding of a hapten suppresses cell-mediated immunity to a subsequent injection with the same hapten.

Moreover, this effect can be abrogated by a prior portocaval anastamosis (Cantor and Dumont, 1967). It has therefore been suggested that alcoholic liver disease damages the physiologic immunosuppressive process of the liver, upsetting the overall immunological balance. Thus, the hypergammaglobulinemia seen in alcoholic liver disease may reflect a failure of the liver to sequester foreign antigens properly (Triger *et al.,* 1972a,b). Such antigenic overload may result from a direct toxic effect on the phagocytic Kupffer cells that populate hepatic tissues, or may possibly result from saturation of the phagocytic abilities of these cells by tissue damage breakdown products. A further possibility is that the antigen that has been sequestered by Kupffer cells may be released into the bloodstream as a result of direct damage caused by alcoholic liver disease. The role of Kupffer cells is to sequester antigen rather than to process it, as do other macrophages. An additional problem may be that the inability of the Kupffer cells to sequester antigen may lead to an increase in the antigen/antibody ratio for a number of antigens, leading to an increase in immune complex formation. In alcoholic liver disease, the ability of the liver to clear such immune complexes may be impaired, leading to the deposition of immune complexes in other organs such as the kidney (Triger and Wright, 1973).

A major school of thought regarding the hypergammaglobulinemia in alcoholic liver disease patients supports the concept of altered antigen clearance by hepatic tissues leading to increased frequency of antigenic encounters, especially with antigens of enteric origin. Many patients with chronic active liver disease had elevated titers to *Salmonella* even though they had negative bacterial cultures for this bacterium (Protell *et al.,* 1971). In another study, patients with active liver disease, especially those with chronic active hepatitis, had significantly elevated titers of antibodies to *E. coli* and *Bacteroides spp.* (Triger *et al.,* 1972a). In contrast, no elevation in the titer of antibodies to *H. influenzae* was observed. These investigators also noted increased γ globulin formation in response to dietary antigens, e.g., gluten fraction III in patients with either cirrhosis or acute hepatitis, and to lactalbumin in patients with cirrhosis (Triger *et al.,* 1972a). However, no patients with such liver disease exhibited elevated antibody titers to ovalbumin or lactoglobulin. The authors suggest that the elevation of antibody titers to these bacterial antigens may be related to pathogenic organisms that originate in the gastrointestinal tract. The elevated titers of antibody to the enteric organisms support the hypothesis that the diseased liver may be defective in sequestering antigens, thereby allowing these antigens to circulate and travel to tissues where significant antibody formation can occur (Triger *et al.,* 1972a). It should be pointed out, however, that only a single nonenteric organism has been tested. Additionally, this hypothesis fails to explain the lack of responsiveness to ovalbumin and lactoglobulin.

Nonetheless, similar findings have been reported by others (Bjorneboe and Prytz, 1972). Patients with alcoholic cirrhosis had particularly high numbers of positive agglutination reactions to a battery of *E. coli* antigens. Moreover, the reactive state was most pronounced in patients with alcoholic cirrhosis and portacaval shunts. These studies support the concept that the alcoholic liver is defective in antigen sequestration function, thereby allowing an increased rate of antigenic encounter and subsequent antibody formation. However, all findings have not supported this hypothesis.

Triger *et al.* (1972b) have found increased titers of antibody to both rubella and measles viruses in patients with a variety of chronic active hepatic diseases. Viral antigens such as these are associated with viremia and therefore may be hepatically sequestered, such sequestration forming an important line of host defense (Triger and Wright, 1973). In contrast, no such increases in titers of antibodies to *Herpes simplex, Mycoplasma pneumoniae,* or enteroviruses were observed (Triger *et al.,* 1972b). Moreover, patients with diagnosed alcoholic cirrhosis did not appear to have elevated antibody titers to any of the pathogenic organisms studied. These results suggest that the influence of alcoholic liver disease on humoral immune responsiveness may be a complex phenomenon. The concept of ineffective hepatic sequestration of antigens originating in the gastrointestinal tract may not necessarily account for most of the observed hypergammaglobulinemia.

The mechanism of hypergammaglobulinemia in alcoholic liver disease has been investigated in other ways. First, the immunoglobulin class or subclass specificity was studied; elevations in the serum concentrations of all types of immunoglobulins were noted (Wilson *et al.,* 1969). While selective deficiency of serum IgA was observed in a limited number of patients with a long history of alcoholism and cirrhosis (Wilson *et al.,* 1968), it was not established that this was related to alcoholism. In most patients with alcoholic liver disease, serum IgA levels are elevated (Wilson *et al.,* 1969). It was noted that, in general, concentrations of serum immunoglobulins increase with the severity of the disease (Wilson *et al.,* 1969). Wilson and co-workers also found that the elevations in the IgG_3 subclass were related to individual genetic differences concerning the Gm system (Gm type refers to a group of genetically determined antigenic differences detectable on the heavy chains of IgG). The authors suggested that this supports the hypothesis of defective immune regulation in these patients, but the data have not received further attention.

The second major means of assessing humoral immunity in patients afflicted with alcoholic liver disease has been to challenge these individuals with a specific antigen. Havens *et al.* presented data supporting the concept of immunological hyperreactivity in alcoholics with chronic liver disease, as demonstrated by increased production of antibodies in response to tetanus toxoid administration. They found persistently high titers of tetanus antitoxin in the peripheral blood of alcoholics. In addition, a very vigorous secondary response to a booster dose of tetanus toxoid was observed (Havens *et al.,* 1957). However, further studies by other investigators utilizing an injection of tetanus toxoid in patients with and without cirrhosis found no difference in the response to this antigen (Cherrick *et al.,* 1959). It should be pointed out, however, that a smaller proportion of these cirrhotic patients were alcoholics than in the previously documented study. In addition, the antigen employed in the latter investigation might have been more highly purified. This lack of difference in response to specific antigenic challenge in patients with alcoholic liver disease favors the hypothesis that the hypergammaglobulinemia is a reflection of increased antigenic load rather than immunological hyperreactivity (Bjorneboe *et al.,* 1970).

ETHANOL AND CELL-MEDIATED IMMUNITY

Confusion regarding the influence of either acute ethanol intake or chronic alcoholism, with or without concomitant liver disease, is also found in studies of alcohol and cell-mediated immunity (Tables V and VI). While numerous clinical studies have been conducted in both acute and chronic ethanolization, few have been adequately controlled and many of the results border on the anecdotal. They provide some knowledge regarding the effects of alcohol on cell-mediated immunity, but there is considerable need for more definitive studies.

A single study in rats, which had developed fatty liver but did not show

Table V

Effect of Prolonged Alcohol Consumption on Delayed Hypersensitivity Responses[a]

		Response (mm)		
Patient	Antigen with greatest response	Control period	Alcohol period	KLH sensitization
1	PPD	35	22	4
2	PPD	21	21	4
3	*Candida*	19	13	0
4	*Candida*	18	29	NT[b]
5	*Candida*	32	18	0
6	*Candida*	52	52	5[c]

[a]Reproduced with permission from Gluckman *et al.* (1977).
[b]Not tested.
[c]Exposed while not consuming alcohol.

Table VI

Correlation of *in Vivo* and *in Vitro* Tests[a]

Antigen	p	Positive skin test		Migration inhibition		Blastogenesis with 2-[^{14}C]thymidine	
		Group A[b]	Group B[c]	Group A	Group B	Group A	Group B
PPD		24 (31)[d]	10 (13)	6 (11)	3 (6)	8 (9)	4 (5)
SK-SD	<.05	14 (31)	11 (13)	5 (13)	4 (7)	6 (9)	3 (5)
Candida		21 (31)	8 (13)	5 (13)	0 (6)	7 (9)	3 (5)
Mumps vaccine	<.05	3 (27)	5 (10)	—	—	—	—
Croton oil		22 (25)	12 (13)	—	—	—	—
DNCB	<.01	6 (25)	9 (9)	—	—	—	—
PHA		—	—	8 (13)	5 (7)	9 (9)	5 (5)

[a]Reproduced with permission from Berenyi *et al.* (1974).
[b]Group A, alcoholic liver disease.
[c]Group B, chronic alcoholism.
[d]Numbers in parentheses, total number of patients tested.

evidence of cirrhosis after 3 months of daily alcoholization, demonstrated a depressed delayed-type hypersensitivity response to 2,4-dinitrofluoroben-zene (Tennenbaum *et al.*, 1969). Marked thymic atrophy and significantly smaller spleens were found in these alcoholized animals. The changes did not appear to be due to hypertrophy of the adrenal cortex and consequent adrenal hyperactivity (Tennenbaum *et al.*, 1969). Beyond this, the influence of alcohol intake, without serious hepatic complications, has not been examined in animal models.

The elevated incidence of a variety of neoplasia led many investigators to suspect that alcoholism might principally affect cell-mediated immunity, a major line of postulated host defense against tumor cells (Hakulinen *et al.*, 1974; Lundy *et al.*, 1975). Lundy *et al.* examined patients who were generally free of alcoholic liver disease, i.e., 71% showed one or fewer indications of hepatic dysfunction. Such patients exhibited a significant decrease in the percentage of circulating T lymphocytes (Lundy *et al.*, 1975). However, such findings have not always been uniform (Bernstein *et al.*, 1974). In these same patients, the blastogenic response of peripheral blood lympho-cytes to the mitogens concanavalin A and phytohemagglutinin was substan-tially reduced (Lundy *et al.*, 1975). Most of these parameters returned to normal ranges when an appropriate therapeutic regimen was introduced. While some of these patients did have significantly low serum folate levels, there was no correlation between these low levels and the observed aber-rant cell-mediated immunological function. Because these patients had either minimal or no liver disease, these data tend to support the hypothesis of a direct toxic effect on the lymphoid system, e.g., ethanol may have either a direct toxic effect on circulating peripheral blood T lymphocytes or a substantial negative impact on the formation and/or maturation of such cells, rather than an intermediate effect via liver disease.

These parameters of cellular immunity have also been investigated by others. Volunteers were given 0.75 liter ethanol per day in the form of 100-proof whiskey (Gluckman *et al.,* 1977) (Table V). In these alcoholized patients, the investigators were unable to establish delayed-type hypersensitivity to the administration of keyhole limpet hemocyanin. Failure to establish delayed-type hypersensitivity to dinitrochlorobenzene has also been noted in chronic alcoholics without liver disease (Berenyi *et al.,* 1974; Gluckman *et al.,* 1977) (Table VI, Fig. 3). The influence of ethanol on the response of mitogens has also been studied by a number of groups. Tisman and Herbert (1973) tested the response of peripheral blood lymphocytes obtained from a variety of patients to both phytohemagglutinin and streptolysin 0 after exposure to ethanol of concentrations in the range of 200–

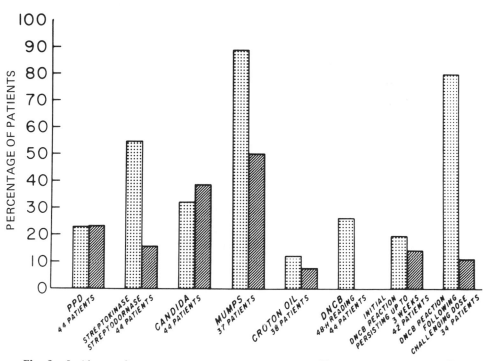

Fig. 3. Incidence of negative response to dermal antigens. ▦, alcoholic liver disease; ▨, chronic alcoholism. (Reproduced with permission from Berenyi *et al.,* 1974.)

300 mg/ml, levels frequently observed in heavily intoxicated individuals. These investigators found a significant suppression of lymphocyte transformation in response to these mitogens when ethanol was introduced (Tisman and Herbert, 1973). Moreover, provision of large quantities of folate and other vitamins failed to correct this immunosuppression, thus supporting the concept of a direct toxic effect of alcohol on T lymphocytes.

However, such results have not been obtained by all groups. Berenyi et al. (1974) found no such decrease in response to phytohemagglutinin in vitro in peripheral blood lymphocytes obtained from chronic alcoholic patients without evidence of concomitant liver disease. A normal lymphocyte transformation response to mitogens was noted even in those patients with a faulty delayed-type hypersensitivity response to dinitrochlorobenzene (Berenyi et al., 1974). Because of the in vitro nature of the test for mitogen responsiveness, these results do not rule out the presence of inhibitory factor(s) in the serum of patients suffering from chronic alcoholism that might alter the expression of cell-mediated immunity in vivo (possibly explaining the disparity between the delayed-type hypersensitivity and mitogen responsiveness results). In addition, these patients were not screened for nutritional status; therefore, either overt or subclinical nutritional deficiencies may have influenced some of the observed results, e.g., the notable degree of anergy. Significant differences in the degree of alcoholization may have contributed to the variation in results obtained in these studies. In addition, tests of lymphocyte transformation are inherently variable, and these discrepancies may reflect significant differences in the culture conditions employed by different groups of investigators. While the overall results are far from conclusive, there is significant evidence that cell-mediated immunity may be strongly affected by ethanol even when alcoholism has not yet resulted in overt liver disease. Further studies will be required to determine the magnitude of the interaction, to define which aspects of cellular immunity are most notably affected, and to determine the locus responsible for such immune dysfunction.

The influence of long-term ethanol intake, with resultant alcoholic liver disease, on cell-mediated immunity has been studied more extensively. The relatively large number of studies reflects the high frequency with which such patients are encountered and their availability for such studies.

In studies of patients with alcoholic liver disease, there was no significant change in the total absolute lymphocyte count but there was a marked and highly significant decrease in peripheral blood T cells (e.g., E rosette–forming cells), whether considered in absolute or relative terms (Bernstein et al., 1974). In contrast, chronic alcoholics without significant liver disease did not manifest such differences in peripheral blood T lymphocyte counts. No correlation was found between the biochemical parameters of liver function and immunodeficiency, but histological examination indicated that those patients with alcoholic hepatitis or stable cirrhosis had reduced numbers of E rosette–forming T lymphocytes (Bernstein *et al.,* 1974). Patients with alcoholic fatty liver did not show such changes. The authors suggested that because a similar reduction in peripheral blood T lymphocytes also occurs in other forms of hepatitis, this may, in fact, be a reflection of hepatic inflammation and eventual necrosis, regardless of the etiology of the liver disease.

As noted above, such a decrease in peripheral blood T lymphocytes might also result from a direct toxic effect of ethanol on T cells, as has been demonstrated clearly for other hematopoietic cell types (Tisman and Herbert, 1973). However, the unaffected numbers of circulating T cells in chronic alcoholics without liver disease would argue against this condition, unless it takes a specified period of time to develop. Another possible mechanism might be hepatic sequestration of these T lymphocytes due to leukocyte infiltration, thereby decreasing the number of circulating T cells. The authors also point out that these results confirm the hypothesis of Triger and Wright (1973) that the immunological abnormalities, e.g., hypergammaglobulinemia, may be the result of imbalanced T- and B-cell function. Others have also found a decreased number of rosette–forming T lymphocytes in alcoholics with liver disease. The mean proportion of E rosette–forming cells in the alcoholic liver disease group was 27.4% compared with 36.2% in controls (Berenyi *et al.,* 1975). According to the authors, these results show that *in vivo* measurement of T-cell rosettes may prove a more valuable indicator of immune status in patients with alcoholic liver disease than *in vitro* assays such as those involving the response to mitogens, which as noted above, are notoriously variable. Thus far, no data have been published quantitating T-cell subsets with monoclonal antibodies.

Another major means of studying cell-mediated immunity in patients with alcoholic liver disease is by observing the response to sensitization with a battery of skin test antigens. Faulty responsiveness to dinitrochlorobenzene has been repeatedly demonstrated in patients with advanced alcoholic liver disease. Nearly 80% of these patients failed to be sensitized to an intradermal injection (Straus *et al.,* 1971; Berenyi *et al.,* 1975). Indeed, many patients with alcoholic liver disease fail to respond to any of the antigens employed including *Candida,* coccidioiden, histoplasmin, intermediate-strength PPD, mumps, and SK-SD (Straus *et al.,* 1971; Berenyi *et al.,* 1974, 1975). In many patients with alcoholic cirrhosis there was a partial impairment of delayed-type hypersensitivity responses, and in a smaller number of these patients there was a complete impairment of such responses (Straus *et al.,* 1971). It is unclear whether the observed defect was the result of an altered inflammatory response or an impaired expression of cellular immu-

Table VII

Variable Responsiveness of Lymphocytes of Patients with (CAH) in the Presence
of Autologous Plasma or Allogeneic Plasma[a]

Case number	Diagnosis	10% autologous whole blood supplemented with:	PWM[b] (10 μl/ml cpm ± SE)[c]	PHA-M[d] (10 μl/ml cpm ± SE)
29 JS	CAH-A	10% autologous plasma	2,416 ± 438	2,523 ± 233
		10% 27 UB normal plasma	2,260 ± 194	16,155 ± 1,130
		10% 28 WW (CAH with cirrhosis) plasma	2,859 ± 89	7,480 ± 1,018
28 WW	CAH-B	10% autologous plasma	7,444 ± 696	5,869 ± 744
		10% 27 UB normal plasma	6,075 ± 455	11,626 ± 824
		10% 29 JS (CAH) plasma	20,150 ± 881	52,778 ± 4,256
27 UB	Healthy donor	10% autologous plasma	48,353 ± 1,222	46,784 ± 900
		10% 29 JS (CAH) plasma	51,100 ± 2,051	63,915 ± 2,264

[a]Reproduced with permission from Behrens et al., 1982.
[b]PWM (pokeweed mitogen).
[c]SE, standard error.
[d]PHA-M, phytohemagglutinin A.

nity. A positive skin test response to croton oil indicated that the lack of delayed-type hypersensitivity was not merely a reflection of a defective inflammatory response but rather faulty recognition of the foreign antigenic material and/or defective cellular responsiveness after such recognition had taken place (Berenyi et al., 1974).

Another means of assessing cell-mediated immunity in patients with alcoholic liver disease has been the study of responsiveness of peripheral blood lymphocytes to T-cell mitogens. These results have proven highly variable due to significant variations in the homogeneity of the patient population. Some investigators have found a significant decrease in response to T-cell mitogens (Hsu and Leevy, 1971; Behrens et al., 1982). Hsu and Leevy (1971) demonstrated the presence of an inhibitory serum factor(s) that was responsible for the depression of responsiveness. There was, however, no such inhibition of the mixed lymphocyte reaction in the same patient population (Hsu and Leevy, 1971). Moreover, the magnitude of serum inhibitory capacity was negatively correlated with serum γ globulin levels. Behrens et al. (1982), while studying lymphocyte responsiveness, expanded these findings to show that a variety of plasma factors inhibited such lymphocyte transformation (Table VII). In contrast, others found no significant effect of chronic alcohol intake in the presence of alcoholic liver disease on the peripheral blood lymphocyte response to mitogens. Lymphocytes from patients with alcoholic liver disease had a normal blastogenic response to phytohemagglutinin *in vitro* and a reduced dinitrochlorobenzene delayed-type hypersensitivity response (Berenyi *et al.,* 1974). Thus, the degree of impairment of cell-mediated immunity that may be observed in alcoholic liver disease remains a matter of controversy. Nonetheless, it would appear that chronic intake of ethanol can have a substantial negative impact on cellular immune responses.

13

Nutritional Modulation of Autoimmune Disease

INTRODUCTION

Nutritional deficiency and associated impaired immunocompetence are recognized as major contributory factors in the vast majority of childhood deaths in Third World nations, particularly because of their complicating influence in measles, respiratory diseases, and diarrhea (Puffer and Serramo, 1973). In addition to the influence of generalized malnutrition on immunity, there is mounting evidence that specific nutrient deficiency can likewise result in compromised immune responsiveness. In fact, as discussed extensively throughout this volume, specific nutrient deficiencies may play a major role in the immunodeficiency syndrome of human PEM (Neumann *et al.,* 1975; Golden *et al.,* 1978). Because of the dramatic effect of nutritional factors on immunological function, attention has been focused on the possibility of utilizing selective nutritional manipulations to regulate the aberrant immune responses of autoimmune disease (Beach *et al.,* 1981b; Hansen *et al.,* 1982; Morrow and Levy, 1983). This is now clinically possible because of major technological advances in food processing and in the development of TPN. In this chapter, we will discuss the empiric observations in experimental models of autoimmunity and demonstrate the feasibility of nutritional immune modulation.

EXPERIMENTAL MODELS OF AUTOIMMUNITY

Autoimmune disease represents a group of syndromes that have in common termination of the naturally occurring unresponsiveness to self components. For many years, Burnet's theory of elimination of all self-reactive clones of lymphocytes during a critical stage of ontogeny dominated thought on the pathogenesis of autoimmunity. However, major new viewpoints have emerged with the knowledge that self-recognition is an essential component of the interaction between T cells, B cells, and macrophages to produce an intact immune response. It is proposed that a balanced system of suppression/control operates to abrogate deleterious forms of self-reactive interactions. Many factors of endogenous and exogenous origin may trigger an imbalance in this intricate synergy, which normally achieves homeostatic control of the self-recognition process.

To date, at least six models of murine lupus have been derived, including (1) New Zealand Black (NZB) mice, (2) (NZB × NZW)F_1 (NZB/W), (3) MRL/Mp-1pr/1pr (MRL/1), (4) BXSB, (5) *kd kd* and (6) *gld,* a newly developed mutant strain (Gershwin and Merchant, 1981). While the end-stage disease present in these animals may seem similar, the pathogenic factors may be quite different in each strain. For instance, development of murine lupus in NZB and NZB/W mice is controlled by several genes and the expression is altered hy an unknown number of secondary factors, while MRL/1 and gld mice carry a single, specific, lymphoproliferative (*1pr*) gene. The final expression of disease, however, is the result of an interaction of only not genetic factors but also of environmental, hormonal, immunological, and viral factors. The most widely used phenotypic marker of these strains of lupus-prone mice is age of onset of autoantibody production and subsequent mortality, which has been found to vary notably among strains. While NZB mice, whether male or female, experience 50% mortality by 15–16 months of age, MRL/1 mice exhibit this rate of mortality by 5–6 months. NZB/W and BXSB mice show significant differences in the timing of mortality based on sex, with male BXSB and female NZB/W mice both dying at a significantly earlier age than their opposite-sex littermates.

Histological examination of all systemic lupus erythematosus (SLE)-prone strains of mice indicate substantial renal deposits of IgG and C3; significant deposits of DNA and the gp70 retroviral envelope antigen are also observed. Deposition of these materials is associated with progressive glomcrular sclerosis and impaired renal function; the latter is the primary cause of death in SLE-prone mice. Lymphoid organs often show similar changes; all strains have premature thymic atrophy. Lymph node hyperplasia is more variable in extent, with a 2-fold increase in NZB/W mice and a 100-fold increase in MRL/1 mice. Approximately 15–30% of SLE-prone strains of mice have myocardial infarcts at autopsy, particularly in the small and medium-sized artcrics and arterioles; myocardial vessels often reveal deposits of IgG, C3, and the gp70 antigen. Furthermore, MRL/1 mice often develop an acute and/or necrotizing polyarteritis, especially in the renal and coronary arteries. Swollen joints of the lower legs and hindfeet also develop in 25% of older MRL/1 mice; these joints exhibit pannus formation, deteriorating articular cartilage, and proliferating synovium. There is thus increasing evidence that MRL/1 mice will provide an appropriate empirical model for the study of rheumatoid arthritis.

All strains of SLE-prone mice present with a number of serological abnormalities, including elevated levels of serum immunoglobulins, antibodies to DNA, and other nuclear antibodies. Strains of mice susceptible to autoimmune disease also have relatively high levels of serum gp70, particularly NZB and NZB/W mice, but elevated serum gp70 is not correlated with the progression of autoimmune disease. At weaning age, all SLE-prone strains are hyperresponsive to challenge with a number of haptens, with a resultant increase in the number of anti-hapten PFC as well as an increased concentration of anti-hapten antibodies in the serum. Additionally, there are a number of striking serological abnormalities that occur in only one or two of the SLE-prone strains of mice. These include anti-erythrocyte antibodies and natural thymocytotoxic antibodies in NZB and NZB/W mice, and anti-Sm (a nuclear glycoprotein) antibody and rheumatoid factor of both the IgG_1 and IgM classes in MRL/1 mice.

Significant levels of circulating immune complexes are found in all such mutant mice. Complexes of DNA—anti-DNA have been shown to be closely associated with lupus nephritis. In addition, gp70—anti-gp70 complexes are found in the serum of older autoimmune mice; the appearance of these complexes parallels the insidious progression of kidney disease in such animals. Renal eluates of diseased kidneys also show significant deposits of IgG-complexed gp70.

Immunological profiles of T- and B-lymphocyte populations in autoimmune strains of mice reveal numerous abnormalities, but few are consistently reproduced in all strains of mice prone to lupus (Milich and Gershwin, 1979). For example, there are no consistently demonstrated abnormalities for T- or B-cell subpopulations with regard to either absolute number or frequency. However, a significant finding that has been repeatedly demonstrated in all of these mutant strains is the early appearance of advanced B-lymphocyte maturity, resulting in B-cell hyperactivity and polyclonal activation (Gershwin et al., 1980, 1982; Ohsugi et al., 1982). The pathological results of such precocious B-cell function are spontaneous polyclonal antibody production, hypergammaglobulinemia, and the secretion of a variety of autoantibodies. Massive amounts of information exist regarding T-cell abnormalities in murine lupus, but much of the evidence has been contradicted by subsequent findings and a consensus is difficult to reach. Some investigators propose that the defect in these mice lies in a failure of antigen-nonspecific suppression as opposed to deficient antigen-specific T-cell suppression. Many studies have demonstrated that T-cell function declines as the lupus-prone strains of mice age; the best evidence for such a depression of immunocompetence was obtained in MRL/1 mice. However, other studies have shown that immune function in older mice expressing autoimmune disease is within normal limits (Milich and Gershwin, 1980). Recently, MRL/1 mice have been demonstrated to have increased helper-cell activity, which might contribute to B-cell hyperactivity. If such aberrations in T-cell function do exist in strains of mice prone to SLE, it is important to determine whether this is a primary immunological deficit or perhaps one of the subsequent factors modulating the expression of the syndrome.

A number of other factors are believed to have a critical influence on the pathogenesis of autoimmune disease. The thymus itself may play a significant role in the progressive development of autoimmunity. For example, deficient production of thymic hormones may result in significant imbalances of T-cell and possibly B-cell function. Similarly, New Zealand mice display an age-dependent loss of morphological and functional characteristics of thymic epithelial cells (Gershwin *et al.,* 1978). Thymectomy has also been shown to inhibit markedly the progression of autoimmune disease under certain circumstances. For instance, the thymus is essential in MRL/1 mice for the development of T-cell function and, therefore, the expression of the autoimmune phenotype. Other experiments have shown, however, that the genotype of the thymic microenvironment in which the T cells develop is irrelevant in the later expression of the disease process. A number of other studies have shown that all strains of mice prone to autoimmunity are relatively resistant to the induction of tolerance by proteins such as human or bovine γ globulin. While viral factors have received significant attention throughout the study of autoimmune disease, little is understood regarding the possible role of viruses or their products in the pathogenesis of autoimmune disease. The notable sex differences in expression of the autoimmune phenotype indicate that sex hormones may also have an important role.

A comprehensive review of the information on the pathogenesis of murine lupus reveals the many differences between the various mutant strains, all of which eventually express a similar pathological syndrome. All strains of mice prone to lupus possess the genetic potential to develop autoimmune disease late in life. However, in some strains, factors may be present that lead to early expression of the autoimmune phenotype. For example in MRL/1 mice, the *lpr* gene represents an accelerating influence that facilitates the expression of the entire range of autoimmune manifestation. Similarly, in NZB/W mice, an X-linked factor promotes early disease expression, and in BXSB mice a Y-linked factor functions in a similar manner. It is now necessary to elucidate the primary processes responsible for the potential expression of autoimmune disease and to distinguish these from secondary factors that facilitate the expression of the autoimmune phenotype.

AMINO ACIDS, PROTEIN, AND AUTOIMMUNE DISEASE

That nutritional factors might be employed to modify the outcome of autoimmune disease was underscored by studies in New Zealand (NZ) mice that utilized diets lacking in phenylalanine and tyrosine (Dubois and Strain, 1973). (NZB × NZW) F_1 (NZB/W) mice fed such diets experienced low body weight gain and a notable delay in the development of lupus-associated immune complex nephritis. As assessed by both light and electron microscopy, kidneys remained normal, with renal glomeruli being neither enlarged nor hypercellular even at 1 year of age. There was no thickening of the mesangial matrix or of the capillary basement membrane, and immunoperoxidase staining indicated that there was a markedly diminished deposition of immunoglobulin in the kidney.

Later studies using diets low in these essential amino acids investigated the possibility that such a deficient diet could be acting via an interaction with viral factors implicated in the etiology of the disease process. It was suggested that a physiological deficit of essential amino acids might alter the course of autoimmune disease by affecting either (1) viral replication and/or virulence or (2) host response to the virus and/or viral products. The results indicated that tissues of control and amino acid–restricted animals released similar levels of x-trophic viruses (Levy, 1977). Moreover, there were no significant differences in the titer of either antibodies or x-trophic virus-neutralizing factor to the AKR-MuLV (endogenous ecotropic virus) when sera from deprived and control mice were compared. Thus, the amelioration of immune complex nephritis and the consequent increase in longevity in NZB/W mice ascribed to a dietary influence of essential amino acid deficiency seemed not to be related to altered levels of endogenous C-type viruses or to an altered host response to these endogenous viruses.

Moderate restriction of total dietary protein early in life is associated with alterations in immunological function in NZB mice and with partial amelioration of the immune complex nephritis in NZB/W mice (Fernandes *et al.,* 1976b,c). NZB mice fed the protein-deficient diet from weaning had significantly lower body weights, did not develop splenomegaly, and did not undergo the customary thymic involution (Fernandes *et al.,* 1972, 1973) (Tables I–IV, Fig. 1). Protein-restricted NZB mice had a lower total serum protein concentration than controls, and experienced less hypergam-

Table I

Hematologic Variations in NZB Mice Maintained on Normal and Low-Protein Diets[a]

Diets	Age (months)	Sex	Hematocrit[b]	WBC/mm³[b]	Total lymphocytes/mm³[b]	Total neutrophils/mm³[b]	Direct Coombs test Positive tested	%
I (protein 22%)	6	F	49.5 ± 2.6	9100 ± 897	6995 ± 689	1688 ± 275	12/15	80
	14	F	39.0 ± 1.4	5703 ± 661	4074 ± 484	1610 ± 213	13/15	87
	6	M	51.9 ± 1.5	8497 ± 401	4201 ± 230	3174 ± 514	7/12	58
	14	M	38.1 ± 1.2	5528 ± 484	3306 ± 317	2237 ± 317	13/15	87
II (protein 6%)	6	F	45.5 ± 0.7	6700 ± 507	5299 ± 307	1354 ± 245	5 15	33
	14	F	38.0 ± 1.0	3673 ± 340	1750 ± 185	1862 ± 247	15/17	88
	6	M	45.9 ± 0.6	6300 ± 1268	4309 ± 436	1391 ± 140	5/12	42
	14	M	38.0 ± 1.2	5697 ± 411	3218 ± 224	2376 ± 265	17/17	100

[a]Reproduced with permission from Fernandes et al. (1976a).
[b]Mean ± SEM.

Table II

Comparison of Spleen and Thymus Weights of NZB Mice on Normal and Low-Protein Diets[a]

Age (months)	Diet I spleen[b]	Diet II spleen[b]	p[c] value	Diet I thymus[b]	Diet II thymus[b]	p[c] value
3–4	404 ± 35 (8)[d]	397 ± 50 (8)	>.05	174 ± 9 (8)	221 ± 27 (8)	>.05
7–10	744 ± 132(10)	425 ± 57 (10)	<.02	66 ± 10 (10)	136 ± 12 (10)	<.001

[a] Reproduced with permission from Fernandes et al. (1976a).
[b] Relative weights ± SE (mg/100 g body weight).
[c] Student t test.
[d] Number of animals per group are listed in parentheses.

Table III

Survival of NZB Mice Maintained on Normal and Low-Protein Diets[a,b]

| Age (months) | Diet I normal protein | | | | | | Diet II low protein | | | | | |
| | Female | | Male | | Total | | Female | | Male | | Total | |
	No.[c]	%	No.	%	No.	%	No.	%	No.	%	No.	%
6	26/26	100	34/36	94.4	60/62	96.8	21/22	95.5	26/27	96.3	47/49	95.9
12	17/26	65.4	22/36	61.1	39/62	62.9	17/22	77.3	20/27	74.1	37/49	75.5
18	8/26	30.8	10/36	27.8	18/62	29.0	10/22	45.5	9/27	33.3	19/49	38.8
24	0/26	0	0/36	0	0/62	0	2/22	9.1	0/27	0	2/49	4.1

[a]Reproduced with permission from Fernandes et al. (1976a).
[b]χ^2 test did not show any statistically significant variations between the groups.
[c]Survivors/total number of mice.

maglobulinemia and a delayed onset of autoimmune hemolytic anemia. Moderate protein deprivation and the associated delay in the onset of autoimmune disease were also correlated with a prolonged maintenance of immune responsiveness (Fernandes et al., 1976c). Protein-restricted NZB mice maintained a more vigorous antibody response to sheep erythrocytes (SRBC) and a higher GVHR than controls. Killer cell activity did not decline with age to the extent observed in control NZB mice, and the decline was moderated in response to T-cell mitogens. In contrast, no effect on responsiveness to the B-cell mitogen, LPS, was observed, and a decrease in the absolute number of θ-positive lymphocytes was seen. However, while these parameters of immunological function were significantly altered when compared with control NZB mice, this particular level and timing of dietary protein restriction did not significantly prolong survival.

NZB/W mice moderately deprived of protein from weaning also experienced notable alterations in autoimmune pathology (Friend et al., 1978). While the beneficial effects of protein restriction were quantitatively less than those of caloric restriction, in many ways they were qualitatively similar. The kidneys of protein-restricted NZB/W mice had significantly less staining by immunofluorescence for immunoglobulin and complement; IgA deposits were notably absent. In addition, there was a substantially different distribution of these deposits, with a predominantly mesangial orientation rather than the glomerular basement membrane—oriented deposition of immunoglobulin and complement observed in NZB/W mice fed adequate protein. In contrast to the glomerular sclerosis and extensive cellular proliferation seen in control NZB/W mice, protein-restricted counterparts experienced almost no cellular proliferation. It is of interest to note that moderate restriction of dietary protein has also been associated with a

Table IV

Influence of Diet on Total Serum Protein and Immunoglobulins in NZB Female Mice[a,b]

Diet	No. of mice	Age (months)	Total protein (g/100 ml)[c]	Concentration of immunoglobulins (mg/100ml)[c]			
				IgG_1	IgG_2	IgM	IgA
Diet I, protein 22%	6	3	4.9 ± 0.2	46 ± 6	228 ± 13	71 ± 3	90 ± 11
Diet II, protein 6%	6	3	4.6 ± 0.1	50 ± 8	240 ± 6	62 ± 3	97 ± 17
			<.05	NS[d]	NS	<.05	NS
Diet I, protein 22%	8	10	5.2 ± 0.4	372 ± 105	877 ± 140	127 ± 10	43 ± 7
Diet II, protein 6%	8	10	4.3 ± 0.3	82 ± 19	650 ± 102	77 ± 4	106 ± 13
			<.05	<.01	NS	<.005	<.0005

[a]Reproduced with permission from Fernandes *et al.* (1976a).

[b]Individual serum samples frozen at −20°C were tested a year later.

[c]Mean ± SE.

[d]Student's *t* test >.05 not significant (NS).

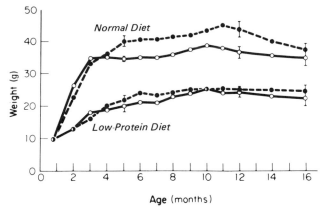

Fig. 1. Average body weights of female (20) and male (20) NZB mice that have been maintained with normal-protein (22%) and low-protein (6%) diets (20 calories/day/mouse). Vertical lines represent ± 1 SEM. The protein alone was manipulated, and the food intake was isocaloric. O———O, males; ●- - - -●, females. (Reproduced with permission from Fernandes *et al.,* 1976a.)

significant prolongation of life in strains of mice not susceptible to autoimmune disease, e.g., DBA/2f mice (Fernandes *et al.,* 1976a).

CALORIES AND AUTOIMMUNE DISEASE

Dietary restriction of total calories has a profound influence on the expression of autoimmune phenomena in murine lupus. Because the influence of a calorie deficit is so pervasive, any study that fails to measure food intake and body weight, and to provide pair-fed and/or weight-matched controls, is suspect on the grounds that a reduced caloric intake might be modulating the expression of autoimmunity. When various combinations of dietary calories, protein, and lipids were fed to NZ mice, the number of calories seemed to be the outstanding feature of diets successful in prolonging life (Fernandes *et al.,* 1972, 1973; Friend *et al.,* 1978) (Fig. 2).

When NZB/W mice were fed a normal protein (20% protein), low calorie (10 calories/day) diet, a significant prolongation of life was achieved. The mean survival time was more than doubled by a 50% reduction in the total number of calories (Fernandes *et al.,* 1976b). The extension of the life span was far greater than that achieved by a restriction of either dietary protein or lipid. Calorie restriction resulted in lower body weight with advancing age and a marked inhibition of the development of renal disease (Fernandes *et al.,* 1978a). Immunological responsiveness was lower at an early age in

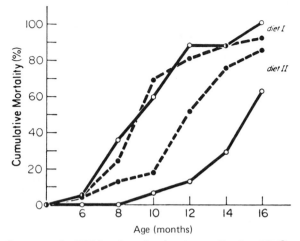

Fig. 2. Mortality curves for NZB female and male mice on diets I and II. ○——○, males; ●- - - -●, females. (Reproduced with permission from Fernandes *et al.,* 1972.) Diet I is high fat—low protein; Diet II is low fat—high protein.

calorically restricted mice than in controls, but was better preserved as the animals aged. Older calorie-restricted mice still had the capacity to generate cytotoxic cells and had a significantly higher response to T-cell mitogens; the B-cell mitogenic response did not differ from that of controls (Fernandes *et al.,* 1978a). Additionally, PFC responses, following either *in vivo* or *in vitro* sensitization to SRBC, were also better maintained in calorically restricted NZB/W mice. Moreover, there appeared to be better preservation of a balanced relationship between helper and suppressor T-cell activity (Fernandes *et al.,* 1978a). The inhibition of progressive renal disease was substantiated by light microscopy, electron microscopy, and immunofluorescence studies, and by all established criteria, disease manifestations were substantially less in the calorically restricted animals (Fernandes *et al.,* 1978a) (Fig. 3). NZB/W mice fed the lower-calorie diet also had significantly less circulating antibody to native DNA (Fernandes *et al.,* 1978a). NZB/W mice fed calorically restricted diets from weaning had significantly lower levels of circulating immune complexes than did control mice. In those renal lesions that did develop, calorically restricted mice had markedly fewer deposits of immunoglobulin and C3 (Safai-Kutti *et al.,* 1980).

Gp70, the retroviral envelope glycoprotein, is found in high concentration in the serum and in deposits in diseased glomeruli (Izui *et al.,* 1979). The appearance of antibodies to gp70 corresponds closely to the onset of autoimmune pathology (Theofilopoulos and Dixon, 1981). NZB/W mice fed low-calorie diets from weaning had 50% lower levels of serum gp70, as well as substantially lower levels of circulating immune complexes to this

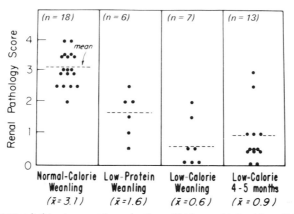

Fig. 3. Quantitative light microscopic evaluation of kidneys obtained from B/W mice in four dietary groups. (Reproduced with permission from Fernandes *et al.,* 1978a.)

glycoprotein (Izui *et al.,* 1981). Notably, serum levels of gp70 immune complexes were decreased to a significantly greater extent than were anti-DNA antibodies (Safai-Kutti *et al.,* 1980). Moreover, renal glomeruli also exhibited significantly less deposition of gp70 antigen and immunoglobulin when renal eluates of calorically restricted mice were studied. Levels of another serum glycoprotein, haptoglobin, were also depressed in NZB/W mice fed low-calorie diets. Because serum glycoproteins such as xenotrophic viral gp70 and haptoglobin are most likely synthesized in the liver, an effect of caloric restriction on hepatic cells may play a key role in this disease process.

Restriction of caloric intake also resulted in a marked inhibition of progressive renal disease and a significant prolongation of the life span in *kdkd* mice (Fernandes *et al.,* 1978b) (Fig. 4). These mice develop a renal disease inherited via an autosomal recessive gene. Histological and immunological abnormalities indicate that this syndrome may have an autoimmune basis. Indeed, such mice exhibit a progressive development of Coomb's positive anemia, a decline with age in lymphocyte proliferation in response to mitogens, a decreased PFC response to SRBC, and an interstitial nephritis; an immune response to tubular basement membrane antigens may be a central pathogenic factor (Fernandes *et al.,* 1978b). *Kdkd* mice fed a calorie-restricted diet (8 calories/day starting at 8–10 weeks of age) did not develop Coombs' positive anemia even by 8 months of age, had higher hematocrits with advancing age, and had relatively normal kidney histology compared with extensive glomerular sclerosis, hyaline casts, round cell interstitial infiltration, increased amounts of connective tissue, marked tubular dilation, and renal damage (Fernandes *et al.,* 1978b). Most importantly, *kdkd* mice fed a low-calorie diet experienced greatly prolonged survival (Fer-

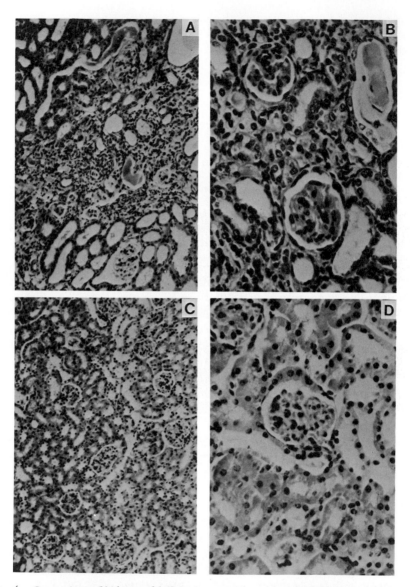

Fig. 4. Comparison of kidneys of *kdkd* mice on high and low food intake. (A) Low-power view of kidney of *kdkd* mouse, aged 7 months, fed a diet containing 16 calories/day. Note tubular dilation, atrophy of tubular cells, hyaline tubular casts, and striking mononuclear interstitial infiltration. (×100.) (B) Higher-power view revealing interstitial infiltration. Glomerular and tubular abnormalities of *kdkd* mice fed higher calorie diet (16 calories/day). (×400.) (C) Kidneys of *kdkd* mouse fed low calorie diet (8 calories/day). (×100.) (D) Kidneys of *kdkd* mouse fed low-calorie diet (8 calories/day). Note lack of interstitial infiltration and normal glomeruli and tubules. (×400.) (Reproduced with permission from Fernandes *et al.*, 1978b.)

nandes *et al.,* 1978b). Whereas all control *kdkd* mice died by 8 months of age, all mice fed calorically restricted diets remained alive. When some of these *kdkd* mice resumed consumption of a normal-calorie control diet, they developed progressive autoimmune disease and died within 60 days.

LIPIDS AND AUTOIMMUNE DISEASE

The initial studies concerning the influence of dietary lipids in NZ mice were very limited and did not provide adequate controls, but nevertheless did serve to point out the possible role of dietary lipid in the modulation of autoimmune disease (Fernandes *et al.,* 1972, 1973). NZB mice were fed either a "high fat-low protein" (11% fat, 17% protein) or a "low fat-high protein" diet (4.5% fat, 23% protein). Mice fed the low fat-high protein diet had lower body weights and poorer reproductive rates, but a delayed and reduced severity of autoimmune hemolytic anemia than mice fed the high fat-low protein diet (Fernandes *et al.,* 1972). Moreover, the low fat-high protein diet resulted in significantly lower titers of antinuclear antibodies and a prolonged maintenance of normal levels of immunological responsiveness, as reflected by an increased cellular cytotoxic response to tumor cell administration and a GVHR. In contrast, antibodies formed in response to SRBC were not affected by this dietary regimen. Most significantly, the life span was significantly greater in NZB mice fed the low fat-high protein diet than in the mice fed the high fat-low protein. More recent data have confirmed these observations (Levy *et al.,* 1982; Kelley and Izui, 1983).

Some studies concerning dietary lipids and autoimmune disease examined fat as a specific dietary component and began to examine the role of individual types of lipids (e.g., saturated versus polyunsaturated). The demonstration that murine lupus could be treated with administration of exogenous prostaglandins (Zurier *et al.,* 1977) further generated interest in the concept that dietary lipids might alter the course of autoimmune disease. Hurd *et al.* (1981) studied the effects of a diet deficient in essential fatty acids (EFA) on the pathogenesis of autoimmune disease in NZB/W mice and found that such a diet prevented the development of glomerulonephritis and significantly prolonged survival. NZB/W mice fed the EFA-deficient diet showed greatly decreased evidence of glomerulonephritis; immunofluorescence studies confirmed less deposition of IgM + IgG in both the capillary loops and mesangium of glomeruli (Hurd *et al.,* 1981). Most notably, prolonged survival was observed in animals fed the EFA-deficient diet; at 10 months of age, only 7% of NZB/W mice fed a control diet remained alive, while 88% of the EFA-deficient mice survived to this age. In addition, 78% of the EFA-deficient mice were still alive at 16 months of age, and a substantial proportion remained alive at 20 months of age.

While treatment with PGE_1 also retarded the appearance of glomerulonephritis and enhanced survival, these effects were not of the magnitude observed in EFA-deficient mice.

One study examined the influence of dietary enrichment with eicosapentanoic acid, a constituent of lipids in murine animal tissues, a fatty acid analog of arachidonic acid (Prickett et al., 1981). NZB/W mice fed the diet high in eicosapentanoic acid experienced notably lower levels of proteinuria, significantly lower levels of antibodies binding native DNA, and a greatly improved rate of survival (Prickett et al., 1981). Measurement of blood lipids and observation of physical appearance indicated that these animals were not EFA deficient; the influence was ascribed to the eicosapentanoic acid, which may have inhibited endogenous PGE_1 synthesis.

VITAMINS AND AUTOIMMUNE DISEASE

Despite substantial evidence that vitamins do influence numerous immune processes (Suskind, 1977), virtually no investigation of the effects of altered vitamin nutriture on autoimmune disease has taken place. A single study has attempted to establish a relationship between autoimmune disease and depressed levels of splenic vitamin C (Leibovitz and Siegel, 1981). Old NZB mice exhibit lower levels of vitamin C in spleen than do normal strains of mice. In addition, NZB mice living to an exceptionally old age, e.g., 24–26 months for females and 16–20 months for males, had significantly higher levels of vitamin C in spleen than did NZB mice experiencing earlier and more severe progression of autoimmune disease (Leibovitz and Siegel, 1981). Considering the major impact that other vitamins such as vitamin A and various synthetic retinoids, pyridoxine, and folate have on immunological function (Nauss et al., 1979; Nauss and Newberne, 1981; Chandra et al., 1981a), the interaction between vitamin nutriture and autoimmune disease is an area that requires more investigation.

Because zinc nutriture influences vitamin A metabolism, it has been postulated that the immunological effects of zinc deficiency are partly mediated by the reduction of vitamin A levels seen in zinc deprivation. To explore this possibility, our group has studied the influence of vitamin A deficiency on autoantibody production in NZB mice (Gershwin et al., 1984). Groups of NZB mice, beginning at 6 months of age, were fed either a vitamin A–deficient diet, a control diet, ad libitum or the pair fed to the deficient group. The diet contained casein as the protein source, as well as adequate levels of trace elements and vitamins. Despite our hypothesis that the reduction of autoantibodies in zinc-deficient NZB mice might be mediated by secondary vitamin A deficiency, we found that vitamin A–deficient animals manifested more severe hypergammaglobulinemia and an earlier onset of both NTA and IgM anti-erythrocyte autoantibodies than did vitamin A— sufficient mice. These results illustrate the importance of rigorous studies of select nutritional parameters and warn of the possibility of clinical harm in feeding inappropriate diets to patients with SLE.

MINERALS AND AUTOIMMUNE DISEASE

As with vitamins, very little investigation of the interactions between dietary minerals and experimental autoimmune disease has been conducted. This is somewhat surprising in light of the substantial literature concerning the alteration of mineral intake, particularly that of calcium and phosphorus in patients with a variety of renal diseases (Holliday et al., 1979). A single study has focused on the influence of altered dietary phosphorus on the subsequent development of nephrotoxic serum nephritis in rats (Karlinsky et al., 1980). Control animals consuming a phosphorus-adequate diet developed a glomerulonephritis characterized by progressive renal failure, elevated serum creatinine concentrations, proteinuria, and early death (Karlinsky et al., 1980). In contrast, animals fed a low-phosphorus diet had significantly lower serum creatinine concentrations, maintained a level of renal function similar to that of normal animals without end-stage renal disease, and did not experience accelerated mortality. Histological examination revealed significantly less renal damage and biochemical analysis indicated less nephrocalcinosis in the phosphorus-deficient mice (Karlinsky et al., 1980). While it did not alleviate disease expression altogether, restriction of dietary phosphorus resulted in a retardation of progressive experimental glomerulonephritis, with prolonged maintenance of renal function and a reduction of histological damage. It should be noted that food intake levels were not monitored in these animals, and thus pair-fed controls were not included. While it is not known if these animals experienced any inanition due to the dietary phosphorus restriction, the possible influence of the caloric restriction that might accompany such inanition cannot be ruled out.

Multiple mechanisms may be responsible for the partial amelioration of experimental immunologic renal disease. Because dietary phosphorus restriction results in a marked reduction of proliferative glomerular lesions and greatly diminished crescent formation, an immunological mechanism seems quite likely. Glomerular infiltration with monocytes and local accumulation of macrophages have both been ascribed a critical role in these processes of renal pathogenesis (Holdsworth et al., 1980). Restriction of dietary phosphorus has been shown to influence adversely the function of PMN leukocytes, which may thereby retard progressive renal damage (Jacob, 1974). Restriction of dietary phosphorus may also alter the pathogenesis of experimental glomerulonephritis through metabolic alterations of the calcium–phosphorus balance and may possibly involve a decrease in parathyroid hormone levels. While the precise mechanism remains to be worked out, it would appear that manipulation of dietary mineral levels has potential therapeutic value.

Compared with other nutrients, the influence of zinc nutriture on the pathogenesis of autoimmune disease has been studied relatively extensively. In initial studies, three different zinc-deficient diets were fed throughout life (i.e., marginally, moderately, and severely deficient) beginning at weaning (Beach *et al.,* 1981b); *ad libitum-* and pair-fed controls were also studied. Mice fed low levels of zinc experienced a significant delay in the onset of autoimmune hemolytic anemia, as reflected by significantly higher hemoglobin levels, higher packed cell volume, lower levels of serum immunoglobulins, and significantly lower titers of anti-erythrocyte autoantibodies (Beach *et al.,* 1981b). Such mice also had lower body weights with advancing age, experienced less splenomegaly, and, most importantly, exhibited a prolonged life span, with over 80% of mice fed the lowest-zinc diets living beyond 10 months of age compared with only approximately 30% of the *ad libitum*-fed control mice. While pair-fed controls also experienced a delay in the progression of autoimmune disease, zinc-deprived NZB mice had higher hemoglobin values and packed cell volumes and lower levels of serum immunoglobulins and anti-erythrocyte autoantibodies than did their pair-fed counterparts, indicating that zinc deprivation per se accounted for a substantial share of the observed retardation in the autoimmune process.

When low-zinc diets were introduced at 6 months of age in mice with established disease, i.e., already showing positive direct antiglobulin test results, further development of the autoimmune syndrome was significantly retarded, but disease manifestations already established were not reversed (Beach *et al.,* 1981b). In contrast to the results of dietary zinc restriction begun early in life, the caloric restriction that accompanied zinc deprivation was most likely responsible for a significant, if not major, share of the observed effects. These results are in accord with those obtained in earlier experiments utilizing NZB/W mice fed calorically restricted but otherwise adequate diets beginning at 4–6 months of age; such mice also experienced a significant retardation of the autoimmune disease process, even when dietary modifications were begun this late in life.

When NZB/W mice were fed the same diets under similar conditions, those fed the lowest-zinc diets experienced a significant delay in the onset of a notable amelioration of the severity of the lupus-like autoimmune syndrome (Beach *et al.,* 1982a). Moderately and severely zinc-deprived mice experienced significantly less proteinuria, a delayed appearance and lower levels of circulating antibodies to dsDNA, lower levels of serum immunoglobulin, a later onset and reduced severity of glomerulonephritis, and a significant prolongation of the life span (Figs. 5–7, Tables, V–VII). Histological examination revealed that while all mice experienced some diffuse glomerulonephritis, *ad libitum*-fed control mice exhibited a severe proliferative immune complex–associated glomerulonephritis. In contrast, renal histology of NZB/W mice fed the lowest levels of zinc was nearly normal (Beach *et al.,* 1982a).

MRL/1 mice deprived of zinc from weaning throughout their life span experienced a significant attenuation of autoimmune disease, as reflected by lower levels of proteinuria, lower levels of circulating antibodies to dsDNA, a notable alleviation of the severe proliferative glomerulonephritis, and a marked prolongation of the life span (Beach *et al.,* 1982b). Indeed, significant numbers of animals lived beyond 12 months of age, even when returned to a control diet at 6 months of age. Moreover, the response to mitogens and the direct PFC response to SRBC immunization were better

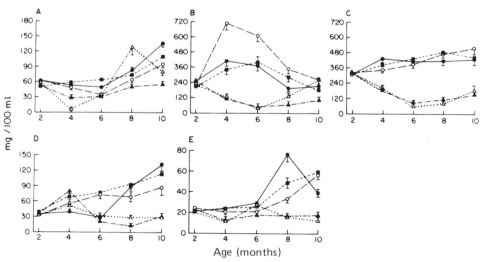

Fig. 5. Total serum immunoglobulin levels of young NZB/W mice (mg/100 ml). A. Serum IgM; B. serum IgG$_1$; C. serum IgG$_{2A}$; D. serum IgG$_{2B}$; E. serum IgA. All data points represent the mean determination for 15 animals, or the number animals remaining alive at that age (see Fig. 6). SEM are included where significant differences exist ($p < .05$). ●, 100 ppm zinc *ad libitum* fed; ○, 100 ppm zinc, inanition controls; ■, 9.0 ppm zinc; ▲, 5.0 ppm zinc; △, 2.5 ppm zinc (Beach *et al.,* 1982a).

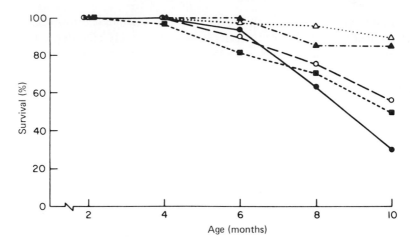

Fig. 6. Survival of young NZB/W mice to 10 months of age, expressed as the percentage of the original animals remaining alive at any age. ●, 100 ppm zinc, *ad libitum* fed; ○, 100 ppm zinc, inanition controls; ■, 9.0 ppm zinc; ▲, 5.0 ppm zinc; △, 2.5 ppm zinc (Beach *et al.,* 1982a).

preserved in the MRL/1 mice deprived of zinc from weaning than in the *ad libitum*-fed controls (Beach *et al.,* 1982b). While the pair-fed controls also experienced a delay in the onset and progression of autoimmunity, the effect on MRL/1 mice deprived of zinc was much more dramatic; as with NZB/W mice, the degree of disease expression was closely correlated with

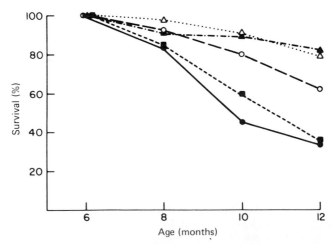

Fig. 7. Survival of old NZB/W mice to 10 months of age, expressed as the percentage of the original animals remaining alive at any age. ●, 100 ppm zinc, *ad libitum* fed; ○, 100 ppm zinc, inanition controls; ■, 9.0 ppm zinc; ▲, 5.0 ppm zinc; △, 2.5 ppm zinc (Beach *et al.,* 1982a).

Table V

DNA Binding of Young NZB/W Mice[a]

Diet	Age									
	2 months		4 months		6 months		8 months		10 months	
	% DNA bound	% increase	% DNA bound	% increase	% DNA bound	% increase	% DNA bound	% increase	% DNA bound	% increase
100 ppm zinc *ad libitum*-fed controls	4.8 ± 0.5[a,b]		15.9 ± 1.8	231	21.1 ± 4.2	548	37.0 ± 4.1	671	41.2 ± 3.9	758
100 ppm zinc inanition controls	4.2 ± 0.3		6.2 ± 0.4[a]	48	9.4 ± 0.6[a]	124	21.2 ± 1.6[a]	405	29.1 ± 3.0[a]	593
9 ppm zinc	3.0 ± 0.5		2.9 ± 0.4[a]	–0–	18.7 ± 2.2	523	29.3 ± 3.1	876	35.4 ± 4.6	1180
5 ppm zinc	3.9 ± 0.3		4.2 ± 0.4[a]	8	3.3 ± 0.4[a]	–0–	11.8 ± 2.7[a,e]	203	21.6 ± 1.8[a,e]	454
2.5 ppm zinc	3.2 ± 0.4		3.3 ± 0.2[a]	3	2.6 ± 0.3[a]	–0–	6.2 ± 0.4[a]	94	18.8 ± 2.4[a]	488

[a]Fifteen mice per group (or number remaining alive; see Table VI).
[b]Mean ± SEM.
[c]Negative control = 5.7%.
[d]$p < .01$ compared to *ad libitum*-fed controls.
[e]$p < .05$ compared to pair-fed controls (Beach *et al.*, 1982a).

Table VI

DNA Binding of Old NZB/W Mice[a,b]

	6 months		8 months		10 months		12 months	
Diet	% DNA bound	% increase	% DNA bound	% increase	% DNA bound	% increase	% DNA bound	% increase
100 ppm zinc *ad libitum*-fed	28.7 ± 3.1[c,d]		36.4 ± 3.8	27	39.7 ± 3.2	38	45.6 ± 6.1	59
100 ppm zinc inanition	26.4 ± 2.9		29.5 ± 3.7	12[e]	31.4 ± 2.8	19[e]	34.2 ± 3.0	30[e]
9 ppm zinc	29.3 ± 2.7		33.4 ± 4.0	14[e]	36.0 ± 3.3	23	41.2 ± 3.7	41
5 ppm zinc	26.8 ± 3.1		27.9 ± 2.8[e]	4[e]	31.6 ± 3.2[e]	18[e]	31.8 ± 2.4[e]	19[e,f]
2.5 ppm zinc	28.3 ± 2.4		29.1 ± 2.6[e]	3[e]	29.4 ± 3.0[e]	4[e]	30.9 ± 2.9[e]	9[e,f]

[a]Beach *et al*, 1982a.
[b]Fifteen mice per group (or number remaining alive; see Table VII).
[c]Mean ± SEM.
[d]Negative control = 5.7%.
[e]$p < .05$ compared to *ad libitum*-fed controls.
[f]$p < .05$ compared to pair-fed controls.

Table VII

Protein Present in the Urine of Old NZB/W Mice[a,b]

Diet	Age			
	6 months	8 months	10 months	12 months
100 ppm zinc, *ad libitum*-fed controls	2 ± 0.2[c,d]	3 ± 0.2	4 ± 0.3	*4 ± 0.1*
100 ppm zinc, inanition controls	2 ± 0.1	2 ± 0.2	2 ± 0.2	*3 ± 0.2*
9 ppm zinc	2 ± 0.2	2 ± 0.1	3 ± 0.2	*4 ± 0.2*
5 ppm zinc	2 ± 0.1	1 ± 0.1	2 ± 0.2[d]	*2 ± 0.2[d]*
2.5 ppm zinc	2 ± 0.1	1 ± 0.1	2 ± 0.2[d]	*2 ± 0.1[d]*

[a]Beach *et al.,* 1982a.
[b]Fifteen mice per group (or number remaining alive; see Fig.7).
[c]Mean ± SEM.
[d]$p < .05$ compared to *ad libitum*-fed controls using geometric means.

plasma zinc values. However, in contrast to both NZB and NZB/W mice, introduction of zinc deficiency at 10 weeks of age (relatively earlier than the introduction of diets at 6 months of age in NZ mice due to the earlier onset of the disease) had virtually no impact on the progression of autoimmune disease. In these MRL/1 mice that were older when dietary restrictions were introduced, caloric restriction had a greater impact than zinc deprivation. In contrast to NZ mice, it would appear that there is a specific age after which the introduction of such dietary restrictions is of litle or no value. Nonetheless, it has been shown that manipulation of trace element intake can have a remarkable impact on the expression of autoimmune disease (Tables VIII–X, Fig. 8).

MECHANISTIC CONSIDERATIONS

The means by which nutritional factors influence the progression of autoimmune disease are complex, with numerous possible mechanisms (Glassock, R. J., 1983; Helliwell *et al.,* 1984). Because human SLE and its empirical animal model, murine lupus, are both diseases of disordered immunological regulation, alterations in the disease process might be ascribed to any of the multiple interactions between the various aspects of the immune response and a range of specific nutrients. The immunological profile, potential modifying factors, and, most certainly, the genetic basis of autoimmune disease may be quite different in each of the models of murine lupus, requiring close comparison between experimental results in each strain (Theofilopoulos and Dixon, 1981). Any nutrient may also actively alter the course of autoimmunity by affecting tissues where end-stage disease actu-

Table VIII

Appearance of Physical Symptoms[a]

Diet	Group	Age (months)	Enlarged lymph nodes	Open sores	Swollen hind legs	Exophthalmia	Necrotic ears	Wasting cachexia
100 ppm zinc; *ad libitum*-fed controls	Young	2	0/13 (0)	0/13 (0)	0/13 (0)	0/13 (0)	0/13 (0)	0/13 (0)
		4	7/8 (88)	5/8 (63)	2/8 (25)	6/8 (75)	5/8 (63)	3/8 (38)
		6	4/4 (100)	4/4 (100)	1/4 (25)	4/4 (100)	4/4 (100)	3/4 (75)
100 ppm zinc; pair-fed controls	Young	2	0/13 (0)	0/13 (0)	0/13 (0)	0/13 (0)	0/13 (0)	0/13 (0)
		4	6/11 (55)	2/11 (18)	1/11 (9)	7/11 (64)	5/11 (45)	2/11 (18)
		6	7/7 (100)	4/7 (57)	1/7 (14)	7/7 (100)	6/7 (86)	3/7 (43)
	Old	2	0/12 (0)	0/12 (0)	0/12 (0)	0/12 (0)	0/12 (0)	0/12 (0)
		4	8/10 (80)	2/10 (20)	2/10 (20)	6/10 (60)	4/10 (40)	3/10 (30)
		6	6/6 (100)	4/6 (67)	2/6 (33)	6/6 (100)	4/6 (67)	2/6 (33)
2.5 ppm zinc	Young	2	0/13 (0)	0/13 (0)	0/13 (0)	0/13 (0)	0/13 (0)	0/13 (0)
		4	2/12 (17)	3/12 (25)	1/12 (8)	7/12 (58)	2/12 (17)	1/12 (8)
		6	4/10 (40)	5/10 (50)	3/10 (30)	9/10 (90)	3/10 (30)	2/10 (20)
	Old	2	0/13 (0)	0/13 (0)	0/13 (0)	0/13 (0)	0/13 (0)	0/13 (0)
		4	3/10 (30)	4/10 (40)	2/10 (20)	6/10 (60)	4/10 (40)	2/10 (20)
		6	3/6 (50)	4/6 (67)	2/6 (33)	6/6 (100)	3/6 (50)	2/6 (33)

[a] Number positive mice/total number of mice remaining alive at that age; percentage is indicated in parentheses (Beach *et al.*, 1982b).

Table IX

Anti-dsDNA Antibodies (Percent Bound)[a,b]

		Age				
		2 months	3 months	4 months	5 months	6 months
100 ppm zinc *ad libitum*-fed controls		9.4 ± 1.1 (13)	15.8 ± 1.2 (11)	25.7 ± 2.0 (8)	35.3 ± 3.4 (5)	39.7 ± 2.7 (4)
100 ppm zinc pair-fed controls	Young	9.1 ± 0.8 (13)	10.6 ± 0.7 (13)	17.4 ± 1.2[c] (11)	23.0 ± 1.4[c] (8)	28.2 ± 2.3[c] (7)
	Old	9.9 ± 1.0 (12)	12.8 ± 0.6 (12)	16.8 ± 0.9[c] (10)	21.9 ± 1.9[c] (7)	30.4 ± 2.6[c] (6)
2.5 ppm zinc	Young	10.6 ± 0.7 (13)	11.1 ± 1.0 (13)	12.4 ± 1.2[c,d] (12)	18.3 ± 1.4[c,d] (10)	21.6 ± 1.8[c,d] (10)
	Old	9.0 ± 0.6 (13)	13.2 ± 1.6 (13)	22.7 ± 1.8[e] (10)	26.9 ± 2.2[e] (7)	34.3 ± 2.7 (6)

[a] Beach *et al.*, 1982b.
[b] Mean ± SEM; number of mice indicated in parentheses.
[c] $p < .01$ compared to *ad libitum*-fed controls.
[d] $p < .05$ compared to pair-fed controls.
[e] $p < .01$ compared to pair-fed controls.

Table X

Survival of MRL/1 Mice[a]

		2 months	3 months	4 months	5 months	6 months
100 ppm zinc *ad libitum*-fed controls		13/13 (100)	11/13 (84)	8/13 (62)	5/13 (38)	4/13 (31)
100 ppm zinc pair-fed controls	Young	13/13 (100)	13/13 (100)	11/13 (84)	8/13 (62)	7/13 (54)
	Old	12/12 (100)	12/12 (100)	10/12 (83)	7/12 (58)	6/12 (50)
2.5 ppm zinc	Young	13/13 (100)	13/13 (100)	12/13 (92)	10/13 (77)	10/13 (77)
	Old	13/13 (100)	13/13 (100)	10/13 (77)	7/13 (54)	6/13 (46)

[a]Number of mice remaining alive at the specified age/total number of mice originally allocated to that diet (percent survival); see text for statistics (Beach *et al.*, 1982b).

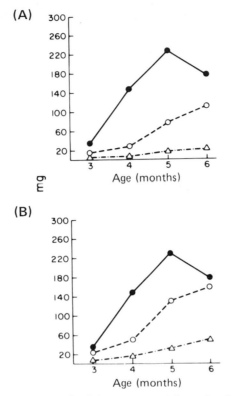

Fig. 8. (A) Lymph node weights (mg) between 3 and 6 months of age for "young" MRL/I mice, i.e., mice started on experimental diet at 4 weeks of age. (B) Lymph node weights (mg) between 3 and 5 months of age for "old" MRL/I mice, i.e., mice started on the experimental diet at 10 weeks of age. ●, 100 ppm zinc, *ad libitum*-fed controls; ○, 100 ppm zinc, pair-fed controls; △, 2.5 ppm zinc (Beach *et al.,* 1982b).

ally occurs. Many nutrients are also capable of modifying the activity of metabolic factors such as hormones and enzymes, and may affect disease by such alteration, e.g., activity levels of sex hormones (Melez *et al.,* 1978). In addition, a multiplicity of interactions between various nutrients, many of which are not even established, may affect autoimmune pathogenesis; for example, zinc deficiency alters vitamin A metabolism (Smith *et al.,* 1973). It is difficult to speculate on many of these interactions, because not only the possible interactions but also the pathogenetic basis of lupus is unclear. It is possible that nutritional studies using the various models of autoimmunity may help to establish the precise nature of the disease process and its underlying mechanisms.

Some reasonable hypotheses can now be advanced, since all five major classes of nutrients (calories, protein, lipids, vitamins, and minerals) have clearly been shown to have a significant impact on pathological consequences and ultimate mortality due to autoimmunity in murine lupus (Beach *et al.,* 1981b, 1982a,b; Levy, 1977; Fernandes *et al.,* 1972, 1973, 1976a,b, 1978a; Friend *et al.,* 1978; Safai-Kutti *et al.,* 1980). Total calories (Malave *et al.,* 1980), dietary protein, lipids (DeWille, *et al.,* 1979), and zinc (Fraker *et al.,* 1977; Fernandes *et al.,* 1979; Beach *et al.,* 1979, 1980d) have all been shown to affect both the development and the maintenance of intact immunocompetence. Since cell-mediated immunity seems to be especially susceptible to nutritional manipulation, any of these nutritional deficiencies might affect the function of specific T-cell subpopulations, whether helper T cells, suppressor T cells, or cytotoxic T cells. In many cases, it seems that T-cell functions are less vigorous at any early age, but subsequently are better preserved in later life (Beach *et al.,* 1982b; Fernandes *et al.,* 1978a). B-cell activity might also be affected by any or all of these nutritional deficiencies. For example, protein deficiency might involve a switch in antibody synthesis to a class of antibody with significantly less potential for immune complex formation and consequent renal deposition (Fernandes *et al.,* 1976a). A deficiency of any of these nutrients might affect the rate of formation of immune complexes (Steward *et al.,* 1981). In addition, accessory cell types might also be affected by nutritional deprivation. For instance, phagocytosis of immune complexes has been shown to be altered in NZ mice (Magilavy *et al.,* 1981). Zinc impairs phagocytosis, and a zinc-deficient diet might enhance the impaired phagocytosis of immune complexes in NZ mice, thereby markedly reducing their pathogenic potential.

A wide range of metabolic factors might be significantly affected by a nutrient deficiency or excess. Levels of sex hormones markedly alter the progression of autoimmune disease (Melez *et al.,* 1978), and because of the close metabolic interaction between lipid metabolism and the synthesis of steroid hormones, it would not be surprising to find alterations in the levels of both simultaneously. Levels of corticosteroids, a major means of therapy in SLE, are affected by altered intake of a variety of nutrients. Elevations of steroids occur in zinc deprivation, and this has been shown to account for many of the observed changes in immune function (DePasquale-Jardieu and Fraker, 1980). It could be that low dietary zinc acts, at least in part, by therapeutically elevating effective levels of serum corticosteroids. This would help to explain the significant effectiveness of dietary zinc in reducing the pathological signs of autoimmune disease even in mice 6 months of age when dietary restriction of zinc was commenced (Beach *et al.,* 1981b, 1982a).

Prostaglandins represent another significant group of compounds that might mediate the effects of some nutrient deficiencies on autoimmunity. Prostaglandins are being recognized as a major regulatory influence on the immune response (Goodwin and Webb, 1980), and their administration to NZB/W mice alters the development of glomerulonephritis and prolongs survival (Zurier et al., 1977), with a pathological course quite similar to that of various nutritionally deprived animals. Prostaglandins are directly metabolized from the free fatty acid arachidonic acid. Deficient EFA intake alters prostaglandin synthesis (Bonta et al., 1976). The effectiveness of eicosapentanoic acid in preventing glomerulonephritis and prolonging survival is quite likely due to an effect on prostaglandin synthesis (Prickett et al., 1981). Zinc deficiency has also been demonstrated to alter prostaglandin synthesis; this may be an important mechanistic consideration in the improved prognosis due to zinc deprivation as well.

The theoretical framework of Theofilopolous and Dixon (1981) is particularly applicable in considering the influence of various nutritional manipulations on the progression of autoimmune disease. The genetic predisposition to autoimmunity is important in all of the accelerating factors that determine the timing of onset of active disease, the pathological complications, the severity of these complications, and ultimately the life span of the animal. Deficiency or excess of specific nutrients should therefore be added to the list of factors that have been demonstrated either to accelerate or to inhibit the progression of the autoimmune disease process through multiple means.

APPLICATIONS IN CLINICAL MEDICINE

Appreciation of the possible utilization of nutrition as a therapeutic tool in clinical medicine has been greatly expanded by the improvement of techniques to detect nutritional deficiencies and by technological advances that have allowed the development of feeding techniques such as TPN. Thus far, attention has been largely focused on the critical influence of nutritional intake on the patient's ability to respond to various states of stress such as infectious diseases, neoplastic challenge, and surgical intervention. For example, a number of studies have shown that malnutrition may be far more prevalent among institutionized and hospitalized patients than was previously surmised. It has also been shown that the immunocompetence and thereby imperiling a successful outcome (Helms et al., 1983; Warnold and Lundholm, 1984). Indeed, impaired indicators of immunological function such as in vitro blast transformation of peripheral blood lymphocytes in response to mitogenic challenge and cutaneous reactivity to a battery of skin test antigens have been suggested as indicators of a patient's nutritional status. Very little thought and even less investigation have been directed toward the aggressive use of nutritional modulation as a means of therapeutic intervention, either through the introduction of limited periods of dietary deficiency or excess or through the use of nutritional synergism and imbalances.

Treatment of autoimmune disorders can be directed either at alleviating the severity of the complications of such autoimmune phenomena or at the immune dysfunction that eventually leads to these fatal complications. SLE in humans is essentially an immune complex disease; the pathological complication of the disorder most incompatible with survival is the end-stage renal disease or glomerulonephritis that develops. Because the renal manifestations of the disease prove fatal so frequently, and because similar types of glomerulonephritis are found in a variety of other pathological conditions, much of the experimental research on potential means of therapy has utilized histological damage in the kidney to assess the effectiveness of any treatment regimen. Many pharmacological agents have frequently been utilized to treat both SLE in humans and murine lupus; foremost among these are immunosuppressive and anti-inflammatory drugs, most notably the corticosteroids. Such drugs seem to be moderately effective in delaying the development of glomerulonephritis and significantly prolonging the life span of the mice to which they are administered. However, these drugs are also associated with myriad side effects such as increased incidence of neoplasms, thus significantly limiting their potential utility. The use of nutritional factors to modulate autoimmune disease is particularly advantageous because such factors are natural constituents and because their toxicity, although not totally absent, is often relatively less than that of drugs.

The use of nutritional therapy to mediate renal disease such as the immune complex glomerulonephritis that accompanies SLE and murine lupus has been based on two basic trends, neither of which even considers the possibility that manipulation of the intake of specific nutrients or combinations of nutrients might significantly alter the pathological basis of such disease processes and therefore might be used to modify the morbid outcome of such pathological processes. The first concept is that the renal insufficiency that accompanies glomerulonephritis, and other such kidney diseases, results in a diminished capacity to excrete the excesses of dietary intake as well as the by-products produced by the metabolism of essential nutrients. The second concept is that renal failure and the accompanying disease process may result in a variety of nutritional deficiencies as a result of dietary restriction, anorexia, simultaneously decreased absorption of nutrients from the gastrointestinal lumen, loss of nutrients or their metabolically active by-products in the urine due to defective glomerular filtration or during dialysis, or as a result of impaired metabolic and synthetic capabilities of the diseased kidney. Therefore, present dietary therapy may involve restriction of certain dietary components and supplementation of other essential nutrients. In addition, the impaired function of the kidney and the inability to excrete large excesses of certain required nutrients must be considered when any nutritional intervention is undertaken in such cases. In addition, the nutritional implications of any other means of therapy must also be considered. For instance, evidence has recently accumulated that plasma levels of trace metals such as zinc may be altered by renal disease and by hemodialysis. This finding is particularly significant in light of the observation that trace element nutriture may significantly alter the pathogenesis of autoimmunity even in late stages of the disease.

It is of interest to note that one of the original observations that led to the attempt to modulate nutritional factors, and thereby to alter the outcome of murine lupus, concerned a diet low in the essential amino acids phenylalanine and tyrosine. However, in the subsequent 20 years, little investigation has been done on the possible beneficial effects of similar types of dietary restriction, and most experiments have bordered on the anecdotal. Perhaps this situation will improve as we increase our understanding of the etiology and pathogenesis of lupus in both humans and murine experimental models.

14

Future Directions

That nutritional status can markedly alter host resistance and response to infectious challenge has been demonstrated repeatedly in this volume. Indeed, associations between food eaten and sickness have been noted throughout history. The interaction between malnutrition and infection was first noted in this century, and the subject gained particular attention regarding children in the Third World. It was generally determined that malnutrition, and its role in the pathogenesis of infectious disease in these children, was the primary contributing factor responsible for the very high childhood mortality rates seen in Third World countries. During the past decade, there has been increasing documentation of nutritional deficiencies in various groups in developed nations as well. At the same time, both clinical and laboratory research has demonstrated the multifaceted interaction between the nutritional status of the host and the immunological response to a wide range of pathogenic insults. While the precise nature of this complex interaction remains to be fully delineated, it is clear from the results obtained thus far that this interplay between nutrition and immunity is of considerable significance for modern medicine and public health.

Perhaps the most notable concept developed from research on nutritional factors and immunological function is that manipulation of individual nutrients, whether through dietary or parenteral means, has a major impact on host immunocompetence. It is now recognized that most early studies, whether in experimental animals or in markedly malnourished children in the Third World, focused on subjects who were quite likely deficient in a wide range of nutrients. In addition, factors such as the timing and/or duration of the nutritional insult and the degree of malnutrition were only rarely defined adequately. Consequently, many studies were principally retrospective (even historical), pointing out the possible importance of such interactions between nutritional and immunological variables, as well as underscoring the pervasive nature and extent of nutritional-immunological disorders in both the Third World and Western nations. In the past decade, much greater emphasis has been placed on the role of individual nutrients in facilitating, and in some cases potentiating, various aspects of the immune response. Future studies must continue this work. The analytical tools and investigative methodologies now exist to define such specific roles. In the past, interpretation of many studies was difficult because of methodological and analytical inconsistencies, thereby invalidating results that were of clinical importance.

Well-designed, carefully controlled studies must be conducted in both experimental and clinical settings to characterize the nature of the interaction between host immunological function and a wide range of essential and nonessential nutrients (Solomons and Allen, 1983). These investigations must focus on the effects of both excess and deficiency and must deal with specific periods of the life cycle: prenatal, neonatal, childhood, adulthood and the aged (Gershwin *et al.,* 1983; Kaminski *et al.,* 1982; Wade *et al.,* 1983). While considerable knowledge already exists, there is an urgent need to extend these findings. As noted earlier, nutrition and immunology are both relatively new scientific disciplines, and are both currently coming to the forefront of science and medicine. As techniques and concepts are refined in both of these rapidly developing specialities, they must be applied to the interaction between nutritional factors and immunity. Many of the studies conducted up to this point have been characterized by sophistication in either nutrition or immunology, and simultaneously by a general lack of expertise in the other discipline. Future endeavors should include more collaboration between experts in the two fields.

A matter for further consideration is the increasing interest of the lay public in these matters. The creation of the United Nations and its specialized agencies, the World Health Organization and the Food and Agriculture Organization, are examples of this trend. Despite the success of some remedial programs, many have failed, and the infant mortality rate has not measurably decreased in many areas. These failures may result from lack of understanding of the problem. At present, we must fill the gaps in our knowledge and then develop effective strategies.

More recently, public interest in personal health has increased in the Western nations, and attention has focused on nutritional intake and food habits. This is one of the major variables that can be readily manipulated by the individual.

Perhaps the most important task facing us at present is how to apply research findings once they are obtained. Prior assessment of the necessary application may help to establish appropriate research directions. While the overall objectives for research programs have been elaborated above, the objectives must be subdivided into those centered on developed nations and those directed principally to developing nations. Within the framework of priorities in these two settings, further subdivision is needed to develop methods to achieve goals at the community as opposed to the individual level.

First, we will consider the less developed nations. The problems facing nations with limited resources for health care were described in Chapter 1. A statistical fact that emphasizes the differences between countries is that the mortality rate from measles is up to 200 fold higher in Third World nations than in the United States or Western Europe (Salomon *et al.,* 1968). Studies throughout the developing world indicate that the interaction between malnutrition and infectious disease is part of the larger ecological context. Strategies that are devised to intercede in this complex synergism must also focus on these interactive influences. Remedial programs that are directed toward only a single causative factor in the high infant and child morbidity and mortality rates will attain only limited success.

Community-level programs in Third World countries must focus on an integrated approach to improving nutritional and health status. A number of pilot studies have shown that the most effective and acceptable intervention took place when remedial programs included multiple interacting objectives such as nutrition, primary health care, and family planning (Rosa, 1967; Omran, 1971; Cassozza and Williams, 1973). Poor sanitation and contaminated water supplies also play a key role in the high morbidity and mortality rates due to infectious disease. Contaminated water supplies and the resultant elevation of bacterial, viral, and parasitic diseases have been noted to have a severe impact on the nutritional status of a large sector of such communities in the Third World (White *et al.,* 1972; World Bank, 1976). In trial intervention studies, it has been found that remedial programs to improve the quality and quantity of the water supply are much more effective if undertaken in conjunction with programs to improve nutritional status and other parameters of public health.

At the individual level in the Third World, considerable progress has been made in decreasing mortality rates due to acute episodes of diarrhea and dehydration, the most common and serious sequelae of malnutrition and infectious disease. Perhaps the most significant progress has been the development of a variety of oral rehydration regimens (Nalin *et al.,* 1970, 1978, 1979, Pizarro *et al.,* 1979a,b; Black *et al.,* 1981). Such methods of rapid rehydration have saved large numbers of infants who would previously have died. Such formulas have now been developed to the extent that treatment regimens are available for various forms of electrolyte imbalance, e.g., hyponatremic versus hypernatremic (Pizarro *et al.,* 1983, 1984). Similar developments have occurred in dietary therapy of children with PEM (B. E. Golden and Golden, 1981, M. H. N. Golden and Golden, 1981).

A serious problem, however, is that once the child is discharged from the hospital with the acute crisis resolved, he or she returns to the home environment, with its many environmental factors that originally contributed to the debilitation. There is thus a need for effective community programs to eliminate these public health hazards.

In the developed nations, the picture is somewhat different. Whereas in the Third World nations nutritional considerations and therapeutic measures are common at the bedside, in the developed countries there has been far less such emphasis, perhaps because of the more subtle nature of the problems. Interest in this area has increased, and several studies now indicate that malnutrition among hospitalized patients, for instance, is far more pervasive than was previously surmised (Bistrian *et al.,* 1974, 1975; Blackburn, 1977).

It is also apparent that specific nutrient deficiencies may be a significant medical problem in hospitalized patients and those with chronic disease (Neumann, 1977; Blackburn and Thornton, 1979; Dickerson, 1984). Our knowledge of nutrient requirements and metabolism has now improved to the extent that it can be brought to the bedside as an important therapeutic tool. This is true of clinical situations that involve acute disease processes such as infectious disease, as well as chronic maladies such as cancer, heart disease, and diabetes. Most studies have focused on the nutritional support measures necessary to maintain the host in reasonably good nutritional condition (Blackburn and Thornton, 1979). Sophisticated use of TPN techniques will make nutritional therapeutic modalities increasingly effective. Our findings need to emphasize the application of basic research and concepts to this clinical situation. In addition, nutritional factors should be explored as potential etiological determinants in these diseases. Considerable effort is currently being expended to determine the role of nutritional factors in the development of a wide variety of malignancies (Willett and Macmahon, 1984). In addition, as new disease processes occur in our rapidly developing societies, appropriate efforts should be made to elucidate the role of nutritional factors in their etiology. For instance, the current acute immunodeficiency syndrome (AIDS) epidemic may include a nutritional component in the development of the full-blown disease (Pitchenik *et al.,* 1983; Gordsmit, 1984; LaPointe *et al.,* 1984; Beach and Laura, 1984).

Public health programs have been largely effective in eliminating the synergistic interaction between malnutrition and infectious disease. However, our major effort in developing new strategies should be focused on chronic diseases We must determine the role that nutrition plays in the development of the disease process, the ways in which nutritional factors can be manipulated to alter the course of the disease, and the role it may play in a therapeutic context (Chandra, R. K., 1984).

Above all, we must continue to develop the basic principles and concepts of the interaction between nutrition and immunity. We know almost nothing about the mechanisms by which nutritional factors can affect both immune function and the ontogeny of the immune response. Elucidation of these mechanisms is an area of research that should prove to be fruitful not only in terms of the basic knowledge, but also in terms of their importance for human health and well-being.

References

Aaskov, J. C., and Halliday, W. J. (1971). Requirement for lymphocyte-macrophage interaction in the response of mouse spleen cultures to pneumococcal polysaccharide. *Cell. Immunol.* **2**, 335.

Abassy, A. S., Badr El-Din, M. K., Hassan, A. I., Aref, G. H., Hammad, S. A., El-Araby, I. I., Badr El-Din, A. A., Soliman, M. H., and Hussein, M. (1974a). Studies of cell-mediated immunity and allergy in protein energy malnutrition. I. Cell-mediated delayed hypersensitivity. *J. Trop. Med. Hyg.* **77**, 13.

Abassy, A. S., Badr El-Din, M. K., Hassan, A. I., Aref, G. H., Hammad, S. A., El-Araby, I. I., and Badr El-Din, A. A. (1974b). Studies of cell-mediated immunity and allergy in protein energy malnutrition. II. Immediate hypersensitivity. *J. Trop. Med. Hyg.* **77**, 18.

Abb, J., and Deinhardt, F. (1980). Effects of retinoic acid on the human lymphocyte response to mitogens. *Exp. Cell Biol.* **48**, 169.

Abb, J., Abb, H., and Deinhardt, F. (1982). Retinoic acid suppression of human leukocyte interferon production. *Immunopharmacology* **4**, 303.

Abdou, N. I., and Richter, M. (1970). The role of bone marrow in the immune response. *Adv. Immunol.* **12**, 201.

Ackerman, S. K., Matter, L., and Douglas, S. D. (1980). Neutrophil chemotaxis and enzyme release competitive inhibition by a diazoacetamide pepsin inhibitor. *Biochim. Biophys. Acta* **629**, 470.

Adams, D. A., Freauff, S. J., and Erickson, K. L. (1983). Biophysical characterization of dietary lipid influences on lymphocytes. *In* "Pharmacological Effects of Lipids" (J. Kabara, ed.), Vol. II (in press).

Alcock, N. W., and Shils, M. E. (1974). Serum immunoglobulin G in the magnesium-depleted rat. *Proc. Soc. Exp. Biol. Med.* **145**, 855–858.

Alexander, F. W., Delves, H. T., and Lay, H. (1972). Plasma copper and zinc in acute leukemia. *Arch. Dis. Child.* **47**, 571.

Alford, R. H. (1970). Metal cation requirements for phytohemagglutinin-induced transformation of human peripheral blood lymphocytes. *J. Immunol.* **104**, 698.

Alleyne, G. A. O. (1966). Cardiac function in severely malnourished Jamaican children. *Clin. Sci.* **30**, 553.

Alleyne, G. A. O. (1967). The effect of severe protein calorie malnutrition on the renal function of Jamaican children. *Pediatrics* **39**, 400.

Alleyne, G. A. O. (1968). Studies on total body potassium in infantile malnutrition: The relation of body fluid spaces and urinary creatinine. *Clin. Sci.* **34**, 199.

Alleyne, G. A. O., and Scullard, G. H. (1969). Alterations in carbohydrate metabolism in Jamaican children with severe malnutrition. *Clin. Sci.* **37**, 631.

Alleyne, G. A. O., and Young, V. R. (1967). Adrenocortical function in children with severe protein-calorie malnutrition. *Clin. Sci.* **33**, 189.

Alleyne, G. A. O., Halliday, D., Waterlow, J. C., and Nicolas, B. L. (1969). Chemical composition of organs of children who died from malnutrition. *Br. J. Nutr.* **23**, 783.

Alleyne, G. A. O., Trust, P. M., Flores, H., and Robinson, H. (1972). Glucose tolerance and insulin sensitivity in malnourished children. *Br. J. Nutr.* **27**, 585.

Alleyne, G. A. O., Hay, R. W., Picou, D. I., Stanfield, J. P., and Whitehead, R. G. (1977). "Protein Energy Malnutrition." Arnold, London.

Al-Rashid, R. A., and Spangler, J. (1971). Neonatal copper deficiency. *N. Engl. J. Med.* **285**, 841.

Alvarado, J., and Luthringer, D. G. (1971). Serum immunoglobulins in edematous protein-calorie malnourished children. *Clin. Pediatr.* (*Philadelphia*) **10**, 174.

Amivaian, K., McKinney, J. A., and Tuchna, L. (1974). Effect of zinc and cadmium on guinea-pig complement. *Immunology* **26**, 1135.

Andrews, G. S. (1979). Studies of plasma zinc, copper, caeruloplasmin, and growth hormone: With special reference to carcinoma of the bronchus. *J. Clin. Pathol.* **32**, 325.

Andvonikashivili, E. L., Mosulishvili, L. M., Belokolsilski, A. I., Khevabaelze, N. E., Ieuzieva, T. K., and Efremova, E. Y. (1974). Content of some trace elements in sarcoma M-1 ONA in dynamics of malignant growth. *Cancer Res.* **34**, 271.

Angyal, A. M., and Archer, G. T. (1968). The zinc content of rat mast cells. *Aust. J. Exp. Biol. Med.* **46**, 119.

Anissimova, V. (1939). Experimental zinc teratomas of the testis and their transplantation. *Am. J. Cancer* **36**, 229.

Antia, A. U., McFarlane, H., and Soothill, J. F. (1968). Serum siderophilin in kwashiorkor. *Arch. Dis. Child.* **43**, 459.

Antonova, M. V., Pristupa, V. A., and Popov, V. P. (1968). Effect of small amounts of trace elements in the diet on immunological responses. *Gig. Sanit.* **33**, 39.

Antony, A., Ramakrishnan, T., Mikelens, P., Jackson, J., and Levinson, W. (1978). Effect of isonicotinic acid hydrazide-copper complex on rous sarcoma virus and its genome RNA. *Bioinorg. Chem.* **9**, 23.

Appledorf, H., and Kelly, L. S. (1979). Proximate trace mineral content of fast foods, pizza, Mexican-American-style foods, and submarine sandwiches. *J. Am. Diet. Assoc.* **74**, 35.

Arai, S., Yamane, I., Tanno, Y., and Takishima, T. (1977). Role of bovine serum albumin in blastoid transformation of lymphocytes by phytohemagglutinin. *Proc. Soc. Exp. Biol. Med.* **154**, 444.

Arakawa, T., Tamura, T., Igarashi, Y., Suzuki, H., and Sandstead, H. H. (1976). Zinc deficiency in two infants during total parenteral alimentation for diarrhea. *Am. J. Clin. Nutr.* **29**, 197.

Araquilla, E. R., Packer, S., Tarmas, W., and Miyamoto, S. (1978). The effect of zinc in insulin metabolism. *Endocrinology* **103**, 1440.

Aref, G. H., Badr El-Din, K., Hassan, A. I., and Draby, I. I. (1970). Immunoglobulins in kwashiorkor. *J. Trop. Med. Hyg.* **73**, 186.

Armstrong-Esther, C. A., Lacey, J. H., Crisp, A. H., and Bryant, T. N. (1978). An investigation of the immune response of patients suffering from anorexia nervosa. *Postgrad. Med. J.* **54**, 395.

Arroyave, G., Viteri, F., and Bèhar, M. (1959). Impairment of intestinal absorption of vitamin A palmitate in severe protein malnutrition (kwashiorkor). *Am. J. Clin. Nutr.* **7**, 185.

Arroyave, G., Wilson, D., de Funes, C., and Bèhar, M. (1962). The free amino acids in blood plasma of children with kwashiorkor and marasmus. *Am. J. Clin. Nutr.* **11**, 517.

Aschkenasy, A. (1979). Prevention of the immuno depressive effects of excess dietary leucine by isoleucine and valine in the rat. *J. Nutr.* **109**, 1214.

Ashkinazi, A., Levin, S., Djaldetti, M., Fishil, E., and Benvenisti, D. (1973). The syndrome of neonatal copper deficiency. *Pediatrics* **52**, 525.

Ashworth, A., Bell, R., James, W. P. T., and Waterlow, J. C. (1968). Calorie requirements of children recovering from protein-calorie malnutrition. *Lancet* **2**, 600.

Asling, C. W., and Hurley, L. S. (1963). The influence of trace elements on the skeleton. *Clin. Orthop. Relat. Res.* **27**, 213.

Atkinson, R. L., Dahms, W. T., Bray, G. A., Jacob, R., and Sandstead, H. H. (1978). Plasma zinc and copper in obesity and after intestinal bypass. *Ann. Intern. Med.* **84**, 491.

Attramadal, A. (1969). The effect of divalent cations in cell adhesion. *J. Periodontal Res.* **4**, 281.

Atukorala, S., Basu, T. K., Dickerson, J. W. T., Donaldson, D., and Sakula, A. (1979). Vitamin A, zinc and lung cancer. *Br. J. Cancer* **40**, 927.

Auld, D. A., Livingston, D. M., and Vallee, B. L. (1974). RNA-dependent DNA polymerase (reverse transcriptase) from avian myoblastosis virus. A zinc metalloenzyme. *Proc. Natl. Acad. Sci. U.S.A.* **71**, 2091.

Avigad, L. S., and Bernheimer, A. W. (1976). Inhibition by zinc of hemolysis induced by bacterial and other cytolytic agents. *Infect. Immun.* **13**, 1378.

Bagg, H. J. (1936). Experimental production of teratoma testis in the fowl. *Am. J. Cancer* **26**, 69.

Bagg, H. J. (1937). Factors involved in the experimental production of teratoma testis in the fowl. *In* "Some Fundamental Aspects of the Cancer Problem," Publ. No. 92, p. 103. Am. Assoc. Adv. Sci., Washington D.C.

Baggs, R. B., and Miller, S. A. (1973). Nutritional iron deficiency as a determinant of host resistance in the rat. *J. Nutr.* **103**, 1554.

Baker, B. L., and Hultquist, D. E. (1978). A copper-binding immunoglobulin from a myeloma patient. Studies of the copper-binding site. *J. Biol. Chem.* **253**, 8444.

Balch, H. H., and Spencer, M. T. (1954). Phagocytosis by human leukocytes. II. Relation of nutritional deficiency in man to phagocytosis. *J. Clin. Invest.* **33**, 1321.

Baly, D. L., Keen, C. L., and Hurley, L. S. (1984a). Pyruvate carboxylase and phosphoenolpyruvate carboxykinase activity in developing rats: Effect of manganese deficiency. *Fed. Proc., Fed. Am. Soc. Exp. Biol.* **43**, 1054.

Baly, D. L. Curry, D. L., Keen, C. L., and Hurley, L. S. (1984b). Effect of manganese deficiency on insulin secretion and carbohydrate homeostasis. *J. Nutr.* (in press).

Baly, D. L., Golub, M. S., Gershwin, M. E., and Hurley, L. S. (1984). Studies of marginal zinc deprivation in rhesus monkeys. III. Effects on vitamin A metabolism. *Am. J. Clin. Nutr.* **40**, 199.

Bang, F. B., Bang, B. G., and Foard, M. (1975). Acute Newcastle virus infection of the upper respiratory tract of the chicken. II. The effect of diets deficient in vitamin A on the pathogenesis of the infection. *Am. J. Pathol.* **78**, 417.

Barak, A. J., Keefer, R. C., and Tuma, D. J. (1971). The possible role of manganese in hepatic lipid transport. *Nutr. Rep. Int.* **3**, 243.

Barbezat, G. D., and Hansen, J. D. L. (1968). The exocrine pancreas and protein-calorie malnutrition. *Pediatrics* **42**, 77.

Barr, D. H., and Harris, J. W. (1973). Growth of P388 leukemia as an ascites tumor in zinc-deficient mice. *Proc. Soc. Exp. Biol. Med.* **144**, 284.

Barry, W. S., and Pierce, N. F. (1979). Protein deprivation causes reversible impairment of mucosal immune response to cholera toxoid/toxin in rat gut. *Nature (London)* **281**, 64.

Battifora, H. A., McCreary, P. A., and Hahnemann, B. M. (1968). Chronic magnesium deficiency in the rat. Studies of chronic myelogenous leukemia. *Arch. Path.* **86**, 610–620.

Bazhora, I. I., Shtefan, E. E., and Timoshevski, I. V. (1974). The effect of microelements—copper, manganese and cobalt—on the antibody-forming function of lymphoid tissue. *Mikrobiol. Zh.* **36**, 771.

Bazzell, K. L., Coleman, R. L., and Mordquist, R. E. (1979). Induction of metallothionein-like protein in human breast tumor cells. *Toxicol. Appl. Pharmacol.* **50**, 199.

Beach, R. S., and Laura, P. F. (1984). Letter to the editor. *Ann. Intern. Med.* **99**, 565.

Beach, R. S., Gershwin, M. E., and Hurley, L. S. (1979). Altered thymic structure and mitogen responsiveness in postnatally zinc-deprived mice. *Dev. Comp. Immunol.* **3**, 725.

Beach, R. S., Gershwin, M. E., and Hurley, L. S. (1980a). Growth and development of postnatally zinc-deprived mice. *J. Nutr.* **110**, 201.

Beach, R. S., Gershwin, M. E., and Hurley, L. S. (1980b). T cell function in the lethal milk (lm/lm) mutant mouse. *Proc. Int. Cong. Immunol. 4th, 1980* p. 171.

Beach, R. S., Gershwin, M. E., and Hurley, L. S. (1980c). Zinc deprivation and the immune response. *Fed. Proc., Fed. Am. Soc. Exp. Biol.* **39**, 888.

Beach, R. S., Gershwin, M. E., Makishima, R. K., and Hurley, L. S. (1980d). Impaired immunologic ontogeny in postnatal zinc deprivation. *J. Nutr.* **110**, 805.

Beach, R. S., Gershwin, M. E., and Hurley, L. S. (1981a). Dietary zinc modulation of moloney sarcoma virus oncogenesis. *Cancer Res.* **41**, 552.

Beach, R. S., Gerhswin, M. E., and Hurley, L. S. (1981b). Nutritional factors and autoimmunity. I. Immunopathology of zinc deprivation in New Zealand mice. *J. Immunol.* **126**, 1999.

Beach, R. S., Gershwin, M. E., and Hurley, L. S. (1982a). Nutritional factors and autoimmunity. II. Prolongation of survival in zinc deprived NZB/W mice. *J. Immunol.* **128**, 308.

Beach, R. S., Gershwin, M. E., and Hurley, L. S. (1982b). Nutritional factors and autoimmunity. III. Zinc deprivation versus restricted food intake in MRL/1 mice; the distinction between interacting dietary influences. *J. Immunol.* **129**, 2686.

Beach, R. S., Gershwin, M. E., and Hurley, L. S. (1982c). Gestational zinc deprivation in mice: Persistence of immunodeficiency for three generations. *Science* **218**, 469.

Beach, R. S., Gershwin, M. E., and Hurley, L. S. (1982d). Zinc copper and manganese in immune function and experimental oncogenesis. *Nutr. Cancer* **3**, 172.

Beach, R. S., Gershwin, M. E., and Hurley, L. S. (1983). Persistent immunological consequences of gestational zinc deprivation. *Am. J. Clin. Nutr.* **38**, 579.

Beas, F., Monckeberg, F., Horwitz, I., and Figueroa, M. (1966). The response of the thyroid gland to thyroid-stimulating hormone (TSH) in infants with malnutrition. *Pediatrics* **38**, 1003.

Beatty, D. W., and Dowdle, E. B. (1979). Deficiency in kwashiorkor serum of factors required for optimal lymphocyte transformation in vitro. *Clin. Exp. Immunol.* **35**, 433.

Behrens, U., Friedrich, I., Vernace, S., Schaffner, F., and Paronetto, F. (1982). Lymphocyte responsiveness per unit volume of blood in patients with chronic nonalcoholic and alcoholic liver disease. Plasma inhibitory factors and functional defects of responder cells. *J. Clin. Lab. Immunol.* **8**, 143.

Beinert, H. (1966). Cytochrome C oxidase: Present knowledge of the state and function of its copper components. *In* "The Biochemistry of Copper" (J. Peisach, P. Aisen, and W. E. Blumberg, eds.), p. 213. Academic Press, New York.

Beisel, W. R. (1976). Trace elements of infectious processes. *Med. Clin. North Am.* **60**, 831.

Beisel, W. R. (1982). Synergism and antagonism of parasitic diseases and malnutrition. *Rev. Infect. Dis.* **4**, 746.

Bell, L. T., and Hurley, L. S. (1973). Ultrastructural effects of manganese deficiency in liver, heart, kidney and pancreas of mice. *Lab. Invest.* **29**, 723.

Bell, L. T., Branstrator, M., Roux, C., and Hurley, L. S. (1975). Chromosomal abnormalities in maternal and fetal tissues of magnesium- or zinc-deficient rats. *Teratology* **12**, 221.

Bell, R. G., and Hazell, L. A. (1975). Influence of dietary protein restriction on immune competence. *J. Exp. Med.* **141**, 127.

Bell, R. G., Turner, R. J., Gracey, M., Suharjono, and Sunoto (1976a). Serum and small intestinal immunoglobulin levels in undernourished children. *Am. J. Clin. Nutr.* **29**, 392.

Bell, R. G., Hazell, L. A., and Price, P. (1976b). Influence of dietary protein restriction on immune competence. II. Effect of lymphoid tissue. *Clin. Exp. Immunol.* **26**, 314.

Bendich, A., Gabriel, E., and Machlin, L. J. (1983). Effect of dietary level of Vitamin E on the immune system of the spontaneously hypertensive (SHR) and normotensive Wistar Kyoto (WKY) rat. *J. Nutr.* **113**, 1920.

Bentwich, Z., and Kunkel, H. G. (1973). Specific properties of human B and T lymphocytes and alterations in disease. *Transplant Rev.* **16**, 29.

Berenyi, M. R., Straus, B., and Cruz, D. (1974). In vitro and in vivo studies of cellular immunity in alcoholic cirrhosis. *Dig. Dis.* **19**, 198.

Berenyi, M. R., Straus, B., and Avilla, L. (1975). T rosettes in alcoholic cirrhosis of the liver. *JAMA, J. Am. Med. Assoc.* **232**, 44.

Berg, T. (1968). Immunoglobulin levels in infants with low birth weights. *Acta Paediatr. Scand.* **57**, 369.

Bernstein, I. M., Webster, K. H., Williams, R. C., and Strickland, R. G. (1974). Reduction in circulating T lymphocytes in alcoholic liver disease. *Lancet* **2**, 488.

Bettger, W. J., Reeves, P. G., Savage, J. E., and O'Dell, B. L. (1980). Interaction of zinc and vitamin E in the chick. *Proc. Soc. Exp. Biol. Med.* **163**, 432.

Bhaskaram, P., and Reddy, V. (1981). Bactericidal activity of human milk leukocytes. *Acta Paediatr. Scand.* **70**, 87.

Bhaskaram, P., Prasad, J. S., and Krishnamachari, K. A. V. R. (1977). Anemia and immune response. *Lancet* **1**, 100.

Bhuyan, U. N., and Ramalingaswami, V. (1972). Responses of the protein-deficient rabbit to staphylococcal bacteremia. *Am. J. Pathol.* **69**, 359.

Bhuyan, U. N., and Ramalingaswami, V. (1973). Immune responses of the protein-deficient guinea pig to BCG vaccination. *Am. J. Pathol.* **72**, 489.

Bhuyan, U. N., and Ramalingaswami, V. (1974). Systemic macrophage mobilization and granulomatous response to BCG in the protein-deficient rabbit. *Am. J. Pathol.* **76**, 313.

Bienia, R., Ratcliff, S., Barbour, G. L., and Kummer, M. (1982). Malnutrition and hospital prognosis in the alcoholic patient. *JPEN, J. Parenter. Enteral Nutr.* **6**, 301.

Bischoff, F., and Long, M. L. (1939). The local effect of zinc upon the develop of the Marsh-Buffalo adenocarcinoma. *Am. J. Cancer* **37**, 531.

Bistrian, B. R., Blackburn, G. L., Hallowell, E., and Heddle, R. (1974). Protein status of general surgical patients. *JAMA, J. Am. Med. Assoc.* **230**, 858.

Bistrian, B. R., Blackburn, G., Scrimshaw, N., and Flatt, J. (1975). Cellular immunity in semi-starved states in hospitalized adults. *Am. J. Clin. Nutr.* **28**, 1148.

Bistrian, B. R., Blackburn, G. L., Vitale, J., Cochran, D., and Naylor, J. (1976). Prevalence of malnutrition in general medical patients. *JAMA, J. Am. Med. Assoc.* **235**, 1567.

Bjorksten, B., Back, O., Gustavson, K. H., Hallmans, G., Hagglof, B., and Tarnvik, A. (1980). Zinc and immune function in Down's syndrome. *Acta Paediatr. Scand.* **69**, 183.

Bjorneboe, M., and Prytz, H. (1972). Antibodies to intestinal microbes in serum of patients with cirrhosis of the liver. *Lancet* **1**, 58.

Bjorneboe, M., Jensen, K. B., Scheibel, I., Thomsen, A. C., and Bentzon, M. W. (1970). Tetanus antitoxin production and gammaglobulin levels in patients with cirrhosis of the liver. *Acta Med. Scand.* **188**, 541.

Black, R. E., Merson, M. H., Taylor, P. R., Yolken, R. H., Yunis, A., and Sack, D. A. (1981). Glucose vs sucrose in oral rehydration solutions for infants and young children with Rotavirus-associated diarrhea. *Pediatrics* **67**, 79.

Blackburn, G. L. (1977). Nutritional assessment and support during infection. *Am. J. Clin. Nutr.* **30,** 1493.

Blackburn, G. L., and Thornton, P. A. (1979). Nutritional assessment of the hospitalized patient. *Med. Clin. North Am.* **63,** 1103.

Blackman, V., Marsden, P. D., Banwell, J., and Hall Craggs, M. (1965). Albumin metabolism in hookworm anaemias. *Trans. R. Soc. Trop. Med. Hyg.* **59,** 472.

Blalock, J. E., and Gifford, G. E. (1975). Inhibition of interferon action by vitamin A. *J. Gen. Virol.* **29,** 315.

Blalock, J. E., and Gifford, G. E. (1976). Comparison of the suppression of interferon production and inhibition of its action by vitamin A and related compounds. *Proc. Soc. Exp. Biol. Med.* **153,** 298.

Blalock, J. E., and Gifford, G. E. (1977). Retinoic acid (vitamin A acid) induced transcriptional control of interferon production. *Proc. Natl. Acad. Sci. U.S.A.* **74,** 5382.

Blaxter, K. L. (1957). The fat soluble vitamins. *Ann. Rev. of Biochem.* **26,** 275.

Blumenthal, I., Lealman, G. T., and Franklyn, P. P. (1980). Fracture of the femur, fish odour, and copper deficiency in a preterm infant. *Arch. Dis. Child.* **55,** 229.

Bois, P. (1963). Effect of magnesium deficiency on mast cells and urinary histamine in rats. *Br. J. Exp. Path.* **44,** 151–155.

Boissonneault, G. A., and Johnston, P. V. (1984). Humoral immunity in essential fatty acid-deficient rats and mice: Effect of route of injection of antigen. *J. Nutr.* **114,** 89.

Boman, B. M., Zachowski, A., and Aubry, J. (1980). Manganese and magnesium dependent properties and inner plasma membrane localization of guanylate cyclase from murine plasmacytoma cells. *Biochimie* **62,** 85.

Bonta, I. L., Bult, H., Ven, L. L. M. V. D., and Noordhook, J. (1976). Essential fatty acid deficiency: A condition to discriminate prostaglandin and non-prostaglandin mediated components of inflammation. *Agents Actions* **6,** 154.

Bowers, T. K., and Eckert, E. (1978). Leukopenia in anorexia nervosa. *Arch Intern. Med.* **138,** 1520.

Bowie, M. D., Brinkman, G. L., and Hansen, J. D. L. (1963). Diarrhea in protein-calorie malnutrition. *Lancet* **2,** 550.

Boyne, R., and Arthur, J. R. (1979). Alterations of neutrophil function in selenium-deficient cattle. *J. Comp. Path.* **89,** 151.

Boynton, L. C., and Bradford, W. L. (1931). Effect of vitamins A and D on resistance to infection. *J. Nutr.* **4,** 323.

Bracha, M., and Schlesinger, M. J. (1976). Inhibition of sindbis virus replication by zinc ions. *Virology* **72,** 272.

Brada, Z., Altman, N. H., and Bulba, S. (1975). The effect of cupric acetate on ethionine metabolism. *Cancer Res.* **35,** 3172.

Brady, F. O., Monaco, M. E., Forman, H. J., Schutz, G., and Fiegelson, P. (1972). On the role of copper in activation of and catalysis by tryptophane-2, 3-dioxygenase. *J. Biol. Chem.* **247,** 7915.

Brenton, D. P., Brown, R. E., and Wharton, B. A. (1967). Hypothermia in kwashiorkor. *Lancet* **1,** 410.

Brewer, G. J., Prasad, A. S., Oelshlegl, F. J., Jr., Schoomaker, E. B., Ortega, J., and Oberlas, D. (1976). Zinc and sickle cell anemia. *In* "Trace Elements in Human Health and Disease" (A. S. Prasad, ed.), Vol. 1, p. 283. Academic Press, New York.

Brinkman, G. L., Bowie, M. D., Friis-Hansen, B., and Hansen, J. D. L. (1965). Body water composition in kwashiorkor before and after loss of edema. *Pediatrics* **36,** 94.

Britton, W. M., Hill, C. H., and Barber, C. W. (1964). A mechanism of interaction between dietary protein levels and coccidiosis in chicks. *J. Nutr.* **82,** 306.

Brook, C. G. D. (1971). Determination of body composition of children from skinfold measurements. *Arch. Dis. Child.* **46**, 182.

Brooke, O. G. (1972). Hypothermia in malnourished Jamaican children. *Arch. Dis. Child.* **47**, 525.

Brooke, O. G. (1973). Thermal insulation in malnourished Jamaican children. *Arch. Dis. Child.* **48**, 901.

Brooke, O. G., and Ashworth, A. (1972). The influence of malnutrition on the postprandial metabolic rate and respiratory quotient. *Br. J. Nutr.* **27**, 407.

Brooke, O. G., and Cocks, T. (1974). Resting metabolic rate in malnourished babies in relation to total body potassium. *Acta Paediatr. Scand.* **63**, 817.

Brooke, O. G., and Salvosa, C. B. (1974). Response of malnourished babies to heat. **Arch. Dis. Child. 49**, 123.

Brooke, O. G., Harris, M., and Salvosa, C. B. (1973). The response of malnourished babies to cold. *J. Physiol. (London)* **233**, 75.

Brown, E. D., McGuckin, M. A., Wilson, M., and Smith, J. C. (1976). Zinc in selected hospital diets. *J. Am. Diet. Assoc.* **69**, 632.

Brown, E. D., Howard, M. P., and Smith, J. C. (1977). The copper content of regular, vegetarian and renal diets. *Fed Proc., Fed. Am. Soc. Exp. Biol.* **36**, 1122.

Brown, F. C., and Ward, D. N. (1959). Studies on mammalian tyrosinase II chemical and physical properties of fractions purified by chromatography. *Proc. Soc. Exp. Biol. Med.* **100**, 701.

Brown, K. H., and Black, R. E. (1981). The nutritional cost of infections. *Prog. Clin. Biol. Res.* **77**, 467.

Brown, K. H., Gilman, R. H., Gaffar, A., Alamagir, S. M., Strife, J. L., Kapikian, A. Z., and Sack, R. B. (1981). Infections associated with severe protein-calorie malnutrition in hospitalized infants and children. *Nutr. Res.* **1**, 33.

Brown, R. D., Brewer, C. F., and Koenig, S. H. (1977). Conformation states of concanavalin A. Kinetics of transitions induced by interaction with Mn^{2+} and Ca^{2+} ions. *Biochemistry* **16**, 3883.

Brown, R. E., and Katz, M. (1965). Antigenic stimulation in undernourished children. *East Afr. Med. J.* **42**, 221.

Brown, R. E., and Katz, M. (1966a). Failure of antibody production to yellow fever vaccine in children with kwashiorkor. *Trop. Geogr. Med.* **18**, 125.

Brown, R. E., and Katz, M. (1966b). Smallpox vaccination in malnourished children. *Trop. Geogr. Med.* **18**, 129.

Brummerstedt, E., Andresen, E., Basse, A., and Flagstad, T. (1974). Lethal trait A-46 in cattle. *Immunol. Invest. Nord. Vet. Med.* **26**, 279.

Brunser, O., Reid, A., Monckeberg, F., Maccioni, A., and Contreras, I. (1968). Jejunal mucosa in infant malnutrition. *Am. J. Clin. Nutr.* **21**, 976.

Bryant, R. E. (1969). Divalent cation requirements for leukocyte adhesiveness. *Proc. Soc. Exp. Biol. Med.* **130**, 975.

Bryant, R. L., and Barnett, J. B. (1979). Adjuvant properties of retinol on IgE production in mice. *Int. Arch. Allergy Appl. Immunol.* **59**, 69.

Buchbinder, N. A., and Roberts, W. C. (1973). An important but unemphasized factor predisposing to infective endocarditis. *Arch. Intern. Med.* **132**, 689.

Buckley, R. H., Whisnant, J. K., Schiff, R. I. *et al.* (1976). Correction of severe combined immunodeficiency by fetal liver cells. *N. Engl. J. Med.* **294**, 1076.

Burnet, F. M. (1974). Invertebrate precusors to immune responses. *Contemp. Top. Immunobiol.* **4**, 13.

Butterworth, B. E., and Korant, B. D. (1974). Characterization of the large picornaviral polypeptides produced in the presence of zinc ion. *J. Virol.* **14**, 282.

Caddell, J. L., and Olson, R. E. (1973). I. An evaluation of the electrolyte status of malnourished Thai children. *J. Pediatr.* **83**, 124.

Caddell, J. L., Suskind, R. M., Sillup, H., and Olson, R. E. (1973). II. Parenteral magnesium load evaluation of malnourished Thai children. *J. Pediatr.* **38**, 129.

Caggiano, V., Schnitzler, R., Strauss, W., Baker, R. K., Carter, A. C., Josephson, A. S., and Wallach, S. (1969). Zinc deficiency in a patient with retarded growth, hypogonadism, hypogammaglobulinemia and chronic infection. *Am. J. Med. Sci.* **257**, 305.

Cannon, P. R. (1945). The relationship of protein metabolism to antibody production and resistance to infection. *Adv. Protein Chem.* **2**, 135.

Cantor, H. M., and Dumont, A. E. (1967). Hepatic suppression of sensitization to antigen absorbed into the portal system. *Nature (London)* **215**, 744.

Caren, L. D., Leveque, J. A., Mandel, A. D. (1983). Effect of ethanol on the immune system in mice. *Dev. Toxicol. Environ. Sci.* **11**, 435.

Carleton, R. L., Friedman, N. P., and Bomze, E. J. (1953). Experimental teratomas of the testis. *Cancer* **6**, 464.

Carleton, W. W., and Price, P. S. (1973). Dietary copper and the induction of neoplasms in the rat by acetylaminoflourine and dimethylnitrosamine. *Food Cosmet. Toxicol.* **11**, 827.

Carlomagno, M. A., O'Brien, B. C., and McMurray, D. N. (1983). Influence of early weaning and dietary fat on immune responses in adult rats. *J. Nutr.* **113**, 610.

Carmichael, L. E., and Barnes, F. D. (1969). Effect of temperature on growth of canine herpesvirus in canine kidney cell and macrophage cultures. *J. Infect. Dis.* **120**, 664.

Carruthers, C., and Suntzeff, V. (1945). Copper and zinc in epidermal carcinogenesis induced by methyl cholanthrene. *J. Biol. Chem.* **159**, 647.

Carryer, H. M., Berman, J. M., and Mason, H. L. (1959). Relative lymphocytosis in anorexia nervosa. *Mayo Clin. Proc.* **34**, 426.

Cassozza, L. J., and Williams, C. D. (1973). Family health versus family planning. *Lancet* **1**, 172.

Catalanatto, F. A. (1978). The trace metal zinc and taste. *Am. J. Clin. Nutr.* **31**, 1098.

Center for Disease Control (1975). "Nutrition Surveillance Sources of Error in Measuring and Weighing Children." U.S. Dept. of Health, Education and Welfare. Washington, D.C.

Chadha, K. C., Grob, P. M., Mikulski, A. J., Davis, L. R., and Sulkowski, E. (1979). Copper chelate affinity chromatography of human fibroblast and leukocyte interferons. *J. Gen. Virol.* **43**, 701.

Chandra, R. K. (1972). Immunocompetence in undernutrition. *J. Pediatr.* **81**, 1194.

Chandra, R. K. (1974). Rosette-forming T lymphocytes and cell-mediated immunity in malnutrition. *Br. Med. J.* **3**, 608.

Chandra, R. K. (1975a). Reduced secretory antibody response to live attenuated measles and poliovirus vaccines in malnourished children. *Br. Med. J.* **2**, 583.

Chandra, R. K. (1975b). Antibody formation in first and second generation offspring of nutritionally deprived rats. *Science* **190**, 289.

Chandra, R. K. (1976). Nutrition as a critical determinant in susceptibility to infection. *World Rev. Nutr. Diet* **25**, 166.

Chandra, R. K. (1977). Lymphocyte subpopulations in human malnutrition: Cytotoxic and suppressor cells. *Pediatrics* **59**, 423.

Chandra, R. K. (1979a). T and B lymphocyte subpopulations and leukocyte terminal deoxynucleotidyl-transferase in energy-protein undernutrition. *Acta Paediatr. Scand.* **68**, 841.

Chandra, R. K. (1979b). Serum thymic hormone activity in protein-energy malnutrition. *Clin. Exp. Immunol.* **38**, 228.

Chandra, R. K. (1980a). Mucosal immunity in nutritional deficiency. *In* "Mucosal Post Defenses in Health and Disease" (Ogra, P. L., and Bienenstock, J., eds.), Ross Laboratories, Columbus, Ohio.

Chandra, R. K. (1980b). "Immunology of Nutritional Disorders." Arnold, London.

Chandra, R. K. (1980c). Cell-mediated immunity in genetically obese (C57BL/6J ob/ob) mice. *Am. J. Clin. Nutr.* **33**, 13.

Chandra, R. K. (1981a). Immunocompetence as a functional index of nutritional status. *Br. Med. Bull.* **37**, 89.

Chandra, R. K. (1981b). Serum thymic hormone activity and cell-mediated immunity in healthy newborns, pre-term, and small-for-gestation infants. *Pediatrics* **64**.

Chandra, R. K. (1981c). Breast feeding, growth and morbidity. *Nutr. Res.* **1**, 25.

Chandra, R. K. (1981d). Interference of malnutrition with specific immune response. *In* "The Impact of Malnutrition on Immune Defense in Parasitic Infestation" (Isliker, H., and Schurch, B., eds.), Huber, Bern, p. 104.

Chandra, R. K. (1984). Parasitic infection, nutrition, and immune response. *Fed. Proc.* **43**, 251.

Chandra, R. K., and Au, B. (1980a). Single nutrient deficiency and cell-mediated immune responses. I. Zinc. *Am. J. Clin. Nutr.* **33**, 736.

Chandra, R. K., and Au, B. (1980b). Spleen hemolytic plaque-forming cell response and generation of cytotoxic cells in genetically obese (C57B1/6J ob/ob) mice. *Int. Arch. Allergy Appl. Immunol.* **62**, 94.

Chandra, R. K., and Au, B. (1981). Single nutrient deficiency and cell-mediated immune responses. III. Vitamin A. *Nutr. Res.* **1**, 181.

Chandra, R. K., and Bhurjwala, R. A. (1977). Elevated serum -fetoprotein and impaired immune response in malnutrition. *Int. Arch. Allergy Appl. Immunol.* **53**, 180.

Chandra, R. K., and Kutty, K. M. (1980). Immunocompetence in obesity. *Acta Paediatr. Scand.* **69**, 25.

Chandra, R. K., Pawa, R. R., and Ghai, O. P. (1968). Sugar intolerance in malnourished infants and children. *Br. Med. J.* **4**, 611.

Chandra, R. K., Au, B., and Geresi, G. (1981a). Single nutrient deficiency and cell-mediated immune responses. II. Pyroidoxine. *Nutr. Res.* **1**, 101.

Chandra, R. K., Heresi, G., and Au, B. (1981b). Serum thymic hormone activity in genetically-obese mice. *Br. J. Nutr.* **45**, 211.

Chandra, R. K., and Saraya, A. K. (1975). Impaired immunocompetence associated with iron deficiency. *J. Pediat,* **86**, 899.

Chang, L. M., and Bollerm, F. J. (1970). Deoxy nucleotide-polymerizing enzymes of calf thymus gland. IV. Inhibition of terminal deoxynucleotidyl transferase by metal ligands. *Proc. Natl. Acad. Sci. U.S.A.* **65**, 1041.

Chapman, H., and Hibbs, J. (1977). Modulation of macrophage tumoricidal capability by components of normal serum: A central role for lipid. *Science* **197**, 282.

Cheney, K. E., Liu, R. K., Smith, G. S., Leung, R. E., Mickey, M. R., and Walford, R. L. (1980). Survival and disease patterns in C57BL/6J mice subjected to undernutrition. *Exp. Gerontol.* **15**, 237.

Cherrick, G. R., Pothier, L., Dufour, J. J., and Sherlock, S. (1959). Immunologic response to tetanus toxoid inoculation in patients with hepatic cirrhosis. *N. Engl. J. Med.* **261**, 340.

Chesters, J. K. (1972). The role of zinc ions in the transformation of lymphocytes by phytohemagglutinin. *Biochem. J.* **130**, 133.

Chesters, J. K., and Will, M. (1973). Some factors controlling food intake by zinc-deficient rats. *Br. J. Nutr.* **30**, 555.

Chevalier, P., and Ashkenasy, A. (1977). Hematological and immunological effects of excess dietary leucine in the young rat. *Am. J. Clin. Nutr.* **30**, 1645.

Chvapil, M. (1976). Effect of zinc on cells and biomembranes. *Med. Clin. North Am.* **60**, 799.

Chvapil, M., Zukoski, C. F., Hattler, B. G., Stankova, L., Montgomery, D., Carlson, E. C., and Ludwig, J. C. (1976). Zinc and cells. *In* "Trace Elements in Human Health and Disease" (A. S. Prasad, ed.), Vol. 1, p. 269. Academic Press, New York.

Chvapil, M., Stankova, L., Bernhard, D. S., Weldy, P. L., Carlson, E. C., and Campbell, J. B. (1977a). Effect of zinc on peritoneal macrophages *in vitro. Infect. Immun.* **16,** 367.

Chvapil, M., Stankova, L., Bernhard, D. S., Zukoski, C. F., and Drach, G. W. (1977b). Effect of prostatic fluid and its fractions on some functions of peritoneal macrophages. *Invest. Urol.* **15,** 173.

Chvapil, M., Stankova, L., Zukoski, C. F., and Zukoski, C. (1977c). Inhibition of some function of polymorphonuclear leukocytes by *in vitro* zinc. *J. Lab. Clin. Med.* **89,** 135.

Chvapil, M., Stankova, L., Bartos, Z., Cox, T., and Nichols, W. (1979). Mobility of peritoneal inflammatory cells after *in vivo* supplementation with zinc. *J. Reticuloendothel. Soc.* **25,** 345.

Ciaparelli, L., Retief, D. H., and Fatti, L. P. (1972). The effect of zinc on 9, 10-dimethyl-1-1,2-benzanthracene (DMBA) induced salivary gland tumours in the albino rat a preliminary study. *S. Afr. Med. J.* **37,** 85.

Cinader, B., Clandinin, M. T., Hosokawa, T., and Robblee, N. M. (1983). Dietary fat alters the fatty acid composition of lymphocyte membranes and the rate at which suppressor capacity is lost. *Immunol. Lett.* **6,** 331.

Clausen, J., and Moller, J. (1967). Allergic encephalomyelitis induced by brain antigen after deficiency in polyunsaturated fatty acids during myelination. *Acta Neurol. Scand.* **43,** 375.

Clayton, C. C., King, H. J., and Spain, J. D. (1953). Effect of dietary copper upon azo dye carcinogenesis and upon some liver components. *Fed. Proc., Fed. Am. Soc. Exp. Biol.* **12,** 190.

Clifford, C. K., Smith, L. M., Erickson, K. L., Hamblin, C. L., Creveling, R. K., and Clifford, A. J. (1983). Effect of dietary triglycerides on lymphocyte transformation in rats. *J. Nutr.* **113,** 669.

Cohen, B. E., and Cohen, I. K. (1973). Vitamin A: Adjuvant and steroid antagonist in the immune response. *J. Immunol.* **111,** 1376.

Cohen, B. E., and Elin, R. J. (1974). Vitamin A-induced nonspecific resistance to infection. *J. Infect. Dis.* **129,** 597.

Cohen, D. I., Illowsky, B., and Linder, M. C. (1979). Altered copper absorption in tumor-bearing and estrogen-treated rats. *Am. J. Physiol.* **236,** E309.

Cohen, S., and Hansen, J. D. L. (1962). Metabolism of albumin and globulin in kwashiorkor. *Clin. Sci.* **23,** 351.

Cohen, N. L., Keen, C. L., Lonnerdal, B., and Hurley, L. S. (1984). Cu deficiency impairs liver Fe mobilization when dietary Fe is low. *Fed. Proc., Fed. Am. Soc. Exp. Biol.* **43,** 681.

Cohn, Z. A. (1972). Some aspects of macrophage membranes. *In* "Inflammation: Mechanisms and Control" (I. M. Lepow and P. A. Ward, eds.), p. 71. Academic Press, New York.

Committee on Nutrition (1976). American Academy of Pediatrics. *Pediatrics* **57,** 278.

Conn, H. O. (1964). Spontaneous peritonitis and bacteremia in Laennec's cirrhosis caused by enteric organisms. *Ann. Intern. Med.* **60,** 568.

Cook, G. C. (1974). Malabsorption in Africa. *Trans. R. Soc. Trop. Med. Hyg.* **68,** 419.

Cooper, E. L. (1970). Transplantation immunity in Helminths and Annelides. *Transplant. Proc.* **2,** 216.

Cooper, M. D., Perey, D. Y., McKneally, M. F., Gabrielsen, A. E., Sutherland, D. E. R., and Good, R. A. (1966). A mammalian equivalent of the avian Bursa of fabricius. *Lancet* **1,** 1388.

Cooper, M. D., Perey, D. Y., and Peterson, R. D. A. (1968). The two-component concept of the lymphoid system. *In* "Immunology Deficiency Diseases in Man," pp. 7–14. National Foundation/March of Dimes, White Plains, New York.

Cooper, W. C., Good, R. A., and Mariani, T. (1974). Effects of protein insufficiency on immune responsiveness. *Am. J. Clin. Nutr.* **27,** 647.

Coovadia, H. M., and Soothill, J. F. (1976). The effect of amino acid restricted diets on the clearance of ^{125}I-labelled polyvinyl pyrolidone in mice. *Clin. Exp. Immunol.* **23,** 562.

Cordano, A. (1978). Copper deficiency in clinical medicine. *In* "Zinc and Copper in Clinical Medicine" (K. M. Hambridge and B. F. Nichols, eds.), p. 119. Spectrum, New York.

Cordano, A., Baertl, J. M., and Graham, G. G. (1964). Copper deficiency in infancy. *Pediatrics* **34,** 324.

Cordano, A., Placko, R. P., and Graham, G. G. (1966). Hypocupremia and neutropenia in copper deficiency. *Blood* **28,** 280.

Corwin, L. M., and Gordon, R. K. (1982). Vitamin E and immune regulation. *Ann. N.Y. Acad. Sci.* **393,** 437.

Corwin, L. M., and Schloss, J. (1980). Influence of vitamin E on the mitogenic response of murine lymphoid cells. *J. Nutr.* **110,** 916.

Cotte, J., Forestier, F., Quero, A. M., Bourrinet, P., and German, A. (1982). The effect of alcohol ingestion on the susceptibility of mice to viral infections. *Alcohol.: Clin. Exp. Res.* **6,** 239.

Cotzias, G. C., Tang, L. C., Miller, S. T., Sladic-Simic, D., and Hurley, L. S. (1972). A mutation influencing the transportation of manganese, L-dopa and L-tryptophan. *Science* **176,** 410.

Cotzias, G. C., Miller, S. T., Papavasiliou, P. S., and Tang, L. C. (1976). Interactions between manganese and brain dopamine. *Med. Clin. North Am.* **60,** 729.

Cowan, M. J., Wara, D. W., Packman, S., and Ammann, A. J. (1979). Multiple biotin-dependent carboxylase deficiencies associated with defects in T-cell and B-cell immunity. *Lancet* **2,** 115.

Coward, D. G., and Whitehead, R. G. (1972). Experimental protein-energy malnutrition in baby baboons. *Br. J. Nutr.* **28,** 223.

Coward, W. A. (1975). Serum colloidal osmotic pressure in the development of kwashiorkor and in recovery: Its relationship to albumin and globulin concentrations and oedema. *Br. J. Nutr.* **34,** 459.

Creamer, B. (1964). Small-intestinal mucosal dynamics and the environment. *Br. Med. J.* **2,** 1373.

Crisp, A. H., Palmer, R. L., and Kalucy, R. S. (1976). How common is anorexia nervosa? A prevalence study. *Br. J. Psychiatry* **128,** 549.

Crompton, D. W. T., Arnold, S., Coward, W. A., and Lunn, P. G. (1978). Nippostrongylus (nematoda) infection in protein-malnourished rats. *Trans. R. Soc. Trop. Med. Hyg.* **72,** 195.

Crowther, D. (1971). L-Asparaginase and human malignant disease. *Nature (London)* **299,** 168.

Cruz, J. R., and Waner, J. L. (1978). Effect of concurrent cytomegaloviral infection and under-nutrition on the growth and immune response of mice. *Infect. Immun.* **21,** 436.

Cunningham-Rundles, C., Cunningham-Rundles, S., Garofalo, J., Iwata, T., Incefy, G., Twomey, J., and Good, R. A. (1979). Increased T lymphocyte function and thymopoietin following zinc repletion in man. *Fed. Proc., Fed. Am. Soc. Exp. Biol.* **38,** 1222.

Cunningham-Rundles, S. (1982). Effects of nutritional status on immunological function. *Am. J. Clin. Nutr.* **35,** 1202.

Cunningham-Rundles, S., Cunningham-Rundles, C., Dupont, B., and Good, R. A. (1980). Zinc-induced activation of human B lymphocytes. *Clin. Immunol. Immunopathol.* **16,** 115.

Curtiss, L. K., DeHeer, D. H., and Edgington, T. S. (1980). Influence of the immunoregulatory serum lipoprotein LDL-In on the *in vivo* proliferation and differentiation of antigen-binding and antibody-secreting lymphocytes during a primary immune response. *Cell. Immunol.* **49,** 1.

Dahlquist, A. (1971). Lactose intolerance and protein malnutrition. *Acta Paediatr. Scand.* **60,** 488.

Dally, P. (1969). "Anorexia Nervosa." Heinemann, London.

Danks, D. M., Campbell, P. E., Stevens, B. J., Mayne, V., and Cartwright, E. (1972). Menkes' kinky-hair syndrome. An inherited defect in copper absorption with widespread effects. *Pediatrics* **50,** 188.

Davies, I. J. T., Musa, M., and Dormandy, T. L. (1968). Measurements of plasma zinc. Part I. In health and disease. *J. Clin. Pathol.* **21,** 359.

Davis, A. J. S. (1969). The thymus and the cellular basis of immunity. *Transplant. Rev.* **1,** 43.

Davis, G. K. (1950). The influence of copper on the metabolism of phosphorus and molybdenum. *In* "A Symposium on Copper Metabolism" (W. D. McElroy and G. Glass, eds.), p. 216. Johns Hopkins Press, Baltimore, Maryland.

Davis, S., Nelson, T., and Shepard, T. (1970). Teratogenicity of Vitamin B_6 deficiency: Omphalocele, skeletal and neural defects, and splenic hypoplasia. *Science* **169,** 1329.

Dawson, C. R., Strothkamp, K. G., and Krul, K. G. (1975). Ascorbate oxidase and related copper proteins. *Ann. N.Y. Acad. Sci.* **258,** 209.

Debes, S. A., and Kirksey, A. (1979). Influence of dietary pyridoxine on selected immune capacities of rat dams and pups. *J. Nutr.* **109,** 744.

Deinard, A. S., Fortuny, I. E., Theologides, A., Anderson, G. L., Boen, J., and Kennedy, B. J. (1974). Studies of the neutropenia of cancer chemotherapy. *Cancer* **33,** 1210.

Dekkers, N. W. H. M. (1981). The Hague.

Dement, P. (1970). Genetic requirements for graft-versus-host reaction in mouse. Different efficacy of incompatibility at D- and K-ends of the H-2 locus. *Folia Biol (Praque)* **16,** 273.

Demerec, M., and Hanson, J. (1951). Mutagenic action of manganous chloride. *Cold Spring Harbor Symp. Quant. Biol.* **16,** 215.

Denckla, W. D. (1974). Role of the pituitary and thyroid glands in the decline of minimal O_2 consumption with age. *J. Clin. Invest.* **53,** 572.

Dennert, G., and Lotan, R. (1978). Effects of retinoic acid on the immune system: Stimulation of T killer cell induction. *Eur. J. Immunol.* **8,** 23.

Dennert, G., Crowley, C., Kouba, J., and Lotan, R. (1979). Retinoic acid stimulation of the induction of mouse killer T-cells in allogeneic and syngeneic systems. *J. Natl. Cancer Inst.* **62,** 89.

Deo, M. G. (1978). Cell biology of protein-calorie malnutrition. *World Rev. Nutr. Diet.* **30,** 32.

DePasquale-Jardieu, P., and Fraker, P. J. (1979). The role of corticosterone in the loss of immune function in the zinc-deficient A/J mouse. *J. Nutr.* **109,** 1847.

DePasquale-Jardieu, P., and Fraker, P. J. (1980). Further characterization of the role of corticosterone in the loss of humoral immunity in zinc-deficient A/J mice as determined by adrenalectomy. *J. Immunol.* **124,** 2650.

DeSousa, M. A. B., Parrott, D. M. V., and Pantelous, E. M. (1969). The lymphoid tissues in mice with congenital aplasia of the thymus. *Clin. Exp. Immunol.* **4,** 637.

Desowitz, R. S., and Barnwell, J. W. (1980). Effect of selenium and dimethyl diocatedecyl ammonium bromide on the vaccine-induced immunity of Swiss—Webster mice against malaria (*Plasmodium berghei*). *Infect. Immun.* **27,** 87.

Dewey, K. G., and Lonnerdal, B. (1983). Milk and nutrient intake of breast-fed infants from 1 to 6 months: Relation of growth and fatness. *J. Pediatr. Gastroenterol. Nutr.* **2,** 497.

DeWille, J. W., Fraker, P. J., and Romsos, D. R. (1979). Effects of essential fatty acid deficiency and various levels of dietary polyunsaturated fatty acids on humoral immunity in mice. *J. Nutr.* **109,** 1018.

DeWille, J. W., Fraker, P. J., and Romsos, D. R. (1981). Effects of dietary fatty acids on delayed-type hypersensitivity in mice. *J. Nutr.* **111,** 2039.

DeWys, W., Pories, W. J., Richter, M. C., and Strain, W. H. (1970). Inhibition of Walker 256 carcinosarcoma growth by dietary zinc deficiency. *Proc. Soc. Exp. Biol. Med.* **135,** 17.

Dianzani, M. U., Torrielli, M. V., Canuto, R. A., Garcea, R., and Feo, F. (1976). The influence of enrichment with cholesterol on the phagocytic activity of rat macrophages. *J. Pathol.* **118**, 193.

Dickerson, J. W. (1984). Nutrition in the cancer patient: A review. *J. R. Soc. Med.* **77**, 309.

DiGeorge, A. M. (1968). Congenital absence of thymus and its immunologic consequences: Concurrence with congenital hypoparathyroidism. *Birth Defects, Orig. Artic. Ser.* **4**, 116.

DiLuzio, N. R., and Blickens, D. A. (1966). Influence of intravenously administered lipids on reticuloendothelial function. *RES, J. Reticuloendothel. Soc.* **3**, 250.

DiLuzio, N. R., and Wooles, W. R. (1964). Depression of phagocytic activity and immune response by methyl palmitate. *Am. J. Physiol.* **206**, 939.

Dion, A. S., Vaidya, A. B., and Fout, G. S. (1974). Cation preferences for poly(rC) Oligo (dG)— Directed DNA synthesis by RNA tumor viruses and human milk particulates. *Cancer Res.* **34**, 3509.

Dionigi, R. (1982). Immunological factors in nutritional assessment. *Proc. Nutr. Soc.* **41**, 355.

DiPaolo, J. A. (1964). The potentiation of lymphosarcomas in the mouse by manganous chloride. *Fed. Proc., Fed. Am. Soc. Exp. Biol.* **23**, 393.

Distasio, J. A., and Niederman, R. A. (1976). Purification and characterization of L-asparaginase with anti-lymphoma activity from *Vibrio* succinogenes. *J. Biol. Chem.* **251**, 6929.

Distasio, J. A., Niederman, R. A., and Kafkewitz, D. (1977). Antilymphoma activity in glutaminase-free L-asparaginase of microbial origin. *Proc. Soc. Exp. Biol. Med.* **155**, 528.

Dixon, J. R., Lowe, D. B., Richards, D. E., Cralley, L. J., and Stokinger, H. E. (1970). The role of trace metals in chemical carcinogenesis. Asbestos cancers. *Cancer Res.* **30**, 1068.

Doisy, E. A. (1972). Micronutrient controls in biosynthesis of clotting proteins and cholesterol. *In* "Trace Substances in Environmental Health" (D. D. Hemphill, ed.), Vol. 1, p. 193. Univ. of Missouri Press, Columbia.

Dolby, J. M., and Honour, P. (1979). Bacteriostasis of escherichia coli by milk. IV. The bacteriostatic antibody of human milk. *J. Hyg.* **83**, 255.

Dorner, M. H., Silverstone, A., Nishiya, A., Sostoa, A., Munn, G., and DeSousa, M. (1980). Ferritin synthesis by human T lymphocytes. *Science* **209**, 1019.

Dossetor, J. F. B., and Whittle, H. C. (1975). Protein-losing enteropathy and malabsorption in acute measles enteritis. *Br. Med. J.* **2**, 592.

Douglas, S. D. (1981). Impact of malnutrition on non-specific defense. *In* "The Impact of Malnutrition on Immune Defense in Parasitic Infestation" (Isliker, H., and Schurch, B., eds.), p. 28, Hans Huber, Bern.

Dowd, P. S., and Heatley, R. V. (1984). The influence of undernutrition on immunity. *Clin. Sci.* **66**, 241.

Dreosti, I. E., and Duncan, J. R. (1975). Proposed site of action for zinc in DNA synthesis. *J. Comp. Pathol.* **86**, 81.

Dreosti, I. E., and Hurley, L. S. (1975). Depressed thymidine kinase activity in zinc deficient rat embryos. *Proc. Soc. Exp. Biol. Med.* **150**, 161.

Dresser, D. W. (1968). Adjuvanticity of vitamin A. *Nature (London)* **217**, 527.

Dubois, E. L., and Strain, L. (1973). Effect of diet on survival and nephropathy of NZB/NZW hybrid mice. *Biochem. Med.* **7**, 336.

Dubos, R., Lee, C. J., and Costell, R. (1969). Lasting biological effects of early environmental influences. *J. Exp. Med.* **130**, 963.

Duncan, J. R., and Dreosti, I. E. (1975). Zinc intake, neoplastic DNA synthesis and chemical carcinogenesis in rats and mice. *J. Natl. Cancer Inst. (U.S.)* **55**, 195.

Duncan, J. R., and Hurley, L. S. (1978). Thymidine kinase and DNA polymerase activity in normal and zinc deficient developing rat embryos. *Proc. Soc. Exp. Biol. Med.* **159**, 39.

Duncan, J. R., Dreosti, I. E., and Albrecht, C. F. (1974). Zinc intake and growth of a transplanted hepatoma induced by 3′-Methyl-4-Dimethylaminoazobenzene in rats. *J. Natl. Cancer Inst.* (*U.S.*) **53**, 277.

Durden, D. L., and Distasio, J. A. (1980). Comparison of the immunosuppressive effects of asparaginases from *Escherichia coli* and *Vibrio succinogenes. Cancer Res.* **40**, 1125.

Eckhert, C. D., and Hurley, L. S. (1977). Reduced DNA synthesis in zinc deficiency: Regulational differences in embryonic rats. *J. Nutr.* **107**, 855.

Edelman, G. M., and Gally, J. A. (1962). The nature of Bence-Jones protein—Chemical similarities to polypeptide chains of myeloma globulin and normal -globulin. *J. Exp. Med.* **116**, 207.

Edelman, R. (1981). Obesity: Does it modulate infectious disease and immunity? "Nutrition, Constraints on our Knowledge," p. 327. New York.

Edwards, J. T. (1937). *Proc. Soc. Med.* **30**, 1046.

Edwards, M. B. (1976). Chemical carcinogenesis in the cheek pouch of syrian hamsters receiving supplementary zinc. *Arch. Oral Biol.* **21**, 133.

Elcoate, P. V., Fischer, M. I., Mawson, C. A., and Millar, M. J. (1955). The effect of zinc deficiency on the male genital system. *J. Physiol. (London)* **129**, 53.

Elin, R. J. (1975). The effect of magnesium deficiency in mice on serum immunoglobulin concentrations and antibody plaque-forming cells. *Proc. Soc. Exp. Biol. Med.* **148**, 620.

Endre, L., Katona, Z., and Gyurkovits, K. (1975). Zinc deficiency and cellular immune deficiency in acrodermatitis interopathica. *Lancet* **1**, 1196.

Erickson, K. L., McNeill, C. J., Gershwin, M. E., and Ossmann, J. B. (1980). Influence of dietary fat concentration and saturation on immune ontogeny in mice. *J. Nutr.* **110**, 1555.

Ermenkova, L., and Ermenkova, K. (1967). Effect of manganese, cobalt and iron on immunobiological reactions in hens. *Zivot Nauki* **4**, 75; *Nutr. Abstr. Rev.* **38**, 888 (1968).

Erway, L. C., Hurley, L. S., and Fraser, A. (1966). Neurological defect: Manganese in phenocopy and prevention of a genetic abnormality of inner ear. *Science* **152**, 1766.

Erway, L. C., Hurley, L. S., and Fraser, A. S. (1970). Congenital ataxia and otolith defects due to manganese deficiency in mice. *J. Nutr.* **100**, 643.

Erway, L. C., Fraser, A., and Hurley, L. S. (1971). Prevention of congenital otolith defect in *Pallid* mutant mice by manganese supplementation. *Genetics* **67**, 97.

Eskeland, T. (1977). The effect of various metal ions and chelating agents on the formation of non-covalently linked and covalently linked IgM polymers. *Scand. J. Immunol.* **6**, 87.

Everson, G. J., and Shrader, R. E. (1968). Abnormal glucose tolerance in manganese-deficient guinea pigs. *J. Nutr.* **94**, 89.

Everson, G. J., Hurley, L. S., and Geiger, J. F. (1959). Manganese deficiency in the guinea pig. *J. Nutr.* **68**, 49.

Faber, K. (1938). Tuberculosis and nutrition. *Acta Tuberc. Scand.* **12**, 287.

Fahim, M. S., and Brawner, T. A. (1980). Treatment of genital herpes simplex virus in male patients. *Arch. Androl.* **4**, 79.

Failla, M. L. (1977). Zinc: Functions and transport in microorganisms. *In* "Microorganisms and Minerals" (E. D. Weinberg, ed.), p. 151. Dekker, New York.

Failla, M. L., and Cousins, R. J. (1978). Zinc accumulation and metabolism in primary cultures of adult rat liver cells. Regulation of gluco corticoids. *Biochim. Biophys. Acta* **543**, 293.

Falchuk, K. H. (1977). Effect of acute disease and ACTH on serum zinc proteins. *N. Engl. J. Med.* **296**, 1229.

Falchuk, K. H., Fawcett, D. W., and Vallee, B. L. (1975). Role of zinc in cell division of *Euglena gracilis. J. Cell Sci.* **17**, 57.

Falin, L. I. (1940). Experimental teratoma testis in the fowl. *Am. J. Cancer* **38**, 199.

Falin, L. I. (1941). Morphologie and differenzcering der nervemelement in der experimentellen teratoiden. *Z. Mikrosk.-Anat. Forsch.* **49**, 193.

Falin, L. I., and Gromzewa, K. E. (1939). Experimental teratoma testis in fowl produced by injections of zinc sulphate solution. *Am. J. Cancer* **36**, 233.

Fare, G. (1966). The effect of cupric oxyacelate on rat liver damage associated with five poisons of unrelated chemical structure. *Br. J. Cancer* **20**, 569.

Fare, G., and Howell, J. S. (1964). The effect of dietary copper on rat carcinogenesis by 3-methoxy dyes. I. Tumors induced at various sites by feeding 3-Methoxy-4-Aminoazobenzene and its N-methyl derivative. *Cancer Res.* **24**, 1279.

Fare, G., and Orr, J. W. (1965). The effect of dietary copper on rat carcinogenesis by 3-Methoxy dyes. II. Multiple skin tumors by painting with 3-Methoxy-4-dimethylaminoazobenzene. *Cancer Res.* **25**, 1784.

Felice, J. H., and Kirksey, A. (1981). Effects of vitamin B-6 deficiency during lactation on the vitamin B_6 content of milk, liver, and muscle of rats. *J. Nutr.* **111**, 610.

Fell, B. F., Dinsdale, D., and Mills, C. F. (1975). Changes in enterocyte mitochondria associated with deficiency of copper in cattle. *Res. Vet. Sci.* **18**, 274.

Fenton, M. R., Burke, J. P., Tursi, F. D., and Arena, F. P. (1980). Effect of a zinc-deficient diet on the growth of IgM-Secreting plasmacytoma (TEPC183). *JNCI, J. Natl. Cancer Inst.* **65**, 1271.

Feo, F., Canuto, R. A., Garcea, R., and Gabriel, L. (1975). Effect of cholesterol content on some physical and functional properties of mitochondria isolated from adult rat liver, fetal liver, cholesterol-enriched liver and hepatomas AH-130, 3924 A and 5123. *Biochim. Biophys. Acta* **413**, 116.

Ferber, E., and Resch, K. (1976). Phospholipid stoffwechsel stimulierter lymphozyten unter suchungen zum molekularen mechanisms der aktivierung. *Naturwissenschaften* **63**, 375.

Ferber, E., DePasquale, G. C., and Resch, K. (1974). Phospholipid metabolism of stimulated lymphocytes composition of phospholipid fatty acids. *Biochim. Biophys. Acta* **398**, 364.

Fergus, E., and Jackson, J. (1959). The tuberculous alcoholic before and during hospitalization. *Am. Rev. Tuberc.* **79**, 659.

Ferguson, A., Lawlor, G., Neumann, L., Oh, W., and Stiehm, E. (1974). Decreased rosette-forming lymphocytes in malnutrition and intrauterine growth retardation. *Trop. Pediatr.* **85**, 717.

Fernandes, G., Yunis, E. J., Smith, J., and Good, R. A. (1972). Dietary influence on breeding behavior, hemolytic anemia, and longevity in NZB mice. *Proc. Soc. Exp. Biol. Med.* **139**, 1189.

Fernandes, G., Yunis, E. J., Jose, D. G., and Good, R. A. (1973). Dietary influence on antinuclear antibodies and cell-mediated immunity in NZB mice. *Int. Arch. Allergy Appl. Immunol.* **44**, 770.

Fernandes, G., Yunis, E. J., and Good, R. A. (1976a). Influence of protein restriction on immune functions in NZB mice. *J. Immunol.* **116**, 782.

Fernandes, G., Yunis, E. J., and Good, R. A. (1976b). Influence of diet on survival of mice. *Proc. Natl. Acad. Sci. U.S.A.* **73**, 1279.

Fernandes, G., Yunis, E., and Good, R. (1976c). Suppression of adenocarcinoma by the immunological consequences of calorie restriction. *Nature (London)* **263**, 504.

Fernandes, G., Friend, P., Yunis, E. J., and Good, R. A. (1978a). Influence of dietary restriction on immunologic function and renal disease in (NZB × NZW) F_1 mice. *Proc. Natl. Acad. Sci. U.S.A.* **75**, 1500.

Fernandes, G., Yunis, E. J., Miranda, M., Smith, J., and Good, R. A. (1978b). Nutritional inhihition of genetically determined renal disease and autoimmunity with prolongation of life in kdkd mice. *Proc. Natl. Acad. Sci. U.S.A.* **75**, 2888.

Fernandes, G., Handwerger, B. S., Yunis, E. J., and Brown, D. M. (1978c). Immune response in the mutant diabetic C57BL/Ks-db + Mouse. *J. Clin. Invest.* **61**, 243.

Fernandes, G., Nair, M., Onoe, K., Tanaka, T., Floyd, R., and Good, R. A. (1979). Impairment of cell-mediated immunity functions by dietary zinc deficiency in mice. *Proc. Natl. Acad. Sci. U.S.A.* **76,** 457.

Firpo, E. J., and Palma, E. L. (1979). Inhibition of foot and mouth disease virus and procapsid synthesis by zinc ions. *Arch. Virol.* **61,** 175.

Fiscina, B., Oster, G. K., Oster, G., and Swanson, J. (1973). Gonococcidal action of copper *in vitro. Am. J. Obstet. Gynecol.* **116,** 86.

Fiser, R. H., Denniston, J. C., McGann, V. G., Kaplan, J., Adler, W. H., III, Kastello, M. D., and Beisel, W. R. (1973). Altered immune functions in hypercholesterolemic monkeys. *Infect. Immun.* **8,** 105.

Fisher, G. L. (1977). Effects of disease on serum copper and zinc values in the beagle. *Am. J. Vet. Res.* **38,** 935.

Fitzgerald, F. T. (1981). The problem of obesity. *Annu. Rev. Med.* **32,** 221.

Flagstad, T., Andersen, S., and Nielsen, K. (1972). The course of experimental *Fosciola hepatica* infection in calves with a deficient cellular immunity. *Res. Vet. Sci.* **13,** 468.

Fleming, C. R., Hodges, R. E., and Hurley, L. S. (1976). A prospective study of serum copper and zinc levels in patients receiving total parenteral nutrition. *Am. J. Clin. Nutr.* **29,** 70.

Flessel, C. P. (1978). Metals mutagens. *Adv. Exp. Med. Biol.* **91,** 117.

Fletcher, J., Mather, J., Lewis, M. J., and Whiting, G. (1975). Mouth lesions in iron deficient anemia: Relationship to *Candida albicans* in saliva and to impairment of lymphocyte transformation. *J. Infec. Dis.* **131,** 44.

Floersheim, G. L., and Bollag, W. (1972). Accelerated rejection of skin homografts by vitamin A acid. *Transplantation* **15,** 564.

Flores, H., Seakins, A., and Monckeberg, F. (1973). p. 115. Raven Press, New York.

Flynn, A. (1977). Copper metabolism in an animal cancer model. *In* "Trace Substances in Environmental Health" (D. D. Hemphill, ed.), Vol. 11, p. 179. Univ. of Missouri Press, Columbia.

Fomon, S. J. (1974). "Infant Nutrition," (second ed.), pp. 35, W. B. Saunders, Co., Philadelphia.

Fomon, S. J. (1978). Nutritional disorders of children: Prevention, screening and follow-up. *Dept. Health Educat. Welfare Public. No. (HSA)* **78,** 5104.

Fong, L. V. Y., Lin, H. J., Chan, W. C., and Newberne, P. M. (1977). Zinc and copper concentrations in tissues from esophageal cancer patients and animals. *In* "Trace Substances in Environmental Health" (D. D. Hemphill, ed.), Vol. 11, p. 184. Univ. of Missouri Press, Columbia.

Fong, L. V. Y., Sivak, A., and Newberne, P. M. (1978). Zinc deficiency and methylbenzylnitrosamine-induced esophageal cancer in rats. *JNCI, J. Natl. Cancer Inst.* **61,** 145.

Foster, C., Jones, J. H., Henle, W., and Dorfman, F. (1944). The effect of vitamin B₁ deficiency and of restricted food intake on the response of mice to the lansing strain of poliomyelitis virus. *J. Exp. Med.* **79,** 221.

Fox, M. P., Bopp, L. H., and Pfau, C. J. (1978). Contact inactivation of RNA and DNA viruses by n-methylisatin p-thiosemicarbazone and $CuSO_4$. *Ann. N.Y. Acad. Sci.* **284,** 533.

Fraker, P. J., Hass, S. M., and Luecke, R. W. (1977). Effect of zinc deficiency on the immune response of the young adult A/J mouse. *J. Nutr.* **107,** 1889.

Fraker, P. J., DePasquale-Jardieu, P., Zwickle, C. M., and Luecke, R. W. (1978). Regeneration of T-cell helper function in zinc-deficient adult mice. *Proc. Natl. Acad. Sci. U.S.A.* **75,** 5660.

Frenk, S., Metcoff, J., Gomez, F., Ramos-Galvan, R., Cravioto, J., and Antonowicz, I. (1957). Intracellular composition and homeostatic mechanisms in severe chronic infantile malnutrition. *Pediatrics* **20,** 105.

Fridlender, B., Chejanovsky, N., and Becker, Y. (1978). Selective inhibition of herpes simplex virs type 1 DNA polymerase by zinc ions. *Virology* **84,** 551.

Fridovich, I. (1975). Superoxide dismutases. *Ann. Rev. Biochem.* **44,** 147.

Friedman, S., and Kaufman, S. (1965). 3,4-dihydroxyphenylethylanimine B-hydroxylase: A copper protein. *J. Biol. Chem.* **240,** 552.

Friend, J. V., Lock, S. O., Gurr, M. I., and Parish, W. E. (1980). Effect of different dietary lipids on the immune responses of Hartley strain guinea pigs. *Int. Arch. Allergy Appl. Immunol.* **62,** 292.

Friend, P. S., Fernandes, G., Good, R. A., Michael, A. F., and Yunis, E. J. (1978). Dietary restrictions early and late. Effects on the nephropathy of the NZB × NZW mouse. *Lab. Invest.* **38,** 629.

Frisancho, A. R. (1974). Triceps skinfold and upper arm muscle size: norms for assessment of nutritional status. *Amer. J. Clin. Nutr.* **27,** 1052.

Frood, J. D. L., Whitehead, R. G., and Coward, W. A. (1971). Relationship between pattern of infection and development of hypoalbuminaemia and hypo- -lipoproteinaemia in rural Ugandan children. *Lancet* **2,** 1047.

Frost, G., Asling, C. W., and Nelson, M. M. (1959). Skeletal deformities in manganese-deficient rats. *Anat. Rec.* **134,** 37.

Fudenberg, H. H., Good, R. A., Goodman, H. C. *et al.* (1971). Primary immunodeficiencies. Report of a World Health Organization committee. *Pediatrics* **47,** 927.

Fushimi, H., Hamison, C. R., and Ravin, H. A. (1971). Two new copper proteins from human brains. *J. Biochem. (Tokyo)* **69,** 1041.

Gainer, J. H. (1977). Effects on interferon of heavy metal excess and zinc deficiency. *Am. J. Vet. Res.* **38,** 869.

Gallagher, C. H., Judah, J. D., and Rees, K. R. (1956). The biochemistry of copper deficiency. I. Enzymological disturbances, blood chemistry and excretion of amino acids. *Proc. R. Soc. London, Ser. B.* **145,** 34.

Gardner, M. B., Ihle, J. N., Pillarisetty, R. J., Talal, N., DuBois, E. L., and Levy, J. A. (1977). Type C virus expression and host response in diet-cured NZB/W mice. *Nature (London)* **268,** 341.

Garrow, J. S. (1965). Total body-potassium in kwashiorkor and marasmus. *Lancet* **2,** 455.

Garrow, J. S. (1967). Loss of brain potassium in kwashiorkor. *Lancet* **2,** 643.

Garrow, J. S., Fletcher, K., and Halliday, D. (1965). Body composition in severe infantile malnutrition. *J. Clin. Invest.* **44,** 417.

Garrow, J. S., Smith, R., and Ward, E. (1968). "Electrolyte Metabolism Severe Infantile Malnutrition." Pergamon, Oxford.

Gatti, R. A., Stutman, O., and Good, R. A. (1970). The lymphoid system. *Annu. Rev. Physiol.* **32,** 529.

Gebhardt, B. M., and Newberne, P. M. (1974). T-cell function in the offspring of lipotrope- and protein-deficient rats. *Immunology* **26,** 489.

Gebrase-DeLima, M., Liu, R. K., Cheney, K. E., Mickey, R., and Walford, R. L. (1975). Immune function and survival in a long-lived mouse strain subjected to undernutrition. *Gerontology* **21,** 184.

Gelfand, E. W., and Pyke, K. W. (1974). Morphological and functional maturation of human thymic epithelium in culture. *Nature (London)* **251,** 421.

Gell, S. G. H. (1948). Discussion on nutrition and resistance to infection. *Proc. R. Soc. Med.* **41,** 323.

Geokas, M. C., Van Lancker, J. L., Kadell, B. M., and Machleder, H. I. (1972). Acute pancreatitis. *Ann. Intern. Med.* **76,** 105.

Georgieff, K. K. (1971). Free radical inhibitory effect of some anticancer compounds. *Science* **173,** 537.

Gershoff, S. N., Gill, T. J., Simonian, S. J., and Steinberg, A. I. (1968). Some effects of amino acid deficiencies on antibody formation in the rat. *J. Nutr.* **95,** 184.

Gershwin, M. E., Ikeda, R. M., Kruse, W. L., Wilson, F., Shifrine, M., and Spangler, W. (1978). Age-dependent loss in New Zealand mice of morphological and functional characteristics of thymic epithelial cells. *J. Immunol.* **120**, 971–979.

Gershwin, M. E., Erickson, K., Montero, J., Abplanalp, H., Eklund, J., Benedict, A. A., and Ikeda, R. M. (1980). The immunopathology of spontaneously acquired dysgammaglobulinemia in chickens. *Clin. Immunol. Immunopathol.* **17**, 15–30.

Gershwin, M. E., Castles, J. J., Saito, W., and Ahmed, A. (1982). Studies of congenitally immunologically mutant New Zealand mice. VII. The ontogeny of thymic abnormalities and reconstitution of nude NZB/W mice. *J. Immunol.* **129**, 2150–2155.

Gershwin, M. E., Beach, R. S., and Hurley, L. S. (1983). Trace metals, aging and immunity. *J. Am. Geriatr. Soc.* **31**, 374.

Gershwin, M. E., Lentz, D. R., Beach, R. S., and Hurley, L. S. (1984). Nutritional factors and autoimmunity. IV. Dietary vitamin A deprivation induces a selective increase in IgM autoantibodies and hypergammaglobulinemia in New Zealand black mice. *J. Immunol.* **133**, 222.

Ghavami, H., Dutz, W., Mohallattee, M., Rossipal, E., and Vessal, K. (1979). Immune disturbances after severe enteritis during the first six months of life. *Isr. J. Med. Sci.* **15**, 364.

Glagov, S., Kent, G., and Popper, H. (1959). Relation of splenic and lymph node changes to hypergammaglobulinemia in cirrhosis. *Arch. Pathol.* **67**, 9.

Glassock, R. J. (1983). Nutrition, immunology, and renal disease. *Kidney Int.* S194.

Glick, B., Chang, T. S., and Jaap, R. J. (1956). The bursa of Fabricius and antibody production. *Poult. Sci.* **35**, 224.

Gluckman, S. J., Dvorak, V. C., and MacGregor, R. R. (1977). Host defenses during prolonged alcohol consumption in a controlled environment. *Arch. Intern. Med.* **137**, 1539.

Golden, B. E., and Golden, M. H. N. (1979). Plasma zinc and the clinical features of malnutrition. *Am. J. Clin. Nutr.* **32**, 2490.

Golden, B. E., and Golden, M. H. N. (1981a). Plasma zinc, rate of weight gain, and the energy cost of tissue deposition in children recovering from severe malnutrition on a cow's milk or soya protein based diet. *Am. J. Clin. Nutr.* **34**, 892.

Golden, M. H. N., and Golden, B. E. (1981b). Effect of zinc supplementation on the dietary intake, rate of weight gain, and energy cost of tissue deposition in children recovering from severe malnutrition. *Am. J. Clin. Nutr.* **34**, 900.

Golden, M. H. N., Jackson, A. A., and Golden, B. E. (1977). Effect of zinc on thymus of recently malnourished children. *Lancet* **2**, 1057.

Golden, M. H. N., Golden, B. E., Harland, P. S. E. G., and Jackson, A. A. (1978). Zinc and immunocompetence in protein-energy malnutrition. *Lancet* **1**, 1226.

Goldfarb, R. H., and Herberman, R. B. (1981). Natural killer cell reactivity: Regulatory interactions among phorbol ester, interferon, cholera toxin and retinoic acid. *J. Immunol.* **126**, 2129.

Goldrick, R. B., Goodwin, R. M., Nestel, P. J., Davis, N. C., and Quinlivan, N. L. (1976). Do polyunsaturated fats predispose to malignant melanoma? *Med. J. Aust.* **1**, 987.

Goldstein, I. M., Kaplan, H. B., Edelson, H. S., and Weisman, G. J. (1979). Ceruloplasmin. A scavenger of superoxide anion radicals. *J. Biol. Chem.* **254**, 4040.

Golla, J. A., Larson, L. A., Anderson, C. F., Lucas, A. R., Wilson, W. R., and Tomasi, T. B. (1981). An immunological assessment of patients with anorexia nervosa. *Am. J. Clin. Nutr.* **34**, 2756.

Golub, M. S., Gershwin, M. E., Hurley, L. S., Hendrickx, A. G., and Baly, D. L. (1982). Induction of marginal zinc deficiency in female rhesus monkeys. *Am. J. Primatol.* **3**, 299.

Golub, M. S., Gershwin, M. E., and Vijayan, V. K. (1983). Passive avoidance performance of mice fed marginally or severely zinc deficient diets during post-embryonic brain development. *Phys. Behav.* **30**, 409.

Golub, M. S., Gershwin, M. E., Hurley, L. S., Baly, D. L., and Hendrickx, A. G. (1984). Studies of marginal zinc deprivation in rhesus monkeys. I. Influence on pregnant dams. *Am. J. Clin. Nutr.* **39**, 265.

Golub, M. S., Gershwin, M. E., Hurley, L. S., Baly, D. L., and Hendrickx, A. G. (1984b). Studies of marginal zinc deprivation in rhesus monkeys. II. Pregnancy outcome. *Am. J. Clin. Nutr.* **39**, 879.

Golub, M. S., Gershwin, M. E., Hurley, L. S., Saito, W. Y., and Hendrickx, A. G. (1984c). Studies of marginal zinc deprivation in rhesus monkeys. IV. Growth of infants in the first year. *Am. J. Clin. Nutr.* **40**, 1290.

Gomez, F., Ramos-Galvan, R., Cravioto, J., Frenk, S., Santanella, J. S., and de la Pena, C. (1956). Fat absorption in chronic severe malnutrition in children. *Lancet* **2**, 121.

Good, R. A., Dalmasso, A. P., Martinez, C. *et al.* (1962). The role of the thymus in development of immunologic capacity in rabbits and mice. *J. Exp. Med.* **116**, 773.

Good, R. A., Fernandes, G., Yunis, E. J., Cooper, W. C., Jose, D. G., Kramer, T. R., and Hansen, M. A. (1976). Nutritional deficiency, immunologic function and disease. *Am. J. Pathol.* **84**, 599.

Goodall, C. M. (1964). Failure of copper to inhibit carcinogenesis by 2-aminofluorine. *Br. J. Cancer* **18**, 777.

Goodman, J. R., Warshaw, J. B., and Dallman, P. R. (1970). Cardiac hypertrophy in rats with iron and copper deficiency: Quantitative contribution of mitochondrial enlargement. *Pediatr. Res.* **4**, 244.

Goodman, S. H., Rodgerson, D. O., and Kauffman, J. (1967). Hypercupremia in a patient with multiple myeloma. *J. Lab. Clin. Med.* **70**, 57.

Goodwin, J. S., and Webb, D. R. (1980). Regulation of the immune response by prostaglandins. *Clin. Immunol. Immunopathol.* **15**, 106.

Gopalan, C. (1968). p. 49. Churchill-Livingstone, Edinburgh and London.

Gopalan, C., and Belvady, B. (1959). Nutrition in maternal and infant feed. *Indian J. Med. Res.* **47**, 177.

Gordon, J. E., and Scrimshaw, N. S. (1965). "Nutrition and the diarrheas of early childhood in the tropics." *Milbank Mem. Food Q.* **43**, 235.

Gordon, J. E., Chitkara, I. D., and Wyon, J. B. (1963). Preventive medicine and epidemiology. *Am. J. Med. Sci.* **245**, 345.

Gordon, J. E., Guzman, M. A., Ascoli, W., and Scrimshaw, N. S. (1964). Acute diarrhoeal disease in less developed countries. *Bull. W. H. O.* **31**, 9.

Gordsmit, J. (1984). Letter to the editor. *N. Engl. J. Med.* **309**, 554.

Gormican, A. (1970). Inorganic elements in foods used in hospital menus. *J. Am. Diet. Assoc.* **56**, 397.

Gotch, F. M., Spry, C. J. F., Mowat, A. G., Beeson, P. B., and Maclennan, I. C. M. (1975). Reversible granulocyte killing defect in anorexia nervosa. *Clin. Exp. Immunol.* **21**, 244.

Grafe, E. (1950). Klinik und forschung. *Dtsch. Med. Wochenschr.* **75**, 441.

Graham, G. G., and Cordano, A. (1969). Copper deletion and deficiency in the malnourished infant. *J. Hopkins Med. J.* **124**, 139.

Grant, J. K., Minguell, J., Taylor, P., and Weiss, M. (1971). A possible role of zinc in the metabolism of testosterone hy the prostate gland. *Biochem. J.* **125**, 21.

Green, H. N. and Mellanby, E. (1930). Carotene and vitamin A: The anti-infective action of carotene. *Br. J. Exp. Pathol.* **11**, 81.

Green, L. H., and Green, G. M. (1968). Differential suppression of pulmonary antibacterial activity as the mechanism of selection of a pathogen in mixed bacterial infection of the lung. *Rev. Respir. Dis.* **98,** 819.

Green, S., and Dobrjansky, A. (1979). *Corynebacterium parvum:* Effects on the biochemistry of mouse serum and liver. *JNCI, J. Natl. Cancer Inst.* **63,** 497.

Greenan, D. M., Knudson, J. M. L., Dunkley, J., MacKinnon, M. J., Myers, D. B., and Palmer, D. G. (1980). Serum copper and zinc in rheumatoid arthritis and osteoarthritis. *N. Z. Med. J.* **91,** 47.

Griffith, K., Wright, E. B., and Dormand, T. L. (1973). Tissue zinc in malignant disease. *Nature (London)* **241,** 60.

Griffith, W.H., and Wade, N. J. (1939). Choline metabolism. I. The occurrence and prevention of hemorrhagenic degeneration in young rats on a low choline diet. *Proc. Soc. Exp. Biol. Med.* **41,** 567.

Griscom, N. T., Craig, J. N., and Neuhauser, E. B. D. (1971). Systemic bone disease developing in small premature infants. *Pediatrics* **18,** 883.

Groziak, S., Kirksey, A., and Hamaker, B. (1984). Effect of maternal vitamin B_6 restriction on pyridoxal phosphate concentrations in developing regions of the central nervous system in rats. *J. Nutr.* **114,** 727.

Gurr, M. I. (1983). The role of lipids in the regulation of the immune system. *Prog. Lipid Res.* **22,** 257.

Gurson, C. T., and Saner, G. (1973). Effects of chromium supplementation on growth in marasmic protein-calorie malnutrition. *Am. J. Clin. Nutr.* **26,** 988.

Gutman, G. A., and Weissman, L. (1972). Lymphoid tissue architecture: Experimental analysis of the origin and distribution of T-cells and B-cells. *Immunology* **23,** 465.

Guy-Grand, D., Griscelli, C., and Vassalli, P. (1975). Peyer's patches, gut IgA plasma cells and thymus function: Study in nude mice bearing thymic grafts. *J. Immunol.* **115,** 361.

Habib, F. K., Hammond, G. L., Lee, I. R., Dawson, J. B., Mason, M. K., Smith, P. H., and Stitch, S. R. (1976). Metal-androgen interrelationships in carcinoma and hyperplasia of the human prostate. *J. Endocrinol.* **71,** 133.

Hadden, D. R. (1967). Glucose, free-fatty acid, and insulin interrelations in kwashiorkor and marasmus. *Lancet* **2,** 589.

Hafez, M., Aref, G. H., Mahareb, S. W., Kassem, A. S., El Tahhan, H., Rizk, Z., Mahfonz, R., and Saad, K. (1977). Antibody production and complement system in protein energy malnutrition. *J. Trop. Med. Hyg.* **80,** 36.

Hakulinen, T., Lehtimaki, L., Lehtonen, M., and Teppo, L. (1974). Cancer morbidity among two male cohorts with increased alcohol consumption in Finland. *J. Natl. Cancer Inst. (U.S.)* **52,** 1711.

Halas, E. S., and Sandstead, H. H. (1975). Some effects of prenatal zinc deficiency on behavior of the adult rat. *Pediatr. Res.* **9,** 94.

Hall, G. A., and Howell, J. M. (1969). The effect of copper deficiency on reproduction in the female rat. *Br. J. Nutr.* **23,** 41.

Hallberg, D., Nilsson, B. S., and Blackman, L. (1976). Immunological function in patients operated on with small intestinal shunts for morbid obesity. *Scand. J. Gastroenterol.* **11,** 41.

Haller, L., Zubler, R. H., and Lambert, P. H. (1978). Plasma levels of complement components and complement haemolytic activity in protein-energy malnutrition. *Clin. Exp. Immunol.* **34,** 248.

Halliday, D. (1967). Chemical composition of the whole body and individual tissues of two Jamaican children whose death resulted primarily from malnutrition. *Clin. Sci.* **33,** 365.

Halsted, J. A., and Smith, J. C. (1970). Plasma zinc in health and disease. *Lancet* **1,** 322.

Halsted, J. A., and Halsted, C. H. (1981). "The Laboratory in Clinical Medicine," p. 321, Saunders, Philadelphia.

Haltalin, K. C., Nelson, J. D., Woodman, E. B., and Allen, A. A. (1970). Fatal Shigella infection induced by folic acid deficiency in young guinea pigs. *J. Infect. Dis.* **121**, 275.

Hambidge, K. M., and Droegemueller, W. (1974). Changes in plasma and hair concentrations of zinc, copper, chromium and manganese during pregnancy. *Obstet. Gynecol.* **44**, 666.

Hambidge, K. M., Hambidge, C., Franklin, M. F., and Baum, D. (1972a). Zinc deficiency in children manifested by poor appetite and growth, impaired taste acuity and low hair zinc levels. *Am. J. Clin. Nutr.* **25**, 453.

Hambidge, K. M., Hambidge, C., Jacobs, M., and Baum, J. D. (1972b). Low levels of zinc in hair, anorexia, poor growth, and hypoguesia in children. *Pediatr. Res.* **6**, 868.

Hambidge, K. M., Walravens, P. A., Brown, R. M., Webster, J., White, S., Anthony, M., and Roth, M. L. (1976). Zinc nutrition of pre-school children in the Denver Head Start program. *Am. J. Clin. Nutr.* **29**, 734.

Hambidge, K. M., Chavez, M. N., Brown, R. M., and Walraven, P. A. (1979a). Zinc nutritional status of young middle-income children and effects of consuming zinc-fortified breakfast cereals. *Am. J. Clin. Nutr.* **32**, 2532.

Hambidge, K. M., Walravens, P. A., Casey, C. E., Brown, R. M., and Bender, C. (1979b). Plasma zinc concentrations of breast-fed infants. *J. Pediatr.* **94**, 607.

Hambraeus, L. (1977). Proprietary milk versus human breast milk in infant feeding: A critical appraisal from the nutritional point of view. *Pediatr. Clin. North Am.* **24**, 17.

Hansen, J. D. L., and Lehmann, B. H. (1969). Serum zinc and copper concentrations in children with protein-calorie malnutrition. *S. Afr. Med. J.* **43**, 1248.

Hansen, J. D. L., Brinkman, G. L., and Bowie, M. D. (1965). Body composition in protein-calorie malnutrition. *S. Afr. Med. J.* **39**, 491.

Hanson, L. A., Ahlstedt, S., Carlsson, B., Goldblum, R. M., Lindblad, B. S., and Kayser, B. (1977). The antibodies of human milk, their origin and specificity. *In* Food and Immunology (Hambreus, L., Hanson, L. A., and McFarlane, H., eds.), p. 148, *Swedish Nutrit. Foundat. Symp. XIII.* Almquist and Wiksell, Internat., Stockholm.

Hardie-Muncy, D. A., and Rasmussen, A. I. (1979). Interrelationships between zinc and protein level and source in weanling rats. *J. Nutr.* **109**, 321.

Harland, P. S. E. G., and Brown, R. E. (1965). Tuberculin sensitivity following B. C. G. vaccination in undernourished children. *East Afr. Med. J.* **42**, 233.

Harmon, B. G., Miller, E. R., Hoeffer, J. A., Ullrey, D. E., and Luecke, R. W. (1963). Relationship of specific nutrient deficiencies to antibody production in swine. II. Patothenic acid, pyridoxine or riboflavin. *J. Nutr.* **79**, 269.

Harris, E. D., and O'Dell, B. L. (1974). Copper and amine oxidases in connective tissue metabolism. *In* "Protein-Metal Interactions" (M. Friedman, ed.), p. 267. Plenum, New York.

Harrison, V. C., and Peat, G. (1972). Significance of milk pH in newborn infants. *Br. Med. J.* **4**, 515.

Hart, D. A., (1978a). Evidence that manganese inhibits an early event during stimulation of lymphocytes by mitogens. *Exp. Cell Res.* **113**, 139.

Hart, D. A. (1978b). Effect of zinc chloride on hamster lymphoid cells. Mitogenicity and differential enhancement of lipopolysaccharide stimulation of lymphocytes. *Infect. Immun.* **19**, 457.

Hass, G. M., Laing, G. H., McCreary, P. A., and Galt, R. M. (1978) Magnesium deprivation in the rat causes loss of induced immunity to malignant lymphoma. *Clin. Res.* **26**, 710A.

Hass, G. M., McCreary, P. A., Laing, G. H., and Galt, R. M. (1980). Lymphoproliferative and immunologic aspects of magnesium deficiency. *In* "Magnesium in Health and Disease." (M. Cantin, and M. Seelig, eds.), pp. 185–200. Spectrum, Jamaica, New York.

Havens, W. P., Shaffer, J. M., and Hopke, C. J. (1951). The production of antibody by patients with chronic hepatic disease. *J. Immunol.* **67**, 347.

Havens, W. P., Dickensheets, J., Bierly, J. N., and Eberhard, T. P. (1954). The half-life of normal human gammglobulin in patients with hepatic cirrhosis. *J. Immunol.* **73**, 256.

Havens, W. P., Myerson, R. M., and Klatchko, J. (1957). Production of tetanus antitoxin by patients with hepatic cirrhosis. *N. Engl. J. Med.* **257**, 637.

Hawley, H. P., and Gordon, G. B. (1976). The effects of long chain free fatty acids on human neutrophil function and structure. *Lab. Invest.* **34**, 216.

Hayes, K. C. (1971). On the pathophysiology of vitamin A deficiency. *Nutr. Rev.* **29**, 3.

Hazuria, R. S., Sarin, G. S., Srivastava, P. N., Misra, R. C., Bhatt, I. N., and Chuttani, H. K. (1974). Intestinal dipeptidases in primary protein malnutrition. *Am. J. Clin. Nutr.* **27**, 760.

Heath, J. C., and Liquier-Milward, J. (1950). The distribution of function of zinc in normal and malignant tissues. Part I. Uptake and distribution of radioactive zinc, ^{65}Zn. *Biochim. Biophys. Acta* **5**, 404.

Heinzerling, R. H., Nockels, C. F., Quarles, C. L., and Tengerdy, R. P. (1974). Protection of chicks against E. coli infection by dietary supplementation with vitamin E. *Proc. Soc. Exp. Biol. Med.* **146**, 279.

Hekker, R. M., Kirchner, S. G., O'Neill, J. A., Hough, A. J., Howard, L., Kramer, S. S., and Green, H. L. (1978). Skeletal changes of copper deficiency in infants receiving prolonged total parenteral nutrition. *J. Pediatr.* **92**, 947.

Helliwell, M. G., Panayi, G. S., and Unger, A. (1984). Delayed cutaneous hypersensitivity in rheumatoid arthritis: the influence of nutrition and drug therapy. *Clin. Rheumatol.* **3**, 39.

Helms, R. A., Miller, J. L., Burckart, G. J., and Allen, R. G. (1983). Clinical outcome as assessed by anthropometric parameters, albumin, and cellular immune function in high-risk infants receiving parenteral nutrition. *J. Pediatr. Surg.* **18**, 564.

Henkin, R. I. (1976). Trace metals in endocrinology. *Med. Clin. North Am.* **60**, 779.

Heyworth, B., and Brown, J. (1975). Jejunal microflora in malnourished Gambian children. *Arch. Dis. Child.* **50**, 27.

Hill, C. H. (1965). Effect of copper deficiency on mortality from fowl typhoid and RPL 12 tumor. *Fed. Proc., Fed. Am. Soc. Exp. Biol.* **24**, 442.

Hill, C. H. (1979). Dietary influences on resistance to salmonella infection in chicks. *Fed. Proc., Fed. Am. Soc. Exp. Biol.* **38**, 2129.

Hirata, F., and Axelrod, J. (1980). Phospholipid methylation and biological signal transmission. *Science* **209**, 1082.

Ho, F. C. S., Wong, R. L. C., and Lawton, J. W. M. (1979). Human colostral and breast milk cells. *Acta Paediatr. Scand.* **68**, 389.

Holdsworth, S. R., Neale, T. J., and Wilson, C. B. (1980). The participation of macrophages and monocytes in experimental immune complex glomerulonephritis. *Clin. Immunol. Immunopathol.* **15**, 510.

Holliday, M. A., McHenry-Richardson, K., and Portale, A. (1979). Nutritional management of chronic renal disease. *Med. Clin. North Am.* **63**, 945.

Holm, G., and Palmblad, J. (1976). Acute energy deprivation in man: Effect on cell-mediated immunological reactions. *Clin. Exp. Immunol.* **26**, 207.

Holmdahl, S. G. (1967). Four population groups with relatively high tuberculosis incidence in Goteborg. *Scand. J. Respir. Dis.* **48**, 308.

Holt, L. E., Snyderman, S. E., Norton, P. M., Roitman, E., and Finch, J. (1963). The plasma aminogram in kwashiorkor. *Lancet* **2**, 1343.

Hook, R. R., and Hutcheson, D. P. (1976). Impairment of the primary immune response in early-onset protein-calorie malnutrition. *Nutr. Rep. Int.* **13**, 541.

Hopkins, A. K., Ransome-Kuti, O., and Majaj, A. S. (1968). Improvement of impaired carbohydrate metabolism by chromium (III) in malnourished infants. *Am. J. Clin. Nutr.* **21**, 203.

Hsu, C. C. S., and Leevy, C. M. (1971). Inhibition of PHA-stimulated lymphocyte transformation by plasma from patients with advanced alcoholic cirrhosis. *Clin. Exp. Immunol.* **8**, 749.

Hungerford, G. F., and Karson, E. F., (1960). The eosinophilia of magnesium deficiency. *Blood* **16**, 1642–1650.

Hurd, E. R., Johnston, J. M., Okita, J. R., MacDonald, P. C., Ziff, H., and Gilliam, J. N. (1981). Prevention of glomuleronephritis and prolonged survival in New Zealand Black/New Zealand White F_1 hybrid mice fed an essential fatty acid-deficient diet. *J. Clin. Invest.* **67**, 476.

Hurley, L. S. (1980). "Developmental Nutrition," p. 270, Prentice Hall, New Jersey.

Hurley, L. S. (1981). Teratogenic aspects of manganese, zinc, and copper nutrition. *Physiol. Rev.* **61**, 249.

Hurley, L. S. (1982). Clinical and experimental aspects of manganese deficiency. *In* "Trace Element Deficiencies and Excesses in World Populations" (A. S. Prasad, ed.), pp. 369–378. Alan R. Liss, Inc., New York.

Hurley, L. S. (1984). Manganese. *In* "Present Knowledge in Nutrition" (R. Olsen, ed.), 5th ed., pp. 558–570. Nutrition Foundation Inc., Washington, D.C.

Hurley, L. S., and Everson, G. J. (1959). Delayed development of righting reflexes in offspring of manganese-deficient rats. *Proc. Soc. Exp. Biol. Med.* **102**, 360.

Hurley, L. S., and Mutch, P. B. (1973). Prenatal and postnatal development after transitory gestational zinc deficiency in rats. *J. Nutr.* **103**, 649.

Hurley, L. S., and Shrader, R. E. (1972). Congenital malformations of the nervous system in zinc-deficient rats. *In* "Neurobiology of the Trace Metals Zinc and Copper" (C. C. Pfeiffer, ed.), pp. 7–51. Academic Press, New York.

Hurley, L. S., and Swenerton, H. (1966). Congenital malformations resulting from zinc deficiency in rats. *Proc. Soc. Exp. Biol. Med.* **123**, 692.

Hurley, L. S., Everson, G. J., and Geiger, J. F. (1958). Manganese deficiency in rats: Congenital nature of ataxia. *J. Nutr.* **66**, 309.

Hurley, L. S., Wooley, D. E., Rosenthal, E., and Timiras, P. S. (1963). Influence of manganese on susceptibility of rats to convulsions. *Am. J. Physiol.* **204**, 493.

Hurley, L. S., Gowan, J., and Swenerton, H. (1971). Teratogenic effects of short-term and transitory zinc deficiency in rats. *Teratology* **4**, 199.

Hurley, L. S., Keen, C. L., and Baly, D. L. (1984). Manganese deficiency and toxicity: Effects on carbohydrate metabolism in the rat. *Neurotoxicology* **5**, 97.

Ifekwunigwe, A. E., Grasset, N., Glass, R., and Foster, S. (1980). Immune response to measles and smallpox vaccinations in malnourished children. *Am. J. Clin. Nutr.* **33**, 621.

Ingenbleek, Y., and Malvaux, P. (1980). Peripheral turnover of thyroxine and related parameters in infant protein-calorie malnutrition. *Am. J. Clin. Nutr.* **33**, 609.

Iwata, T., Incefy, G. S., Tanaka, T., Fernandes, G., Menendez-Botet, C. J., Pih, K., and Good, R. A. (1979). Circulating thymic hormone levels in zinc deficiency. *Cell. Immunol.* **47**, 100.

Izui, S., McConahey, P. J., Theofilopoulos, A. N., and Dixon, F. J. (1979). Association of circulating retroviral gp70-anti-gp70 immune complexes with murine systemic lupus erythematosus. *J. Exp. Med.* **149**, 1099.

Izui, S., Fernandes, G., Hara, T., McConahey, P. J., Jensen, F. C., Dixon, F. J., and Good, R. A. (1981). Low-calorie diet selectively reduces expression of retroviral envelope glycoprotein gp70 in sera of NZB × NZW F_1 hybrid mice. *J. Exp. Med.* **15**, 1116.

Jackson, C. M. (1925). McGraw-Hill (Blakiston), New York.

Jackson, D. W., Law, G. R. J., and Nockels, C. F. (1978). Maternal vitamin E alters passively acquired immunity of chicks. *Poult. Sci.* **57**, 70.

Jackson, T. M., and Zaman, S. N. (1980). The in vitro effect of the thymic factor thymopoietin on a subpopulation of lymphocytes from severely malnourished children. *Clin. Exp. Immunol.* **39,** 717.

Jacob, H. S. (1974). Acquired phagocytic dysfunction. A complication of the hypophosphatemia at parenteral hyperalimentation. *N. Engl. J. Med.* **290,** 1403.

James, W. P. T. (1971). Jejunal disaccharidase activities in children with marasmus and with kwashiorkor. *Arch. Dis. Child.* **46,** 218.

James, W. P. T., and Hay, A. M. (1968). Albumin metabolism: Effect of the nutritional state and the dietary protein intake. *J. Clin. Invest.* **47,** 1958.

Jelliffe, D. B. (1953). Clinical notes on kwashiorkor in western Nigeria. *J. Trop. Med. Hyg.* **56,** 104.

Jelliffe, D. B. (1966). "The Assessment of the Nutritional Status of the Community," W. H. O. Monogr. No. 53. World Health Organ., Geneva.

Jelliffe, D. B. (1976). World trends in infant feeding. *Am. J. Clin. Nutr.* **29,** 1227.

Jelliffe, D. B., and Jelliffe, E. F. P. (1978). The volume and composition of human milk in poorly nourished communities. A review. *Am. J. Clin. Nutr.* **31,** 492.

Jelliffe, D. B., and Jelliffe, E. F. P. (1979). Midarm muscle volume: A suggestion. *Am. J. Clin. Nutr.* **32,** 2170.

Jelliffe, D. B., and Jelliffe, E. F. P. (1982). "Assessment of Nutrition Status." Oxford Univ. Press, London and New York.

Johansson, S. G. O., Mellbin, T., and Vahlquist, B. (1968). Immunoglobulin levels in Ethiopian preschool children with special reference to high concentrations of immunoglobulin E. (IgND). *Lancet* **1,** 1118.

Jones, H. W., Roberts, J., and Brantner, J. (1954). Incidence of tuberculosis among homeless men. *JAMA, J. Am. Med. Assoc.* **155,** 1222.

Jose, D. G., and Good, R. (1971). Absence of enhancing antibody in cell mediated immunity to tumour heterografts in protein deficient rats. *Nature (London)* **231,** 323.

Jose, D. G., and Good, R. A. (1973). Quantitative effects of nutritional protein and calorie deficiency upon immune responses to tumors in mice. *Cancer Res.* **33,** 807.

Jose, D. G., Welch, J. S., and Doherty, R. L. (1970). Humoral and cellular immune responses to streptococci, influenza and other antigens in Australian aboriginal school children. *Aust. Paediatr. J.* **6,** 192.

Jose, D. G., Stutman, O., and Good, R. (1973). Long term effects on immune function of early nutritional deprivation. *Nature (London)* **241,** 57.

Joynson, D. H. M., Walker, D. M., Jacobs, A., and Dolby, A. E. (1972). Defect of cell mediated immunity in patients with iron deficiency anemia. *Lancet* **2,** 1058.

Julius, R., Schulkind, M., Sprinkle, T., and Rennert, O. (1973). Acrodermatitis enteropathica with immune deficiency. *J. Pediatr. (St. Louis)* **83,** 1007.

Jurin, M., and Tannock, I. F. (1972). Influence of vitamin A on immunological response. *Immunology* **23,** 283.

Kahlau, G. (1937). Zur Experimentellen erzeugung von hoderteratomen beim hahn durch injektion von zinklosungen. *Frankf. Z. Pathol.* **50,** 281.

Kamamoto, Y., Makiura, S., Sugihara, S., Hiasa, Y., Arai, M., and Ito, N. (1973). The inhibitory effect of copper on DL-ethionine carcinogenesis in rats. *Cancer Res.* **33,** 1129.

Kaminski, M. V., Jr., Nasr, N. J., Freed, B. A., and Sriram, K. (1982). The efficacy of nutritional support in the elderly. *J. Am. Coll. Nutr.* **1,** 35.

Kaplan, S. S., and Basford, R. E. (1976). Effect of vitamin B_{12} and folic acid deficiencies on neutrophil function. *Blood* **47,** 801.

Kar, S., and Day, A. J. (1978). Composition and metabolism of lipid in macrophages from normally fed and cholesterol-fed rabbits. *Exp. Mol. Pathol.* **28,** 65.

Karcioglu, Z. A., Sarper, R. M., VanRinsvelt, H. A., Guffey, J. A., and Fink, R. W. (1978). Trace element concentration in renal cell carcinoma. *Cancer* **42,** 1330.

Karlinsky, M. L., Haut, L., Buddington, B., Schrier, N. A., and Alfrey, A. C. (1980). Preservation of renal function in experimental glomerulonephritis. *Kidney Int.* **17,** 293.

Karpel, J. T., and Peden, U. H. (1972). Copper deficiency in long-term parenteral nutrition. *J. Pediatr. (St. Louis)* **80,** 32.

Katz, M., and Steihm, E. R. (1977). Host defense in malnutrition. *Pediatrics* **59,** 495.

Kay, R. G., Tasman-Jones, C., Pybus, J., Whiting, R., and Black, H. (1976). A syndrome of acute zinc deficiency during total parenteral alimentation in man. *Ann. Surg.* **183,** 331.

Kazimierczak, W., and Maslinksi, C. (1974). The effect of zinc ions on selective and nonselective histamine release *in vitro. Agents Actions* **4,** 1.

Kazuna, S., Morimoto, S., and Kawai, K. (1979). Effects of some anti-rheumatic agents on copper-catalyzed thermal aggregation of gammaglobulin. *Agents Actions* **9,** 375.

Keele, B. B., McCord, J. M., and Fridovich, I. (1970). Superoxide dismutase from *Escherichia coli* B: A new manganese-containing enzyme. *J. Biol. Chem.* **245,** 6176.

Keen, C. L., Lonnerdal, B., and Hurley, L. S. (1984). Metabolism and biochemistry of manganese. *In* "Biochemistry of the Elements" (E. Frieden, ed.). Plenum, New York (in press).

Keet, M. P., and Thom, H. (1969). Serum immunoglobulins in kwashiorkor. *Arch. Dis. Child.* **44,** 600.

Kelley, V. E., and Izui, S. (1983). Enriched lipid diet accelerates lupus nephritis in NZB × NZW mice. Synergistic action of immune complexes and lipid in glomerular injury. *Am. J. Pathol.* **111,** 288.

Kelly, J. P., and Parker, C. W. (1979). Effects of arachidonic acid and other unsaturated fatty acids on mitogenesis in human lymphocytes. *J. Immunol.* **122,** 1556.

Kemmerer, A. R., Elvehjeim, C. A., and Hart, E. B. (1931). Studies on the relation of manganese to the nutrition of the mouse. *J. Biol. Chem.* **92,** 623.

Kendall, A. C., and Nolan, R. (1972). Polymorphonuclear leukocytic activity in malnourished children. *Cent. Afr. J. Med.* **18,** 73.

Kenney, M. A., Roderuck, C. E., Arnrich, L., and Piedad, F. (1968). Effect of protein deficiency on the spleen and antibody formation in rats. *J. Nutr.* **95,** 173.

Kenney, M. A., Magee, J. L., and Piedad-Pascual, F. (1970). Dietary amino acids and immune response in rats. *J. Nutr.* **100,** 1063.

Kerpel-Fronius, E., and Kaiser, E. (1967). Hypoglycaemia in infantile malnutrition. *Acta Paediatr. Scand.* **172,** 119.

Keusch, G. T. (1977). The consequences of fever. *Am. J. Clin. Nutr.* **30,** 1211.

Keusch, G. T. (1981). Host defense mechanisms in protein energy malnutrition. *Adv. Exp. Med. Biol.* **135,** 183.

Keusch, G. T., Urrutia, J. J., Fernandez, R., and Kovacs, I. B. (1976). Protein-calorie malnutrition (PCM) in a Mayan community: Effects on neutrophil function at birth. *Am. J. Clin. Nutr.* **29,** 472.

Keusch, G. T., Douglas, S. D., Braden, K., and Geller, S. A. (1978a). Antibacterial functions of macrophages in experimental protein-calorie malnutrition. I. Description of the model, morphologic observations, and macrophage surface IgG receptors. *J. Infect. Dis.* **138,** 125.

Keusch, G. T., Douglas, S. D., Hammer, G., and Braden, K. J. (1978b). Antibacterial functions of macrophages in experimental protein-calorie malnutrition. II. Cellular and humoral factors for chemotaxis, phagocytosis, and intracellular bactericidal activity. *J. Infect. Dis.* **138,** 134.

Keys, A. (1950). Energy requirement of adults. *JAMA, J. Am. Med. Assoc.* **142,** 333.

Khalil, M., Kabiel, A., El-Khateelw, S., Aref, K., El Lozy, M., Jahin, S., and Nasr, F. (1974). Plasma and red cell water and elements in protein-calorie malnutrition. *Am. J. Clin. Nutr.* **27,** 260.

Kim, Y., and Michael, A. F. (1975). Hypocomplementemia in anorexia nervosa. *J. Pediatr.* (*St. Louis*) **87**, 582.

King, H. J., Spain, J. D., and Clayton, C. C. (1957). Dietary copper salts and azo dye carcinogenesis. *J. Nutr.* **63**, 301.

Kirchner, H., and Ruhl, H. (1970). Stimulation of peripheral lymphocytes by Zn^{2+} *in vitro.* *Exp. Cell Res.* **61**, 229.

Kjosen, B., Bassoe, H. H., and Mykind, O. (1975). The glucose oxidation in isolated leukocytes from female patients suffering from overweight or anorexia nervosa. *Scand. J. Clin. Lab. Invest.* **35**, 447.

Klevay, L. M. (1975). The ratio of zinc to copper of diets in the United States. *Nutr. Rep. Int.* **11**, 237.

Klevay, L. M., Reck, S., and Barcome, D. F. (1979). Evidence of dietary copper and zinc deficiencies. *JAMA, J. Am. Med. Assoc.* **241**, 1916.

Klevay, L. M., Reck, S. H., Jacob, R. A., Logan, G. M., Munoz, J. M., and Sandstead, H. H. (1980). The human requirement for copper. I. Healthy men fed conventional, American diets. *Am. J. Clin. Nutr.* **33**, 45.

Klurfield, D. M., Allison, M. J., Gerszten, E., and Dalton, H. P. (1979). Alterations of host defenses paralleling cholesterol-induced atherogenesis. II. Immunologic studies of rabbits. *J. Med.* **10**, 49.

Kollmorgen, G. M., Sansing, W. A., Leghman, A. A., Fischer, G., Longley, R. A., Alexander, S. S., King, M. M., and McCay, P. B. (1979). Inhibition of lymphocyte function in rats fed high-fat diets. *Cancer Res.* **39**, 3458.

Kolomitseva, M. G., Voznesenskaia, F. M., and Isaeva, E. A. (1969). Immunobiologic reactivity of the animal organism with regard to various concentrations of copper in its rations. *Zh. Mikrobiol. Epidemiol. Immunobiol.* **46**, 99.

Kon, S. K., and Cowie, A. T. (1961). "Milk: The Mammary Gland and Its Secretion," Vol. II, p. 150. Academic Press, New York.

Korsnt, B. D., and Butterworth, B. E. (1976). Inhibition by zinc of rhino-virus protein cleavage. Interaction of zinc with capsiel polypeptides. *J. Virol.* **18**, 298.

Kos, W. L., Loria, R. M., Snodgrass, M. J., Cohen, D., Thorpe, T. G., and Kaplan, A. M. (1979). Inhibition of host resistance by nutritional hypercholesteremia. *Infect. Immun.* **26**, 658.

Koster, F. T., Curlin, G. C., Aziz, K. M. A., and Haque, A. (1981). Synergistic impact of measles and diarrhoea on nutrition and mortality in Bangladesh. *Bull. W. H. O.* **59**, 901.

Kraeuter, S. L., and Schwartz, R. (1980). Blood and mast cell histamine levels in magnesium-deficient rats. *J. Nutr.* **110**, 851–858.

Kramer, T. R., and Good, R. A. (1978). Increased in vitro cell-mediated immunity in protein-malnourished guinea pigs. *Clin. Immunol. Immunopathol.* **11**, 212.

Krause, L., Williams, M., and Broitman, S. A. (1980). Relationship of diet high in lipid and cholesterol on immune function in rats given 1,2,dimethyl hydrazine (DMH). *Am. J. Clin. Nutr.* **33**, 937.

Krishnan, S., Bhuyan, U. N., Talwar, G. P., and Ramalingaswami, V. (1974). Effect of vitamin A and protein-calorie undernutrition on immune responses. *Immunology* **28**, 383.

Kroes, J., and Ostwald, R. (1971). Erythrocyte membranes-effect of increased cholesterol content on permeability. *Biochim. Biophys. Acta* **249**, 647.

Kulapongs, P., Edelman, R., Suskind, R., and Olson, R. E. (1977a). Defective local leukocyte mobilization in children with kwashiorkor. *Am. J. Clin. Nutr.* **30**, 367.

Kulapongs, P., Suskind, R., Vithayasai, V., and Olson, R. E. (1977b). *In vitro* cell mediated immune response in Thai children with protein-calorie malnutrition. *In* "Malnutrition and Immune Response." p. 99, Raven Press, New York.

Kulapongs, P., Vithayassi, V., Suskind, R., and Olson, R. E. (1974). Cell mediated and phagocytosis and killing function in children with severe iron deficiency anemia. *Lancet* **2**, 689.

Kung, J. T., Mackenzie, C. G., and Talmage, D. W. (1979). The requirement for biotin and fatty acids in the cytotoxic T-cell response. *Cell. Immunol.* **48,** 100.

Kuvibidila, S. R., Nauss, K.M., Baliga, B. S., and Suskind, R. M. (1983). Impairment of blastogenic reasponse of splenic lymphocytes from iron deficient mice. *In vitro* repletion by hemin, transferrin, and ferric chloride. *Am. J. Clin. Nutr.* **37,** 557.

Lahey, M. E., Behar, M., Viteri, F., and Scrimshaw, N. S. (1958). Values for copper, iron, and iron-binding capacity in serum in Kwashiorkor. *Pediatrics* **22,** 72.

Lahey, M. F., Gubler, C. J., Chase, M. S., Cartwright, G. E., and Wintrobe, M. M. (1952). Studies on copper metabolism. II. Hematologic manifestations of copper deficiency in swine. *Blood* **7,** 1053.

Lansdown, A. B. G. (1977). Histological observations on thymic development in fetal and newborn mammals subject to intrauterine growth retardation. *Biol. Neonate* **31,** 252.

LaPointe, *et al.* (1984). Reply to letter to the editor. *N. Engl. J. Med.* **309,** 555.

Leach, R. M., and Lilburn, M. S. (1978). Manganese metabolism and its function. *World Rev. Nutr. Diet.* **32,** 123.

Leach, R. M., and Muenster, A. M. (1962). Studies of the role of manganese in bone formation. I. Effect upon mucopolysaccharide content of chick bone. *J. Nutr.* **78,** 51.

Ledbetter, J. A., Rouse, R. V., Spedding, H., Micklem, S., and Herzenberg, L. A. (1980). T cell subsets defined by expression of Lyt-1,2,3 and Thy-1 antigens. Two-parameter immunofluorescence and cytotoxicity analysis with monoclonal antibodies modifies current views. *J. Exp. Med.* **152,** 280.

Lederer, W. H., Kumar, M., and Axelrod, A. E. (1975). Effects of pantothenic acid deficiency on cellular antibody synthesis in rats. *J. Nutr.* **105,** 17.

Leek, J. C., Vogler, J. B., Gershwin, M. E., Golub, M. S., Hurley, L. S., and Hendrickx, A. G. (1984). Studies of marginal zinc deprivation in rhesus monkeys. V. Fetal and infant skeletal effects. *Am. J. Clin. Nutr.* **40,** 1203.

Leibovitz, B., and Siegel, B. V. (1981). Ascorbic acid and the immune response. *Adv. Exp. Med. Biol.* **135,** 1.

Lemmi, C. A., Cooper, E. L., and Moore, T. C. (1974). An approach to studying evolution of cellular immunity. *Contemp. Top. Immunobiol.* **4,** 109.

Lennard, E. S., Bjornson, A. B., Petering, H. G., and Alexander, J. W. (1974). An immunologic and nutritional evaluation of burn neutrophil function. *J. Surg. Res.* **16,** 286.

Leonard, P. J., and MacWilliam, K. M. (1964). Cortisol binding in the serum in kwashiorkor. *J. Endocrinol.* **29,** 273.

Levine, S., and Sowinski, R. (1980). Effect of essential fatty acid deficiency on experimental allergic encephalomyelitis in rats. *J. Nutr.* **110,** 891.

Levinson, W., Rhode, W., Mikelens, P., Jackson, J., Antony, A., and Ramakrishnan, T. (1977). Inactivation and inhibition of rous sarcoma virus by copper-binding ligands. Thiosemicarbazones, 8-hydroxyquinolones, and isonicotinic acid hydrazide. *Ann. N.Y. Acad. Sci.* **284,** 525.

Levy, J. A. (1977). Type C virus expression and host response in diet-cured NZB/W mice. *Nature (London)* **268,** 341.

Levy, J. A., Ibrahim, A. B., Shirai, T., Ohta, K., Nagasawa, R., Yoshida, H., Estes, J., and Gardner, M. (1982). Dietary fat affects immune response, production of antiviral factors, and immune complex disease in NZB/NZW mice. *Proc. Natl. Acad. Sci.* **79,** 1974.

Lewis, B., Wittmann, W., Krut, L. H., Hansen, J. D. L., and Brock, J. F. (1966). Free fatty acid flux through plasma in protein malnutrition of infants. *Clin. Sci.* **30,** 371.

Lewis, R. A., Hultquist, D. E., Bker, B. L., Falls, H. F., Gershowitz, H., and Penner, J. A. (1976). Hypercupremeia associated with a monoclonal immunoglobulin. *J. Lab. Clin. Med.* **88,** 375.

Lim, T. S., Putt, N., Safranski, D., Chung, C., and Watson, R. R. (1981). Effect of vitamin E on cell-mediated immune responses and serum corticosterone in young and maturing mice. *Immunology* **44**, 289.

Lipsky, P. E., and Ziff, M. (1980). Inhibition of human helper T cell function in vitro by D-penicillamine and $CuSO_4$. *J. Clin. Invest.* **65**, 1069.

Lipschitz, D. A., Simpson, K. M., Cook, J. D., and Morris, E. R. (1979). Absorption of monoferric phylate by dogs. *J. Nutrit.* **109**, 1154.

Ljvraga, P. (1934). Sui cosidetti teratomi sperimentali del testicolo da zinco. *Pathologica* **26**, 726.

Lloyd, A. V. C. (1968). Tuberculin test in children with malnutrition. *Br. Med. J.* **3**, 529.

Locniskar, M., Nauss, K. M., and Newberne, P. M. (1983). The effect of quality and quantity of dietary fat on the immune system. *J. Nutr.* **113**, 951.

Lomnitzer, R., Rosen, E. U., Geefhuysen, J., and Rabson, A. R. (1976). Defective leukocyte inhibitory factor (LIF) production by lymphocytes in children with kwashiorkor. *S. Afr. Med. J.* **50**, 1820.

Long, E. R. (1941). Constitution and related factors in resistance to tuberculosis. *Arch. Pathol.* **32**, 122.

Loomis, R. J., Marshall, L. A., and Johnston, P. V. (1983). Sera fatty acid effects on cultured rat splenocytes. *J. Nutr.* **13**, 1292.

Lubovici, P. P., and Axelrod, A. E. (1951). Circulating antibodies in vitamin-deficiency states. Pteroylglutamic acid, niacin-tryptophan, Vitamins B_{12}, A, and D deficiencies. *Proc. Soc. Exp. Biol. Med.* **77**, 526.

Luhby, A. L. (1959). Megaloblastic anemia in infancy. III. Clinical considerations and analysis. *J. Pediatr.* (*St. Louis*) **54**, 617.

Lundy, J., Raaf, J. H., Deakins, S., Wanebo, H. J., Jacobs, D. A., Lee, T., Jacobowitz, D., Spear, C., and Oettgen, H. F. (1975). The acute and chronic effects of alcohol on the human immune system. *Surg., Gynecol. Obstet.* **14**, 212.

Lunn, P. G., Whitehead, R. G., Hay, R. W., and Baker, B. A. (1973). Progressive changes in serum cortisol, insulin and growth hormone concentrations and their relationship to the distorted amino acid pattern during the development of kwashiorkor. *Br. J. Nutr.* **29**, 399.

Lunn, P. G., Whitehead, R. G., and Baker, B. A. (1976a). The relative effects of a low protein high carbohydrate diet on the free amino acid composition of liver and muscle. *Br. J. Nutr.* **36**, 219.

Lunn, P. G., Whitehead, R. G., Baker, B. A., and Austin, S. (1976b). The effect of cortisone acetate on the course of development of experimental protein energy malnutrition in rats. *Br. J. Nutr.* **36**, 537.

Lunn, P. G., Whitehead, R. G., Cole, T. J., and Austin, S. (1979a). The relationship between hormonal balance and growth in malnourished children and rats. *Br. J. Nutr.* **41**, 73.

Lunn, P. G., Whitehead, R. G., and Coward, W. A. (1979b). Two pathways to kwashiorkor? *Trans. R. Soc. Trop. Med. Hyg.* **73**, 438.

Lyon, T. D. B., Smith, H., and Smith, L. B. (1979). Zinc deficiency in the west of Scotland? A dietary intake study. *Br. J. Nutr.* **42**, 413.

McCann, J., Choi, E., Yamasaki, E., and Ames, B. (1975). Detection of carcinogens as mutagens in the salmonella/microsome test: Assay of 300 chemicals. *Proc. Natl. Acad. Sci. U.S.A.* **72**, 5135.

McCollester, D. L. (1979). Manganese and autologous-membrane-dependent anticancer autologous antigen preparation ('AAP') for treating established cancer. *Trans. Biochem. Soc.* **7**, 1068.

McCord, J. M., and Fridovich, J. (1969). Superoxide dismutase: An enzymatic function for erythrocuprein. *J. Biol. Chem.* **250**, 6049.

McCoy, J. H., and Kenney, M. A. (1975). Depressed immune response in the magnesium-deficient rat. *J. Nutr.* **105**, 791–797.

McCoy, J. H., Kenney, M. A., and Gillham, B. (1979). Immune response in rats fed marginal, adequate and high intakes of manganese. *Nutr. Rep. Int.* **19**, 165.

McCreary, P. A., Battifora, H. A., Laing, G. H., and Hass, G. M. (1966). Protective effect of magnesium deficiency on experimental allergic encephalomyelitis in the rat. *Proc. Soc. Exp. Biol. Med.* **121**, 1130–1133.

McCreary, P. A., Battifora, H. A., and Hahnemann, B. M. (1967). Leukocytosis, bone marrow hyperplasia, and leukemia in chronic magnesium deficiency in the rat. *Blood* **29**, 683–690.

McCreary, P. A., Laing, G., and Hass, G. (1973). Susceptibility of normal and magnesium deficient rats to weekly subtumorigenic doses of liver lymphoma cells. *Am. J. Path.* **70**, 89a–90a.

MacCuish, A. C., Urbaniak, S. J., Goldstone, A. H., and Irvine, W. J. (1974). PHA responsiveness and subpopulations of circulating lymphocytes in pernicious anemia. *Blood* **44**, 849.

McDermott, M. R., Mark, D. A., Befus, A. D., Baliga, B. S., Suskind, R. M., and Bienenstock, J. (1982). *J. Immunol.* **45**, 1.

McEwen, C. M. (1965). Human plasma monoamine oxidase. I. Purification and identification. *J. Biol. Chem.* **240**, 2003.

McFarland, W., and Libre, E. P. (1963). Abnormal leukocyte response in alcoholism. *Ann. Intern. Med.* **59**, 865.

McFarlane, H., Reddy, S., Adcock, K. J., Adeshina, H., Cooke, A. R., and Akene, J. (1970). Immunity, transferrin, and survival in kwashiorkor. *Br. Med. J.* **4**, 268.

McGregor, I. A. (1982). Malaria: Nutritional implications. *Rev. Infect. Dis.* **4**, 798.

McHugh, M. I., Wilkinson, R., Elliott, R. W., Field, E. J., Dewar, P., Hall, R. R., Taylor, R. M. R., and Uldall, P. R. (1977). Immunosuppression with polyunsaturated fatty acids in renal transplantation. *Transplantation* **24**, 263.

Mackie, B. S. (1974). Malignant melanoma and diet. *Med. J. Aust.* **1**, 810.

Mackowiak, P. A., Jones, S. R., Martin, R. M., and Smith, J. W. (1976). Oropharyngeal colonization of chronic alcoholics (CA) by gram negative bacilli (GNB) and other potential pathogens. *Clin. Res.* **24**, 349a.

McLaren, D. S., Tchalian, M., and Ajans, Z. A. (1965). Biochemical and hematologic changes in the vitamin A-deficient rat. *Am. J. Clin. Nutr.* **17**, 131.

McLaren, D. S., Pellett, P. S., and Read, W. W. C. (1967). A simple scoring system for classifying the severe forms of protein-calorie malnutrition of each childhood. *Lancet* **1**, 533.

McLaren, D. S., and Burman, D. (1976). "Textbook of Pediatric Nutrition," p. 91, Churchill Livingstone, Edinburgh.

McLeod, B. E., and Robinson, M. F. (1972). Metabolic balance of manganese in young women. *Br. J. Nutr.* **27**, 221.

McMahon, L. J., Montgomery, D. W., Guschewsky, A., Woods, A. H., and Zukoski, C. F. (1976). In vitro effects of $ZnCl_2$ on spontaneous sheep red blood cells (E) rosette formation by lymphocytes from cancer patients and normal subjects. *Immunol. Commun.* **5**, 53.

McMurray, D. N., Rey, H., Casazza, L. J., and Watson, R. R. (1977). Effect of moderate malnutrition on concentrations of immunoglobulins and enzymes in tears and saliva of young Colombian children. *Am. J. Clin. Nutr.* **30**, 1944.

McQuitty, J. T., DeWyes, W. D., Monaco, L., Strain, W. H., Rob, C. G., Apgar, J., and Pories, W. J. (1970). Inhibition of tumor growth by dietary zinc deficiency. *Cancer Res.* **30**, 1387.

Magilavy, D. B., Rifai, A., and Plotz, P. H. (1981). An abnormality of immune complex kinetics in murine lupus. *J. Immunol.* **126**, 770.

Mahler, H. R. (1963). Uricase. *In* "The Enzymes" (P. D. Boyer, H. Lardy, and F. Myrbäck, eds.), 2nd rev. ed. Vol. 8, Part, B, p. 285. Academic Press, New York.

Malave, I., and Layrisse, M. (1976). Immune response in malnutrition. Differential effect of dietary protein restriction on the IgM and IgG response to alloantigens. *Cell. Immunol.* **21**, 337.

Malave, I. B., and Pocino, M. (1980). Abnormal regulatory control of the antibody response to heterologous erythrocytes in protein-calorie malnourished mice. *Clin. Immunol. Immunopathol.* **16**, 19.

Malave, I., Nemeth, A., and Blanca, I. (1978). Immune response in malnutrition. Effect of protein deficiency on the DNA synthetic response to alloantigens. *Int. Arch. Allergy Appl. Immunol.* **56**, 128.

Malave, I., Nemeth, A., and Pocino, M. (1980). Changes in lymphocyte populations in protein-calorie-deficient mice. *Cell. Immunol.* **49**, 235.

Malkovsky, M., Edwards, A. J., Hunt, R., Palmer, L., and Medawar, P. B. (1983). T-cell-mediated enhancement of host-versus-graft reactivity in mice fed a diet enriched in vitamin A acetate. *Nature (London)* **302**, 338.

Mangal, P. C., and Verma, K. B. (1979). Effect of induced skin cancer on the concentrations of some trace elements in the mouse. *Indian J. Med. Res.* **69**, 290.

Mann, G. V. (1974a) The influence of obesity on health. *N. Engl. J. Med.* **291**, 178.

Mann, G. V. (1974b). The influence of obesity on health. *N. Engl. J. Med.* **291**, 226.

Marks, H. H. (1959). Influence of obesity on mobidity and mortality. *Bull. N.Y. Acad. Med.* [2] **36**, 296.

Maro, B., and Bornens, M. (1979). The effect of zinc chloride on the redistribution of surface immunoglobulins in rat B lymphocytes. *FEBS Lett.* **97**, 116.

Mason, K. E. (1979). A conspectus of research on copper metabolism and requirements of man. *J. Nutr.* **109**, 1979.

Mata, L. J., and Urrutia, J. J. (1971). Intestinal colonization of breast-fed children in a rural area of low socioeconomic level. *Ann. N.Y. Acad. Sci.* **176**, 93.

Mata, L. J., Urrutia, J. J., and Lechtig, A. (1971). Infection and nutrition of children of a low socioeconomic rural community. *Am. J. Clin. Nutr.* **24**, 249.

Mata, L. J., Jimenez, F., Cordon, M., Rosales, R., Prera, E., Schneider, R. E., and Viteri, F. E. (1972a). Gastrointestinal flora of children with protein-calorie malnutrition. *Am. J. Clin. Nutr.* **25**, 1118.

Mata, L. J., Urrutia, J. J., Albertazzi, C., Pellecer, O., and Arellano, E. (1972b). Influence of recurrent infections on nutrition and growth of children in Guatemala. *Am. J. Clin. Nutr.* **25**, 1267.

Mathews, J. D., Whittingham, S., Mackay, I. R., and Malcolm, L. A. (1972). Protein supplementation and enhanced antibody-producing capacity in new guinean school-children. *Lancet* **2**, 675.

Mathur, A., Wallenius, K., and Abdulla, M. (1979). Influence of zinc on onset and progression of oral carcinogenesis rats. *Acta Odontol. Scand.* **37**, 277.

Mathur, M., Ramalingaswami, V., and Deo, M. G. (1972). Influence of protein deficiency on 19S antibody-forming cells in rats and mice. *J. Nutr.* **102**, 841.

Matoth, Y., Zamir, R., Bar-Shani, S., and Grossowicz, N. (1964). Studies on folic acid in infancy. II. Folic and folinic acid blood levels in infants with diarrhea malnutrition, and infection. *Pediatrics* **33**, 694.

Meade, C. J., and Mertin, J. (1976). The mechanism of immunoinhibition by arachidonic and linoleic acid: Effects on the lymphoid and reticuloendothelial systems. *Int. Arch. Allergy Appl. Immunol.* **51**, 2.

Meade, C. J., and Mertin, J. (1978). Fatty acids and immunity. *Adv. Lipid Res.* **16**, 127.

Meade, C. J., Mertin, J., Sheena, J., and Hunt, R. (1978). Reduction by linoleic acid of the severity of experimental allergic encephalomyelitis in the guinea pig. *J. Neurol. Sci.* **35**, 291.

Meade, C. J., Sheena, J., and Merin, J. (1979). Effects of the obese (ob/ob) genotype on spleen cell immune function. *Int. Arch. Allergy Appl. Immunol.* **58**, 121.

Meares, E. M. (1975). Factors that influence surgical wound infections. *Urology* 6, 535.

Medawar, P. B., and Hunt, R. (1981). Anti-cancer action of retinoids. *Immunology* 42, 349.

Melez, K. A., Reeves, J. P., and Steinberg, A. D. (1978). Regulation of the expression of autoimmunity in NZB × NZW F_1 mice by sex hormones. *J. Immunopharmacol.* 1, 27.

Menkes, J. H., Alter, M., Steigleder, G. K., Weakley, D. R., and Sung, J. H. (1962). A sex-linked recessive disorder with retardation of growth, peculiar hair, and focal cerebellar degeneration. *Pediatrics* 29, 764.

Meredith, P. J., and Walford, R. L. (1977). Effect of age on response to T- and B-cell mitogens in mice congenic at the H-2 locus. *Immunogenetics* 5, 109.

Meredith, P. J., and Walford, R. J. (1979). Autoimmunity, histocompatibility, and aging. *Mech. Ageing Dev.* 9, 61.

Merritt, R. J., Blackburn, G. L., Bistrian, B. R., Palombo, J., and Suskind, R. M. (1981). Consequences of modified fasting in obese pediatric and adolescent patients: Effect of a carbohydrate-free diet on serum proteins. *Am. J. Clin. Nutr.* 34, 2752.

Mertin, J., and Hughes, D. (1975). Specific inhibitory action of polyunsaturated fatty acids on lymphocyte transformation induced by PHA and PPD. *Int. Arch. Allergy Appl. Immunol.* 48, 203.

Mertin, J., and Hunt, R. (1976). Influence of polyunsaturated fatty acids on survival of skin allografts and tumor incidence in mice. *Proc. Natl. Acad. Sci. U.S.A.* 73, 928.

Mertin, J., Hughes, D., Shenton, B. K., and Dickinson, J. P. (1974). In vitro inhibition by unsaturated fatty acids of the PPD- and PHA-induced lymphocyte response. *Klin. Wochenschr.* 52, 248.

Mertin, J., Meade, C. J., Hunt, R., and Sheena, J. (1977). Importance of the spleen for the immuno-inhibitory action of linoleic acid in mice. *Int. Arch. Allergy Appl. Immunol.* 53, 469.

Michael, J. G., Ringenback, R., and Hottenstein, S. (1971). The antimicrobial activity of human colostral antibody in the newborn. *J. Infect. Dis.* 124, 445.

Michalowsky, I. (1928). Eine experimentelle erzeugung teratoider geschwulste der hoden beim hahn. Zweite mitteilung. *Virchows Arch. Pathol. Anat. Physiol.* 267, 27.

Michalowsky, I. (1929). Das 10. Experimentelle Zinkteratom. II. Mitteilung. *Virchows Arch. Pathol. Anat. Physiol.* 274, 319.

Mihas, A. A., Gibson, R. G., and Hirschowitz, B. I. (1975). Suppression of lymphocyte transformation by 16, (16) dimethyl prostaglandin E_2 and unsaturated fatty acids. *Proc. Soc. Exp. Biol. Med.* 149, 1026.

Milanino, R., Conforte, A., Fracasso, M. E., Frano, L., Leone, R., Passarella, E., Tarter, G., and Velo, G. P. (1979). Concerning the role of endogenous copper in the acute inflammatory process. *Agents Actions* 9, 581.

Milich, D. R., and Gershwin, M. E. (1979). Murine autoimmune hemolytic anemia induced via xenogenic erythrocyte immunization. I. Qualitative characteristics and strain variation, susceptibility to induction. *Clin. Immunol. Immunopath.* 14, 172.

Mildvan, A. S., Scrutton, M. C., and Utter, M. F. (1966). Pyruvate carboxylase. VII. A possible role for tightly bound manganese. *J. Biol. Chem.* 241, 3488.

Miller, E. R., Lueche, R. W., Ullrey, D. E., Baltzer, B. V., Bradley, B. L., and Hoefer, J. A. (1968). Biochemical, skeletal and allometric changes due to zinc deficiency in the baby pig. *J. Nutr.* 95, 273.

Miller, J. F. A. P. (1964). The thymus and the development of immunologic responsiveness. *Science* 144, 1544.

Mills, C. F., and Williams, R. B. (1962). Copper concentration and cytochrome oxidase and ribonuclease activities in the brains of copper deficient lambs. *Biochem. J.* 85, 629.

Millward, D. J., Garlick, P. J., Stewart, R. J. C., Nnanyelugo, D. O., and Waterlow, J. C. (1975). Skeletal-muscle growth and protein turnover. *Biochem. J.* **150**, 235.

Minkel, D. T., Dolhun, P. J., Calhoun, B. L., Saryan, L. A., and Petering, D. H. (1979). Zinc deficiency and growth of Erlich ascites tumor. *Cancer Res.* **39**, 2451.

Moffit, A. E., Dixon, J. R., Phipps, F. C., and Stokinger, H. E. (1972). The effect of benzpyrene, phenobarbital, and carbon tetrachloride to subcellular metal distribution and microsomal enzyme activity. *Cancer Res.* **32**, 1148.

Moller, G. (1973). T and B lymphocytes in humans. *Transplant. Rev.* **16**, 1.

Montgomery, D. W., Don, L., Zukoski, C. F., and Chvapil, M. (1974). The effect of zinc and other metals on complement hemolysis of sheep red blood cells in vitro. *Proc. Soc. Exp. Biol. Med.* **145**, 263.

Montgomery, D. W., Chvapil, M., and Zukoski, C. F. (1979). Effects of zinc chloride on guinea pig complement component activity in vitro. Concentration-dependent inhibition and enhancement. *Infect. Immun.* **23**, 424.

Montgomery, R. D. (1960). Magnesium metabolism in infantile protein malnutrition. *Lancet* **2**, 74.

Montgomery, R. D. (1962). Changes in the basal metabolic rate of the malnourished infant and their relation to body composition. *J. Clin. Invest.* **41**, 1653.

Moore, D. L., Heyworth, B., and Brown, J. (1974). PHA-Induced lymphocyte transformations in leukocyte cultures from malarious, malnourished and control gambian children. *Clin. Exp. Immunol.* **17**, 647.

Morley, D. C. (1962). Measles in Nigeria, *Am. J. Dis. Child.* **103**, 230.

Morrison, D. B., and Nash, T. P. (1930). The copper content of infant livers. *J. Biol. Chem.* **88**, 479.

Morrow, W. J. W., and Levy, J. A. (1983). Dietary regulation of the autoimmune process in murine lupus. *Immunology Today* **4**, 249.

Moscatelli, P., Bricarelli, F. D., Piccinini, A., Tomatis, C., and Dufour, M. A. (1976). Defective immunocompetence in foetal undernutrition. *Helv. Paediatr. Acta* **31**, 241.

Mulhern, S. A., Morris, V. C., Vessey, A. R., and Levander, O. A. (1981). Influence of selenium and chow diets on immune function in first and second generation mice. *Fed. Proc., Fed. Am. Soc. Exp. Biol.* **40**, 935.

Murphy, E. W., Page, L., and Watt, B. K. (1971). Trace minerals in type A school lunches. *J. Am. Diet. Assoc.* **58**, 115.

Murray, M. J., and Murray, A. B. (1977). Starvation suppression and refeeding activation of infection. *Lancet* **1**, 123.

Murray, M. J., and Murray, A. B. (1981). Toward a nutritional concept of host resistance to malignancy and intracellular infection. *Perspect. Biol. Med.* **24**, 290.

Murray, M. J., Murray, A. B., Murray, M. B., and Murray, C. J. (1976). Anomali food shelters in the ogaden famine and their impact on health. *Lancet* **1**, 1283.

Mutch, P. B., and Hurley, L. S. (1974). Effect of zinc deficiency during lactation on postnatal growth and development of rats. *J. Nutr.* **104**, 828.

Naeye, R. L., Diener, M. M., Harcke, H. T., and Blanc, W. A. (1971). Relation of poverty and race to birth weight and organ and cell structure in the newborn. *Pediatr. Res.* **5**, 17.

Nakayama, E., Dippold, W., Shiku, H., Oettgen, H. F., and Old, L. J. (1980). Alloantigen-induced T-cell-proliferation: Lyt phenotype of responding cells and blocking of proliferation by Lyt antisera. *Proc. Natl. Acad. Sci. U.S.A.* **77**, 2890.

Nalin, D. R., Cash, R. A., and Rohman, M. (1970). Oral (or nasogastric) maintenance therapy for cholera patients in all age groups. *Bull. W.H.O.* **43**, 361.

Nalin, D. P., Mata, L., Vargas, W., Loria, A. R., Levins, M. M., Lizano, C., Simhan, A., and Mahs, E. (1978). Comparison of sucrose with glucose in oral therapy of infant diarrhea. *Lancet* **2**, 277.

Nalin, D. R., Levine, M. M., Mata, L., Cespedes, C., Vargas, W., Lizano, C., Loria, A. R., Simhon, A., and Urohs, E. (1979). Oral rehydration and maintenance of children with rotavirus and bacterial diarrhea. *Bull. W.H.O.* **57,** 453.

Nash, L., Iwata, T., Fernandes, G., Good, R. A., and Incefy, G. (1979). Effect of zinc deficiency on autologous rosette forming cells. *Cell. Immunol.* **48,** 238.

Nauss, K. M., and Newberne, P. M. (1981). Effects of dietary folate, vitamin B_{12} and methionine/choline deficiency on immune function. *Adv. Exp. Med. Biol.* **135,** 63.

Nauss, K. M., Mark, D. A., and Suskind, R. M. (1979). The effect of vitamin A deficiency on the in vitro cellular immune response of rats. *J. Nutr.* **109,** 1815.

Nelson, J. D., and Haltalin, K. C. (1972). Effect of neonatal folic acid deprivation on later growth and susceptibility to Shigella infection in the guinea pig. *Am. J. Clin. Nutr.* **25,** 992.

Nelson, W. E. (1962). "Textbook of Pediatrics," (7th ed.), Saunders, Philadelphia.

Neumann, C. G. (1977). Interaction of malnutrition and infection. *Arch. Intern. Med.* **137,** 1364.

Neumann, C. G. (1979). Reference data. *In* "Nutrition and Growth" (D. B. Jelliffe and E. F. P. Jelliffe, eds.), Vol. 2, pp. 299–327. Plenum, New York.

Neumann, C. G., and Alpaugh, M. (1976). Birthweight doubling time: A fresh look. *Pediatrics* **57,** 469.

Neumann, C. G., Lawlor, G. J., Stiehm, E. R., Swendseid, M. E., Newton, C., Herbert, J., Ammann, A. J., and Jacob, H. S. (1975). Immunologic responses in malnourished children. *Am. J. Clin. Nutr.* **28,** 89.

Neumann, C. G., Stiehm, E. R., and Swenseid, M. (1977). "Malnutrition and the Immune Response," p. 191. Raven Press, New York.

Neumann, C. G., Jelliffe, D. B., Zerfas, A. J., and Jelliffe, E. F. P. (1982). Nutritional assessment of the child with cancer. *Cancer Res.* **42,** 699S.

Newberne, P. M. (1966). Overnutrition on resistance of dogs to distemper virus. *Fed. Proc., Fed. Am. Soc. Exp. Biol.* **25,** 1701.

Newberne, P. M., and Gebhardt, B. M. (1973). Pre and postnatal malnutrition and responses to infection. *Nutr. Int.* **7,** 407.

Newberne, P. M., Hunt, C. E., and Young, V. R. (1968). The role of diet and the reticuloendothelial system in the response of rats to salmonella typhimurium infection. *Br. J. Exp. Pathol.* **49,** 448.

Nichols, B. L., Alvarado, J., Kimzey, S. L., Hazelwood, C. F., and Viteri, F. E. (1973). p. 363. Raven Press, New York.

Nichols, B. L., Alvarado, J., Rodriguez, J., Hazelwood, C. F., and Viteri, F. E. (1974). Therapeutic implications of electrolyte, water, nitrogen losses during recovery from protein-calorie malnutrition, *J. Pediatr.* **84,** 759.

Nielsen, K. (1976). p. 23. Academic Press, New York.

Nishioka, H. (1975). Mutagenic activities of metal compounds in bacteria. *Mutat. Res.* **31,** 185.

Nockels, C. F. (1979). Protective effects of supplemental vitamin E against infection. *Fed. Proc., Fed. Am. Soc. Exp. Biol.* **38,** 2134.

Nolen, G. A. (1972). Effect of various restricted dietary regimens on the growth, health and longevity of albino rats. *J. Nutr.* **102,** 1477.

Nordenstrom, J., Jarstrand, C., and Wiernik, A. (1979). Decreased chemotactic and random migration of leukocytes during intralipid infusion. *Am. J. Clin. Nutr.* **32,** 2416.

Nostrand, I. F., and Glantz, M. D. (1973). Purification and properties of human liver monoamine oxidase. *Arch. Biochem. Biophys.* **158,** 1.

Oberley, L. W., and Buettner, G. R. (1979). Role of superoxide dismutase in cancer: A review. *Cancer Res.* **39,** 1141.

O'Dell, B. L., Reeves, P. G., and Morgan, R. F. (1976). Interrelationships of tissue copper and zinc in rats nutritionally deficient in one or the other of these elements. *In* "Trace

Substance in Environmental Health" (D. D. Hemphill, ed.), Vol. 10, p. 411. Univ. of Missouri Press, Columbia.

Offner, H., and Clausen, J. (1974). Inhibition of lymphocyte response to stimulants induced by unsaturated fatty acids and prostaglandins. *Lancet* **2**, 400.

Offner, H., and Clausen, J. (1978). The enhancing effect of unsaturated fatty acids on E rosette formation. *Int. Arch. Allergy Appl. Immunol.* **56**, 376.

Ogra, P. L., Fishaut, M., and Theodore, C. (1979). Immunology of breast milk: Maternal neonatal interactions. *In* "Human Milk: Its Biological and Social Value" (S. Freier and A. I. Eidelman, eds.), p. 115. Excerpta Medica, Amsterdam.

Ohsugi, Y., Gershwin, M. E., Ahmed, A., Skelly, R. R., and Milich, D. R. (1982). Studies of congenitally immunologic mutant New Zealand mice. VI. Spontaneous and induced auto-antibodies to red cells and DNA occur in New Zealand x-linked immunodeficient (X^{id}) mice without phenotypic. *J. Immunol.* **128**, 2220.

Oleske, J. M., Westphal, M. L., Starr, S. S., Shore, S., Gorden, D., Bogden, J., Coplen, D. B., and Nahmias, A. (1979). Correction with zinc therapy of depressed cellular immunity in acrodermatitis enteropathica. *Am. J. Dis. Child.* **133**, 915.

Olusi, S. O., Wallwork, J. C., and McFarlane, H. (1976). Intrauterine malnutrition and IgG allotypes in the rat. *Biol. Neonate* **30**, 187.

Olusi, S. O., Thurman, G. B., and Goldstein, A. L. (1980). Effect of thymosin on T-lymphocyte rosette formation in children with kwashiorkor. *Clin. Immunol. Immunopathol.* **15**, 687.

Omole, T. A., and Onawunmi, O. A. (1979). Effect of copper on growth and serum constituents of immunized and non-immunized rabbits infected with trypanosoma brucei. *Ann. Parasitol. Hum. Comp.* **54**, 495.

Omran, A. (1971). "The Health Theme in Family Planning." Carolina Population Center, Clin. of North Carolina, Chapel Hill.

Orent, E. R., and McCollum, E. V. (1931). Effects of deprivation of manganese in the rat. *J. Biol. Chem.* **92**, 651.

Orgel, A., and Orgel, L. (1965). Induction of mutations in bacteriophage T4 with divalent manganese. *J. Mol. Biol.* **14**, 453.

Osaki, S., Johnson, D. A., and Frieden, E. (1966). The possible significance of the ferrous oxidase activity of ceruloplasmin in normal human serum. *J. Biol. Chem.* **241**, 2746.

Owen, J. J. T., and Ritter, M. A. (1969). Tissue interaction in the development of thymus lymphocytes. *J. Exp. Med.* **129**, 431.

Pakhomov, Y. N. (1970). The significance of various microelements in the general immunologic reactivity of the animal body. *Zh. Mikrobiol. Epidemiol. Immunobiol.* **47**, 128.

Palan, P. R., and Eidenoff, M. L. (1978). Specific effect of zinc ions on DNA polymerase activity of avian myeloblastosis virus. *Mol. Cell. Biochem.* **21**, 67.

Palmblad, J. (1976). Fasting (acute energy deprivation) in Man: Effect on polymorphonuclear granulocyte functions, plasma iron and serum transferrin. *Scand. J. Haematol.* **17**, 217.

Palmblad, J. (1979). Plasma levels of complement factors 3 and 4, orosomucoid and opsonic functions in anorexia nervosa. *Acta Paediatr. Scand.* **68**, 617.

Palmblad, J., Cantell, K., Holm, G., Norberg, R., Stranders, H., and Sunblad, L. (1977). Acute energy deprivation in man: Effect on serum immunoglobulins antibody response, complement factors 3 and 4, acute phase reactants and interferon-producing capacity of blood lymphocytes. *Clin. Exp. Immunol.* **30**, 50.

Palmblad, J., Hallberg, D., and Engsteed, L. (1980). Polymorphonuclear (PMN) function after small intestinal shunt operation for morbid obesity. *Br. J. Haematol.* **44**, 101.

Palmer, C. E., Jablon, S., and Edwards, P. Y. (1957). Tuberculosis morbidity of young men in relation to tuberculun sensitivity and body build. *Am. Rev. Tuberc.* **76**, 517.

Palmer, E. L., Gary, G. W., Black, R., and Martin, M. L. (1980). Antiviral activity of colostrum and serum immunoglobulins A and G. *J. Med. Virol.* **5**, 123.

Panda, B., and Combs, G. F. (1963). Impaired antibody production in chicks fed diets low in vitamin A, Patothenic acid or riboflavin, *Proc. Soc. Exp. Biol. Med.* **113**, 530.

Papavasilou, P. S., Kutt, H., Miller, S. T., Rosal, V., Wang, Y. Y., and Aronson, R. B. (1979). Seizure disorders and trace metals: Manganese tissue levels in treated epileptics. *Neurology* **29**, 1466.

Passmore, R. (1947). Mixed deficiency diseases in India: A clinical description. *Trans. R. Soc. Trop. Med. Hyg.* **41**, 189.

Patrick, J., Golden, B. E., and Golden, M. H. N. (1980). Leukocyte sodium transport and dietary zinc in protein energy malnutrition. *Am. J. Clin. Nutr.* **33**, 617.

Pedrero, E., and Kozelka, F. L. (1951). Effect of copper on hepatic tumors produced by 3'-methyl-4-dimethylaminoazobenzene. *AMA Arch. Pathol.* **52**, 455.

Pedroni, F., Bianchi, F., Vgazio, A. G., and Burgio, G. R. (1975). Immunodeficiency and steely hair. *Lancet* **1**, 1303.

Pekarek, R. S., Powanda, M. C., and Wannemacher, R. W. (1972). The effect of leukocytic endogenous mediator (LEM) on serum copper and ceruloplasmin concentrations in the rat. *Proc. Soc. Exp. Biol. Med.* **141**, 1029.

Pekarek, R. S., Hoagland, A. M., and Powanda, M. C. (1977). Humoral and cellular immune responses in zinc deficient rats. *Nutr. Rep. Int.* **16**, 267.

Pekarek, R. S., Sandstead, H. H., Jacob, R. A., and Barcome, D. F. (1979). Abnormal cellular immune responses during acquired zinc deficiency. *Am. J. Clin. Nutr.* **32**, 1466.

Pelus, L. M., and Strausser, H. R. (1977). Prostaglandins and the immune response. *Life Sci.* **20**, 903.

Petering, H. G., Buskirk, H. H., and Crim, J. A. (1967). The effect of dietary mineral supplements of the rat of the antitumor activity of 3-ethoxy-2-oxobutraldehyde Bis (thiosemicarbaxone). *Cancer Res.* **27**, 1115.

Petro, T. M., and Bhattacharjee, J. K. (1981). Effect of dietary essential amino acid limitations upon the susceptibility to salmonella typhimurium and the effect upon humoral and cellular immune responses in mice. *Infect. Immun.* **32**, 251.

Phillips, J. L. (1976). Specific binding of zinc transferrin to human lymphocytes. *Biochem. Biophys. Res. Commun.* **72**, 634.

Phillips, J. L., and Azaki, P. (1974). Zinc transferrin enhancement of nucleic acid synthesis in phytohemagglutinin-stimulated human lymphocytes. *Cell. Immunol.* **10**, 31.

Phillips, J. L., and Sheridan, P. J. (1976). Effect of zinc administration on the growth of L1210 and BW5147 tumors in mice. *J. Natl. Cancer Inst. (U.S.)* **57**, 361.

Phillips, J. L., Tuley, J. A., and Bowman, R. P. (1979). Zinc uptake in normal and leukemic lymphocytes: Effect of poly-L-ornithine. *J. Natl. Cancer Inst. (U.S.)* **58**, 1229.

Pickart, L., and Thaler, M. M. (1980). Growth-modulating tripeptide (Glycylhist-idyllsine): Association with copper and iron in plasma, and stimulation of adhesiveness and growth of hepatoma cells in culture by tripeptide-metal ion complexes. *J. Cell. Physiol.* **102**, 129.

Picou, D., and Phillips, M. (1972). Urea metabolism in malnourished and recovered children receiving a high or low protein diet. *Am. J. Clin. Nutr.* **25**, 1261.

Picou, D., and Taylor-Roberts, T. (1969). The measurement of total protein synthesis and catabolism and nitrogen turnover in infants in different nutritional states and receiving different amounts of dietary protein. *Clin. Sci.* **36**, 283.

Picou, D., and Waterlow, J. C. (1962). The effect of malnutrition on the metabolism of plasma albumin. *Clin. Sci.* **22**, 459.

Pimstone, B. L., Barbezat, G., Hansen, J. D. L., and Murray, P. (1968). Studies on growth hormone secretion in protein-calorie malnutrition. *Am. J. Clin. Nutr.* **21**, 482.

Pitchenik, A. E., Fischl, M. A., Dickinson, G. M., Becker, D. M., Fournier, A. M., O'Connell, M. T., Colton, R. M., and Spira, T. J. (1983). Opportunistic infections and Kaposis sarcoma among

Haitians: Evidence of a newly acquired immunodeficiency state. *Ann. Intern. Med.* **98,** 277.

Pittard, W. B. (1979). Breast milk immunology. A frontier in infant nutrition. *Am. J. Dis. Child.* **133,** 83.

Pittard, W. B., and Bill, K. (1979). Immunoregulation by breast milk cells. *Cell. Immunol.* **42,** 437.

Pizarro, D., Posada, G., Mohs, E., Levine, M. M., and Nalin, D. R. (1979a). Evaluation of oral therapy for infant diarrhea in an emergency room setting; the acute episode as an opportunity for instructing mothers in home treatment. *Bull. W.H.O.* **57,** 983.

Pizarro, D., Mata, L., Posada, G., Nalin, D., and Mohs, E. (1979b). Oral rehydration of neonates with dehydrating diarrheas. *Lancet* **2,** 1209.

Pizarro, D., Posada, G., Villavicencio. N., Mohs, E., and Levine, M. (1983). Oral rehydration in hypernatremic and hyponatremic diarrheal dehydration. *Am. J. Dis. Child.* **137,** 730.

Pizarro, D., Posada, G., and Levine, M. (1984). Hypernatremic diarrheal dehydration treated with "slow" (12-hour) oral rehydration therapy: A preliminary report. *J. Pediatr.* **104,** 316.

Pories, W. J., DeWys, W. D., Flynn, A., Mansour, E. G., and Strain, W. H. (1978a). Implications of the inhibition of animal tumors by dietary zinc deficiency. *Adv. Exp. Med. Biol.* **91,** 243.

Pories, W. J., Van Rij, A. M., and Bray, J. T. (1978b). Does zinc cause cancer? *In* "Trace Substances and Environmental Health" (D. D. Hemphill, ed.), Vol. 12, p. 164. Univ. of Missouri Press, Columbia.

Porter, H., Sweeney, M., and Porter, E. M. (1964). Neonatal hepatic mitochondrocuprein. II. Isolation of the copper-containing subfraction from mitochondria of newborn human liver. *Arch. Biochem. Biophys.* **104,** 97.

Poskitt, E. M. E. (1971). Effect of measles on plasma-albumin levels in Ugandan village children. *Lancet* **2,** 68.

Poskitt, E. M. E. (1972). Seasonal variation in infection and malnutrition at a rural paediatric clinic in Ugandia. *Trans. R. Soc. Trop. Med. Hyg.* **66,** 931.

Poswillo, D. E., and Cohen, B. (1971). Inhibition of carcinogenesis by dietary zinc. *Nature (London)* **231,** 447.

Poznansky, M., Kirkwood, D., and Solomon, A. K. (1973). Modulation of red cell K+ transport by membrane lipids. *Biochim. Biophys. Acta* **330,** 351.

Prasad, A. S., Halsted, J. A., and Nadimi, M. (1961). Syndrome of iron deficiency anemia, hepatosplenomegaly, hypogonadism, dwarfism and geophagia. *Am. J. Med.* **31,** 532.

Prasad, A. S., Miale, A., Farid, Z., Schulert, A., and Sandstead, H. H. (1963). Zinc metabolism in patients with the syndrome of iron deficiency anemia, hypogonadism and dwarfism. *J. Lab. Clin. Med.* **61,** 537.

Prasad, K. N., Ahrens, C. R., and Barrett, J. M. (1969). Homeostasis of zinc and iron in mouse B16 melanoma. *Cancer Res.* **29,** 1019.

Pretorius, P. J., and de Villers, L. S. (1962). Antibody response in children with protein malnutrition. *Am. J. Clin. Nutr.* **10,** 379.

Pretorius, P. J., and Weymeyer, A. S. (1966). Nutritional marasmus in Bantu infants in the Pretoria area. Part III. The effect of caloric intake on nitrogen and fat balance, certain serum constituents and the rate of recovery. *S. Afr. Med. J.* **40,** 240.

Price, P. (1978a). Responses of polyvinyl pyrrolidone and pneumococcal polysaccharide in protein-deficient mice. *Immunology* **34,** 87.

Price, P. (1978b). The elevation of adoptive responses to sheep erythrocytes in protein-deficient mice. *Immunology* **35,** 531.

Price, P., and Bell, R. G. (1975). The toxicity of inactivated bacteria and endotoxin in mice suffering from protein malnutrition. *J. Reticuloendothel. Soc.* **18,** 230.

Price, P., and Bell, R. G. (1976). The effects of nutritional rehabilitation on antibody production in protein-deficient mice. *Immunology* **31,** 953.

Price, P., and Bell, R. G. (1977). Factors determining the effects of chronic protein-deficiency on antibody responses to sheep red blood cells and brucella abortus vaccine in mice. *Aust. J. Exp. Biol. Med. Sci.* **55**, 59.

Prickett, J. D., Robinson, D. R., and Steinberg, A. D. (1981). Dietary enrichment with the polyunsaturated fatty acid eicosopentaneoic acid prevents proteinuria and prolongs survival in NZB × NZW F₁ mice. *J. Clin. Invest.* **68**, 556.

Prohaska, J., and Lukasewycz, O. (1981). Copper deficiency suppresses the immune response of mice. *Science* **213**, 559.

Protell, R. L., Soloway, R. D., Martin, W. J., Schoenfield, L. J., and Summerskill, W. H. J. (1971). Anti-salmonella agglutinins in chronic active liver disease. *Lancet* **2**, 330.

Puffer, R. R., and Serrano, C. V. (1973). The role of nutritional deficiency in mortality findings of the inter-American investigation of mortality in childhood. *Pan. Am. Health Organ.* **7**, 1.

Purkayastha, S., Kapoor, B. M. L., and Deo, M. G. (1975). Influence of protein deficiency on homograft rejection and histocompatibility antigens in rats. *Indian J. Med. Res.* **63**, 1150.

Purtilo, D. T., Riggs, R. S., Evans, R., and Neafie, R. C. (1976). Humoral immunity of parasitized, malnourished children. *Am. J. Trop. Med. Hyg.* **25**, 229.

Putrament, A., Baranowake, H., Ejchart, A., and Prazmo, W. (1975). Manganese mutagenesis in yeast. A practical application of manganese for the induction of mitochondrial antibiotic-resistant mutations. *J. Gen. Microbiol.* **90**, 265.

Quarterman, J., and Humphries, W. R. (1979). Effect of zinc deficiency and zinc supplementation on adrenals, plasma steroids and thymus in rats. *Life Sci.* **24**, 177.

Rabinovitch, M., and Destefano, M. J. (1973). Macrophage spreading in vitro. II. Manganese and other metals as inducers or as cofactors for induced spreading. *Exp. Cell Res.* **79**, 423.

Ranade, S. S., Shah, S., and Haria, P. (1979). Transition metals in an experimental tumor system. *Experientia* **35**, 460.

Rao, K. M. K., Schwartz, S. A., and Goods, R. A. (1979). Age-dependent effects of zinc on the transformation response of human lymphocytes to mitogens. *Cell. Immunol.* **42**, 270.

Ratcliffe, H. L., and Merrick, J. V. (1957a). Tuberculosis induced by droplet nuclei infection its developmental pattern in hamsters in relation to levels of dietary protein. *Am. J. Pathol.* **33**, 107.

Ratcliffe, H. L., and Merrick, J. V. (1957b). Tuberculosis induced by droplet nuclei infection its developmental pattern in guinea pigs and rats in relation to dietary protein. *Am. J. Pathol.* **33**, 1121.

Rath, E., and Thenen, S. W. (1980). Influence of age and genetic background on in vivo fatty acid synthesis in obese (ob/ob) mice. *Biochim. Biophys. Acta* **618**, 18.

Reddy, V., and Srikantia, S. G. (1964). Antibody response in kwashiorkor. *Indian J. Med. Res.* **52**, 1154.

Reddy, V., Jagadeesan, V., and Ragharamulu, N. (1976a). Functional significance of growth retardation in malnutrition. *Am. J. Clin. Nutr.* **29**, 3.

Reddy, V., Raghuramulu, N., and Bhaskaram, C. (1976b). Secretory IgA in protein-calorie malnutrition. *Arch. Dis. Child.* **51**, 871.

Reed, D. W., Passon, P. G., and Hultquist, D. E. (1970). Purification and properties of a pink copper protein from human erythrocytes. *J. Biol. Chem.* **245**, 2954.

Reinhardt, M. C., and Stewart, N. W. (1979). Antibody affinity and clearance function studies in high and low antibody affinity mice. The effect of protein deficiency. *Immunology* **38**, 735.

Resch, K., and Ferber, E. (1974). The role of phospholipids in lymphocyte activation. *Proc. Leucocyte Cult. Conf.* **9**, 281.

Reynolds, J. A., Harrington, D. G., Crabbs, C. L., Peters, C. J., and DiLuzio, N. R. (1980). Adjuvant activity of a novel metabolizable lipid emulsion with inactivated viral vaccines. *Infect. Immun.* **28**, 937.

Rigas, D. A., Eginitis-Rigas, C., and Head, C. (1979). Biphasic toxicity of diethyldithiocarbamate, a metal chelator, to T lymphocytes and polymorphonuclear granulocytes: Reversal by zinc and copper. *Biochem. Biophys. Res. Commun.* **88**, 373.

Ring, J., Seifert, J., Mertin, J., and Brendel, W. (1974). Prolongation of skin allografts in rats by treatment with linoleic acid. *Lancet* **2**, 1331.

Ristori, C., Boccardo, H., Borgono, J. M., and Armijo, E. (1962). Medical importance of measles in Chile. *Am. J. Dis. Child.* **103**, 236.

Rivière, M., Chouroulinkov, J., and Guérin, M. (1960). Production de tumeurs par injections intratesticulaires de chlorure de zinc chez le rat. *Bull. Assoc. Fr. Etude Cancer* **47**, 55.

Robak, J., Panczenko, B., and Gryglewski, R. (1975). The influence of saturated fatty acids on prostaglandin synthetase activity. *Biochem. Pharmacol.* **24**, 2057.

Roberts, R. B., and Aldous, E. (1951). Manganese metabolism of *Escherichia coli* as related to its mutagenic action. *Cold Spring Harbor Symp. Quant. Biol.* **15**, 229.

Robson, L. C., and Schwarz, M. R. (1975). Vitamin B_6 deficiency and the lymphoid system. I. Effects on cellular immunity and in vitro incorporation of ^{3}H-Uridine by small lymphocytes. *Cell. Immunol.* **16**, 135.

Rodin, A. E., and Goldman, A. S. (1969). Autopsy findings in acrodermatitis enteropathica. *Am. J. Clin. Pathol.* **51**, 315.

Rogers, H. J., and Synge, C. (1978). Bacteriostatic effect of human milk on *Escherichia coli:* The role of IgA. *Immunology* **34**, 19.

Ronaghy, H. A., Reinhold, J. G., Mahloudji, M., Ghavami, P., Fox, M. R. S., and Halsted, J. A. (1974). Zinc supplementation of malnourished school-boys in Iran: Increased growth and other effects. *Am. J. Clin. Nutr.* **27**, 112.

Room, G., Roffe, L., and Maini, R. N. (1979). The inhibitory effects of D-penicillamine on hyman lymphocyte cultures stimulated by phytohemagglutinin, the antagonistic action of L-cysteine and synergistic inhibition by copper sulphate. *Scand. J. Rheumatol.* **28**, 47.

Rosa, F. W. (1967). Impact of new family planning approaches on rural maternal and child health coverage in developing countries: India's example. *Am. J. Public Health* **57**, 1327.

Rose, A. H., and Turner, K. J. (1978). Effect of a low protein diet on the capacity of mice to express a type I hypersensitivity response. *Int. Arch. Allergy Appl. Immunol.* **56**, 344.

Rosen, F. S. (1968). The lymphocyte and the thymus gland genetic and hereditary abnormalities. *N. Engl. J. Med.* **279**, 643.

Rosenberg, I. H., Solomons, N. W., and Schneider, R. E. (1977). Malabsorption associated with diarrhea and intestinal infections. *Am. J. Clin. Nutr.* **30**, 1248.

Rous, P. (1911). A sarcoma of the fowl transmissible by an agent separable from the tumor cells. *J. Exp. Med.* **13**, 397.

Ruben, F. L., Smith, E. A., Foster, S. O., Casey, H. L., Pifer, J. M., Wallace, R. B., Atta, A. I. *et al.* (1973). Simultaneous administration of smallpox, measles, yellow fever, and diphtheria-pertussis-tetanus antigens to Nigerian children. *Bull. W.H.O.* **48**, 175.

Ruben, L. N., and Balls, N. (1967). Further studies of a transmissible amphibian lymphosarcoma. *Cancer Res.* **27**, 293.

Rucker, R. B., Parker, H. E., and Rogler, J. C. (1969). Effect of copper deficiency on chick bone collagen and selected bone enzymes. *J. Nutr.* **98**, 57.

Ruhl, J., and Bochert, G. (1971). Kinetics of the Zn^{2+}-stimuation of human peripheral lymphocytes in vitro. *Proc. Soc. Exp. Biol. Med.* **137**, 1089.

Ruhl, J., and Kirchner, H. (1978). Monocyte-dependent stimulation of human T cells by zinc. *Clin. Exp. Immunol.* **32**, 484.

Safai-Kutti, S., Fernandes, G., Wang, Y., Safai, B., Good, R. A., and Day, N. K. (1980). Reduction of circulating immune complexes by calorie restriction in (NZB × NZW) F_1 mice. *Clin. Immunol. Immunopathol.* **15**, 293.

Salimonu, L. S., and Osunkoya, B. O. (1980). Lymphocytes in protein-calorie malnutrition. *Am. J. Clin. Nutr.* **33**, 2699.

Salimonu, L. S., Johnson, A. O. K., Williams, A. I. O., Adeleye, G. I., and Osunkoya, B. O. (1982a). The occurrence and properties of E rosette inhibitory substance in the sera of malnourished children. *Clin. Exp. Immunol.* **47**, 626.

Salimonu, L. S., Ojo-Amaize, E., Williams, A. I. O., Johnson, A. O. K., Cooke, A. R., Adekunle, F. A., Alm, G. V., and Wigzell, H. (1982b). Depressed natural killer cell activity in children with protein-calorie malnutrition. *Clin. Immunol. Immunopathol.* **24**, 1.

Salomon, J. B., Mata, L. J., and Gordon, J. E. (1968). Malnutrition and the common communicable diseases of childhood in rural Guatemala. *Am. J. Public Health* **58**, 505.

Sandstead, H. H. (1973). Zinc nutrition in the United States. *Am. J. Clin. Nutr.* **25**, 1251.

Sandstead, H. H., Prasad, A. S., Schulert, A. R., Farid, Z., Miale, A., Bassily, S., and Darby, W. J. (1977). Human zinc deficiency, endocrine manifestations and response to treatment. *Am. J. Clin. Nutr.* **30**, 422.

Sandstead, H. H., Vo-Khactu, K. P., and Solomons, N. W. (1976). Conditioned zinc deficiencies. *In* "Trace Elements in Human Health and Disease" (A. S. Prasad, ed.), Vol. 1, p. 33. Academic Press, New York.

Saryan, L. A., Minkel, D. T., Dolhun, P. J., Calhoun, B. L., Wielgus, S., Schaller, M., and Petering, D. G. (1979). Effects of zinc deficiency on cellular processes and morphology or Erlich ascites tumor cells. *Cancer Res.* **39**, 2457.

Schlage, C., and Wortberg, B. (1972a). Zinc in the diet of healthy preschool and school children. *Acta Paediatr. Scand.* **51**, 421.

Schlage, C., and Wortberg, B. (1972b). Dietary manganese in diet of healthy preschool and school children. *Acta Paediatr. Scand.* **61**, 648.

Schlesinger, L., and Stekel, A. (1974). Impaired cellular immunity in marasmic infants. *Am. J. Clin. Nutr.* **27**, 615.

Schlesinger, L., Ohlbaum, A., Grez, L., and Stekel, A. (1976). Decreased interferon production by leukocytes in marasmus. *Am. J. Clin. Nutr.* **29**, 758.

Schlossmann, S. F. (1972). Antigen recognition: The specificity of T cells involved in the cellular immune response. *Transplant. Rev.* **10**, 97.

Schonland, M. M., Shanley, B. C., Loening, W. E. K., Parent, Ml. A., and Coovadia, H. M. (1972). Plasma-cortisol and immunosuppression in protein-calorie malnutrition. *Lancet* **2**, 435.

Schopfer, K., and Douglas, S. D. (1976a). In vitro studies of lymphocytes from children with kwashiorkor. *Clin. Immunol. Immunopathol.* **5**, 21.

Schopfer, K., and Douglas, S. D. (1976b). Neutrophil function in children with kwashiorkor. *J. Lab. Clin. Med.* **88**, 450.

Schrauzer, G. N. (1976). Cancer mortality correlation studies. I. Statistical associations between cancers at anatomically unrelated sites and some epidemiological implications. *Med. Hypotheses* **2**, 31.

Schrohenloher, R. E. (1978). Copper-catalysed reoxidation of human monoclonal IgM. *Scand. J. Immunol.* **8**, 443.

Schroit, A. J., and Gallily, R. (1979). Macrophage fatty acid composition and phagocytosis: Effect of unsaturation on cellular phagocytic activity. *Immunology* **36**, 199.

Schuhmacher, J., Mattern, J., Volm, N., and Wayss, K. (1979). *In vivo* uptake of ^{57}Co, ^{54}Mn, and ^{65}Zn by peripheral lymphocytes, tumor and various organs of rats bearing Walker 256 Carcinosarcoma. *Eur. J. Cancer* **15**, 1365.

Schwartz, M. K. (1975). Role of trace elements in cancer. *Cancer Res.* **35**, 3481.

Scrimshaw, N. S. (1981). Significance of the interactions of nutrition and infection in children. *In* "Textbook of Pediatric Nutrition" (Suskind, R. M., ed.), p. 229. Raven Press, New York, 1981.

Scrimshaw, N. S., Taylor, C. E., and Gordon, J. E. (1959). Interactions of nutrition and infection. *Am. J. Med. Sci.* **237**, 367.

Scrimshaw, N. S., Salamon, J. B., Bruch, H. A., and Gordon, J. E. (1966). Studies of diarrheal disease in central America. VIII. Measles, diarrhea, and nutritional deficiency in rural Guatemala. *Am. J. Trop. Med. Hyg.* **15**, 625.

Scrimshaw, N. S., Taylor, C. E., and Gordon, J. E. (1968). World Health Organ. Monogr. Ser. No. 57. W.H.O., Geneva.

Scrutton, M. C., Utter, M. F., and Mildvan, A. S. (1972). Pyruvate carboxylase. IV. The presence of a tightly bound manganese. *J. Biol. Chem.* **241**, 3480.

Seely, J. R., Humphrey, G. B., and Matter, J. (1971). Copper deficiency in a premature infant fed an iron-fortified formula. *N. Engl. J. Med.* **285**, 109.

Selivonchick, D. P., and Johnston, P. V. (1975). Fat deficiency in rats during development of the central nervous system and susceptibility to experimental allergic encephalomyelitis. *J. Nutr.* **105**, 288.

Sellmeyer, E., Bhettay, E., Truswell, A. S., Meyers, O. L., and Hansen, J. D. L. (1972). Lymphocyte transformation in malnourished children. *Arch. Dis. Child.* **47**, 429.

Selvaraj, R. J., and Bhat, K. S. (1972a). Metabolic and bactericidal activities of leukocytes in protein-calorie nutrition. *Am. J. Clin. Nutr.* **25**, 166.

Selvaraj, R. J., and Bhat, K. S. (1972b). Phagocytosis and leucocyte enzymes in protein-calorie malnutrition. *Biochem. J.* **127**, 255.

Sempos, C. T., Johnson, N. E., Elmer, P. J., Allington, J. K., and Matthews, M. E. (1982). A dietary survey of 14 Wisconsin Nursing Homes. *J. Amer. Diet. Assoc.* **81**, 35.

Seth, V., and Chandra, R. K. (1972). Opsonic activity, phagocytosis, and bactericidal capacity of polymorphs in undernutrition. *Arch. Dis. Child* **47**, 282.

Sever, J. L., Fuccillo, D. A., Ellenberg, J., and Gilkeson, M. R. (1975). Infection and low birth weight in an industrialized society. *Am. J. Dis. Child.* **129**, 557.

Sever, L. E. (1975). Zinc and human development: A review. *Hum. Ecol.* **3**, 43.

Sharpless, G. R. (1946). The effects of copper on liver tumor induction by p-dimethylaminoazobenzene. *Fed. Proc., Fed. Am. Soc. Exp. Biol.* **5**, 239.

Shaw, J. C. L. (1979). Trace elements in the fetus and young infant. I. Zinc. *Am. J. Dis. Child.* **133**, 1250.

Shaw, J. C. L. (1980). Trace elements in the fetus and young infant. II. Copper, manganese, selenium, and chromium. *Am. J. Dis. Child.* **134**, 74.

Sheffy, B. E., and Schultz, R. D. (1979). Influence of vitamin E and selenium on immune response mechanisms. *Fed. Proc.* **38**, 2139.

Shenken, B. J., Matarazzo, W. J., Hirsch, R. L., and Gray, I. (1977). Trace metal modification of immunocompetence. I. Effect of trace metals in the cultures of *in vitro* transformation of B lymphocytes. *Cell. Immunol.* **34**, 19.

Shields, G. S., Coulson, W. F., Kimball, D. A., Carnes, W. H., Cartwright, G. E., and Wintrobe, M. M. (1962). Studies on copper metabolism. XXXII. Cardiovascular lesions in copper deficient swine. *Am. J. Pathol.* **41**, 603.

Shilotri, P. G. (1977). Glycolytic, hexose monophosphate shunt and bactericidal activities of leukocytes in ascorbic acid deficient guinea pigs. *J. Nutr.* **107**, 1507.

Shimkin, M. B., Stoner, G. D., and Theiss, J. C. (1978). Lung tumor response in mice to metals and metal salts. *Adv. Exp. Med. Biol.* **91**, 85.

Shrader, R. E., and Everson, G. J. (1967). Anomalous development of otoliths associated with postural defects in manganese deficient guinea pigs. *J. Nutr.* **91**, 453.

Shrader, R. E., Erway, L., and Hurley, L. S. (1973). Mucopolysaccharide synthesis in the developing inner ear of manganese-deficient and pallid mutant mice. *Teratology* **8**, 257.

Siegel, R. C., Pinnell, S. R., and Martin, G. R. (1970). Cross-linking of collagen and elastin properties of lysyl oxidase. *Biochemistry* **9**, 4486.

Slonecker, C. E., and Osmanski, P. (1974). The effects of protein deficiency on acute inflammatory responses in rats. *J. Reticuloendothel. Soc.* **16**, 239.

Smith, A. G., and Powell, L. (1957). Genesis of teratomas of the testis. A study of normal and zinc-injected testes of roosters. *Am. J. Pathol.* **33**, 653.

Smith, J. C., McDaniel, E. G., Farr, F. F., and Halsted, J. A. (1973). Zinc: A trace element essential in vitamin A metabolism. *Science* **181**, 954.

Smith, R. (1960). Total body water in malnourished rats. *Clin. Sci.* **19**, 275.

Smith, S. E., and Ellis, G. H. (1947). Copper deficiency in rabbits. Achromotrichia, alopecia and dermatosis. *Arch. Biochem.* **15**, 81.

Smith, W. B., Shohet, S. B., Zagajeski, E., and Lubin, B. H. (1975). Alteration in human granulocyte function after in vitro incubation with L-asorbic acid. *Ann. N.Y. Acad. Sci.* **258**, 329.

Symthe, P. M., Schonland, M., Brereton-Stiles, G. G., Grace, H. J., Mafoyane, AS., Schonland, M., Coovadia, H. M., Loennig, W. E., Parent, M. A., and Vos, G. H. (1971). Thymolympathic deficiency and depression of cell-mediated immunity in protein-calorie malnutrition. *Lancet* **2**, 939.

Soli, A. H., Goldfine, I. D., Roth, J., and Kahn, C. R. (1974). Thymic lymphocytes in obese (ob/ob) mice. *J. Biol. Chem.* **13**, 4127.

Solomons, N. W., and Allen, L. H. (1983). The functional assessment of nutritional status: principles, practice and potential. *Nutr. Rev.* **41**, 33.

Solomons, N. W., Layden, T. J., Rosenberg, I. l., Vo-Khactu, K., and Sandstead, H. H. (1976). Plasma trace metals during total parenteral alimentation. *Gastroenterology* **70**, 1022.

Solsocinski, P. Z., Canterbury, W. J., and Porsanda, M. C. (1977). Differential effect of parenteral zinc in the course of various bacterial infections. *Proc. Soc. Exp. Biol. Med.* **156**, 334.

Sorenson, J. R. J., and Hangarter, W. (1977). Treatment of rheumatoid and degenerative disease with copper complexes. A review with emphasis on coppersalicylate. *Inflammation* **2**, 217.

Spectur, A. A. (1968). Part III. Lipids, hormones and atherogenesis. The transport and utilization of free fatty acid. *Ann. N.Y. Acad. Sci.* **149**, 768.

Spitznagel, J. K., and Allison, A. C. (1970). Mode of action of adjuvants: Retinol and other lysosome-labilizing agents in adjuvants. *J. Immunol.* **104**, 119.

Sprunt, D. H. (1942). The effect of undernourishment on the susceptibility of the rabbit to infection with vaccinia. *J. Exp. Med.* **75**, 297.

Srivastava, U. S., Rakshit, A. K., Seebag, M., Omoloko, C., and Thakur, M. L. (1981). Metabolism of adenine nucleosides and nucleotides, nucleic acids and proteins in the thymus and spleen of neonatal progeny of dietary restricted rats. *Nutr. Rep. Int.* **23**, 1035.

Srouji, M. N., Balistreri, W. F., Caleb, M. H., South, M. A., and Starr, S. (1978). Zinc deficiency during parental nutrition: Skin manifestations and immune imcompetence in a premature infant. *J. Pediatr. Surg.* **13**, 570.

Stankova, L., Gerbhardt, N. B., Nagel, L., and Bigley, R. H. (1975). Ascorbate and phagocyte function. *Infect. Immun.* **12**, 252.

Steim, G. M. (1972). Membrane transition: Some aspects of structure and function. In: mitochondria biogenesis and bioenergetics. *In* "Biomembranes: Molecular Arrangements and Transport Mechanisms" (S. G. Van Denberg, P. Borst, L. L. M. Van Deenen, J. C. Riemersma, E. C. Slater, and J. M. Targer, eds.), FEBS, Stn Meet., p. 195. North-Holland Publ., Amsterdam.

Steward, M. W., Devey, M. E., and Reinhardt, M. C. (1981). Antibody affinity: Its relationship to immune complex disease and the effect of malnutrition. *In* "The Immunology of Infant Feeding" (A. W. Wilkinson, ed.), pp. 997–106. Plenum Press, New York.

Stich, H. F., and Kuhnlein, U. (1979). Chromosome breaking activity of human feces and its enhancement by transition metals. *Int. J. Cancer* **24**, 284.

Stillman, E. G. (1924). Persistence of inspired bacteria in the lungs of alcoholized mice. *J. Exp. Med.* **40,** 353.

Stoolmiller, A. C. (1977). Manganese stimulation of complex carbohydrate synthesis in cultured NB2a mouse neuroblastoma cells. *Fed. Proc., Fed. Am. Soc. Exp. Biol.* **35,** 2791.

Straus, B., Berenyi, M. R., Huang, J. M., and Straus, E. (1971). Delayed hypersensitivity in alcoholic cirrhosis. *Dig. Dis.* **16,** 509.

Strober, S. (1975). Immune function cell surface characteristics and maturation of B cell populations. *Transplant. Rev.* **24,** 84.

Stroder, J., and Kasal, P. (1970). Evaluation of phagocytosis in rickets. *Acta Paediatr. Scand.* **59,** 288.

Strom, T., Bear, R., and Carpenter, C. (1975). Insulin-induced augmentation of lymphocyte-mediated cytotoxicity. *Science* **187,** 1206.

Strunk, R. C., Payne, C. M., Nagle, R. B., and Kunke, K. (1979). Alteration of the structure and function of guinea pig peritoneal macrophages by a soybean oil emulsion. *Am. J. Pathol.* **96,** 755.

Sullivan, J. L., and Ochs, H. D. (1978). Copper deficiency and the immune system. *Lancet* **2,** 686.

Suskind, R., Sirisinha, S., Vithayasai, V., Edelman, R., Damrongsak, D., Charapatana, C., and Olson, R. E. (1976a). Immunoglobulins and antibody response in children with protein-calorie malnutrition. *Am. J. Clin. Nutr.* **29,** 836.

Suskind, R., Edelman, R., Kulapongs, P., Pariyanonda, A., and Sirisinha, S. (1976b). Complement activity in children with protein-calorie malnutrition. *Am. J. Clin. Nutr.* **29,** 1089.

Suskind, R. M. (1977). "Malnutrition and the Immune Response," p. 378, Raven Press, New York.

Suttle, N. F., Field, A. C., and Barlow, R. M. (1970). Experimental copper deficiency in sheep. *J. Comp. Pathol.* **80,** 151.

Suzuki, M. (1968). Transport of cholesterol by blood leukocytes and plasma in rabbits. *J. Nutr.* **97,** 203.

Swenerton, H., and Hurley, L. S. (1968). Severe zinc deficiency in male and female rats. *J. Nutr.* **95,** 8.

Swenerton, H., Shrader, R., and Hurley, L. S. (1969). Zinc-deficient embyros. Reduced thymidine incorporation. *Science* **166,** 1014.

Tanaka, Y., Hatano, S., Nishi, Y., and Usui, T. (1980). Nutritional copper deficiency in a Japanese infant on formula. *J. Pediatr.* **96,** 225.

Taneja, P. N., Ghai, O. P., and Bhakoo, O. N. (1962). Importance of measles to India. *Am. J. Dis. Child.* **103,** 226.

Tanner, J. M. (1952). The assessment of growth and development in children. *Arch. Dis. Child.* **27,** 10.

Tapper, M. L. (1980). Infections complicating the alcoholic host. *In* "Infections in the Abnormal Host," (Grieco, M. H., ed.), p. 474.

Taub, R. N., Krantz, A. R., and Dresser, D. W. (1970). The effects of localized injection of adjuvant material on the draining lymph node. *Immunology* **18,** 171.

Tennenbaum, J. I., Ruppert, R. D., St. Pierre, R. L., and Greenberger, N. J. (1969). The effect of chronic alcohol administration on the immune responsiveness of rats. *J. Allergy* **44,** 272.

Tennican, P. O., Carl, G. Z., and Chvapil. M. (1979). Diverse effects of topical and systemic zinc on the virulence of herpes simplex genitalis (HSV-2). *Life Sci.* **24,** 1877.

Theofilopoulos, A. N., and Dixon, F. J. (1981). Etiopathogenesis of murine SLE. *Immunol. Rev.* **55,** 179.

Thomson, A. M., and Black, A. E. (1965). Nutritional aspects of human lactation. *Bull. W.H.O.* **52,** 163.

References

Tisdale, W. (1961). Spontaneous colon bacillus bacteremia in laennec's cirrhosis. *Gastroenterology* **40**, 141.

Tisman, G., and Herbert, V. (1973). In vitro myelosuppression and immunosuppression by Ethanol. *J. Clin. Invest.* **52**, 1410.

Todd, W. R., Elvehjem, C. A., and Hart, E. B. (1934). Zinc nutrition in the rat. *Am. J. Physiol.* **107**, 145.

Tonkin, C. H., and Brostoff, J. (1978). Do fatty acids exert a specific effect on human lymphocyte transformation in vitro? *Int. Arch. Allergy Appl. Immunol.* **57**, 171.

Triger, D. R., and Wright, R. (1973). Hyperglobulinemia in liver disease. *Lancet* **1**, 1494.

Triger, D. R., Alp, M. H., and Wright, R. (1972a). Bacterial and dietary antibodies in liver disease. *Lancet* **1**, 60.

Triger, D. R., Kurtz, J. B., MacCallum, F. O., and Wright, R. (1972b). Raised antibody titers to measles and rubella viruses in chronic active hepatitis. *Lancet* **1**, 665.

Truswell, A. S. (1975). p. 125. Academic Press, New York.

Tsan, M.-F., and Chen, J. W. (1980). Oxidation of methionine by human polymorphonuclear leukocytes. *J. Clin. Invest.* **65**, 1041.

Tsang, W. M., Belin, J., Monro, J. A., Smith, A. D., Thompson, R. H. S., and Zilkha, K. J. (1976). *J. Neurol., Neurosurg. Psychiatry* **39**, 767.

Tui, C., Kuo, N. H., and Schmidt, L. (1954). The protein status in pulmonary tuberculosis. *Am. J. Clin. Nutr.* **2**, 252.

Turner, R. G., and Loew, E. R. (1931). Effect of withdrawal of vitamin A on leukocyte and differential count in the albino rat. *Proc. Soc. Exp. Biol. Med.* **28**, 506.

Uhr, J. W., Weissmann, G., and Thomas, L. (1963). Acute hypervitaminosis A in guinea pigs. II. Effects of delayed-type hypersensitivity. *Proc. Soc. Exp. Biol. Med.* **112**, 287.

Underwood, E. J. (1977). "Trace Elements in Human and Animal Nutrition," 4th ed., Academic Press, New York.

Urrutia, J. J., Mata, L. J., Trent, F., Cruz, J. R., Villatoro, E., and Alexander, R. E. (1975). Infection and low birth weight in a developing country. *Am. J. Dis. Child.* **129**, 558.

Vallee, B. L. (1976). Zinc biochemistry in the normal and neoplastic growth processes. *In* "Cancer Enzymology" (J. Schultz and F. Ahmad, eds.), p. 159. Academic Press, New York.

Van Rensburg, S. J. (1972). Failure of low protein and zinc intakes to influence nitrosamine-induced oesophageal carcinogenesis. *S. Afr. Med. J.* **46**, 1137.

Van Wyk, J. J., Baxter, J. H., Akeroyd, J. H., and Motulsky, A. G. (1953). The anemia of copper deficiency in dogs compared with that produced by iron deficiency. *Bull. Johns Hopkins Hosp.* **93**, 41.

Vasantha, N., and Freese, E. (1979). The role of manganese in growth and sporulation of *Bacillus subtilis. J. Gen. Microbiol.* **112**, 329.

Vaughn, V. J., and Weinberg, E. D. (1978). *Candida albicans* dimorphism and virulence: Role of copper. *Mycopathologia* **64**, 39.

Vilter, R. W., Bozian, R. C., Hess, E. V., Zellner, D. C., and Petering, H. G. (1974). Manifestations of copper deficiency in a patient with systemic sclerosis on intravenous hyperalimentation. *N. Engl. J. Med.* **291**, 188.

Vir, S. C., and Love, A. H. G. (1979). Zinc and copper status of the elderly. *Am. J. Clin. Nutr.* **32**, 1472.

Viteri, F. E., and Schneider, R. E. (1974). Gastrointestinal alterations in protein-calorie malnutrition. *Med. Clin. North Am.* **58**, 1487.

Viteri, F. E., Béhar, M., Arroyave, G., and Scrimshaw, N. S. (1964). *In* "Mammalian Protein Metabolism" (H. N. Munro and J. B. Allison, eds.), Vol. 2, p. 523. Academic Press, New York.

Viteri, F. E., Flores, J. M., Alvarado, J., and Béhar, M. (1973). Intestinal malabsorption in malnourished children before and during recovery. *Am. J. Dig. Dis.* **18**, 201.

Vuori, E., Makinen, S. M., Kara, R., and Kuitunen, P. (1980). The effects of the dietary intakes of copper, iron, manganese, and zinc on the trace element content of human milk. *Am. J. Clin. Nutr.* **33**, 227.

Wacker, W. E. C. (1978). Biochemistry of zinc—role in wound healing. *In* "Zinc and Copper in Clinical Medicine" (K. M. Hambidge and B. L. Nichols, eds.), p. 15. S. P. Medical and Scientific Books/Spectrum Publications, Inc., New York.

Waddell, C. C., Taunton, O. D., and Twomey, J. J. (1976). Inhibition of lymphoproliferation by hyperlipoproteinemia plasma. *J. Clin. Invest.* **58**, 950.

Wade, S., Lemonnier, D., Bleiberg, F., and Delorme, J. (1983). Early nutritional experiments: effects on the humoral and cellular immune responses in mice. *J. Nutr.* **113**, 1131.

Wagner, W. H., and Silberman, H. (1984). Lipid-based parenteral nutrition and the immunosuppression of protein malnutrition. *Arch. Surg.* **119**, 809.

Waldmann, R. A. (1969). Disorders of immunoglobulin metabolism. *N. Engl. J. Med.* **281**, 1170.

Walford, R. L. (1974). Immunologic theory of aging: Current status. *Fed. Proc., Fed. Am. Soc. Exp. Biol.* **33**, 2020.

Walford, R. L., Liu, R. K., Gebrase-DeLima, M., Mathies, M., and Smith, G. S. (1973). Longterm dietary restriction and immune function in mice: Response to sheep red blood cells and to mitogenic agents. *Mech. Ageing Dev.* **2**, 447.

Walford, R. L., Gottesman, S. R. S., and Weindruch, R. H. (1981). Immunopathology of aging. *Ann. Rev. Gerontol. Geriatr.* **2**, 3.

Walker, M. A., and Page, L. (1977). Nutritive content of college meals. *J. Am. Diet. Assoc.* **7**, 260.

Wallenius, K., Mathur, A., and Abdulla, M. (1979). Effect of different levels of dietary zinc on development of chemically induced oral cancer in rats. *Int. J. Oral Surg.* **8**, 56.

Walravens, P. A., and Hambidge, K. M. (1976). Growth of infants fed a zinc-supplemented formula. *Am. J. Clin. Nutr.* **29**, 1114.

Waltens, M., and Roe, F. J. C. (1975). A study of the effects of zinc and tin administered orally to mice over a prolonged period. *Food Cosmet. Toxicol.* **3**, 272.

Warnold, L., and Lundholdm, K. (1984). Clinical significance of preoperative nutritional status in 215 noncancer patients. *Ann. Surg.* **199**, 299.

Warshaw, A. L. (1972). Pancreatic abcesses. *N. Engl. J. Med.* **287**, 1234.

Waszewska-Czyzewska, M., Wesierska-Gadek, J., and Leguthko, L. (1978). Immunostimulatory effect of zinc in patients with acute lymphoblastic leukemia. *Folia Haematol. (Leipzig)* **105**, 727.

Waterlow, J. C. (1963). The partition of nitrogen in the urine of malnourished jamaican infants. *Am. J. Clin. Nutr.* **12**, 235.

Waterlow, J. C. (1968). Observations on the mechanism of adaptation to low protein intakes. *Lancet* **2**, 1091.

Waterlow, J. C. (1976). *In* "Nutrition in Preventive Medicine" (G. H. Boston and J. M. Bengoa, eds.), p. 530. World Health Organ., Geneva.

Waterlow, J. C., and Alleyne, G. A. O. (1971). Protein malnutrition in children: Advances in knowledge in the last ten years. *Adv. Protein Chem.* **25**, 117.

Waterlow, J. C., and Stephen, J. M. L. (1968). The effect of low protein diets on the turnover rates of serum, liver and muscle protein in the rat, measured by continuous infusion of [C]Lysine. *Clin. Sci.* **35**, 287.

Watson, C. E., and Freesemann, D. (1970). Immunoglobulins in protein-calorie malnutrition. *Arch. Dis. Child.* **45**, 282.

Watson, R. R., and Haffer, K. (1980). Modifications of cell-mediated immune responses by moderate dietary protein stress in immunologically immature and mature BALB/c mice. *Mech. Ageing Dev.* **12**, 269.

Watson, R. R., Rister, M., and Baehner, R. L. (1976). Superoxide dismutase activity in poly-morphonuclear leukocytes and alveolar macrophages of protein malnourished rats and guinea pigs. *J. Nutr.* **103**, 1801.

Watson, R. R., Reyes, M. A., and McMurray, D. N. (1978). Influence of malnutrition on the concentration of IgA, lysozyme, amylase, and aminopeptidase in children's tears. *Proc. Soc. Exp. Biol. Med.* **157**, 215.

Watson, E. S., Murphy, J. C., ElSohly, H. N., ElSohly, M. A., and Turner, C. E. (1983). Effects of the administration of coca alkaloids on the primary immune responses of mice: interaction with delta 9-tetrahydrocannabinol and ethanol. *Toxicol. Appl. Pharmacol.* **71**, 1.

Watts, T. (1969). Thymus weights in malnourished children. *J. Trop. Pediatr.* **115**, 155.

Wayburne, S. (1968). p. 7. Churchill-Livingston, Edinburgh and London.

Wedgewood, J. R., Ochs, H. D., and Davis, S. D. (1975). The recognition and classification of immunodeficiency diseases with bacteriophage X 174. *Birth Defects, Orig. Artic. Ser.* **11**, 331.

Weindruch, R. H., and Suffin, S. C. (1980). Quantitative histologic effects on mouse thymus of controlled dietary restriction. *J. Gerontol.* **4**, 525.

Weindruch, R. H., and Walford, R. L. (1982). Dietary restriction in mice beginning at 1 year of age: Effect on life-span and spontaneous cancer incidence. *Science* **215**, 1415.

Weindruch, R. H., Kristie, J. A., Cheney, K. E., and Walford, R. L. (1979). Influence of controlled dietary restriction on immunologic function and aging. *Fed. Proc., Fed. Am. Soc. Exp. Biol.* **38**, 2007.

Weindruch, R. H., Gottesman, S. R. S., and Walford, R. L. (1982). Modification of age-related immune decline in mice dietarily restricted from or after midadulthood. *Proc. Natl. Acad. Sci. U.S.A.* **79**, 898.

Weindruch, R. H., Devens, B. H., Raff, H. V., and Walford, R. L. (1983). Influence of dietary restriction and aging on natural killer cell activity in mice. *J. Immunol.* **130**, 993.

Weissman, N., Shields, G. S., and Carnes, W. H. (1963). Cardiovascular studies on copper-deficient swine. IV. Contents and solubility of the aortic elastin, collagen, and hexosamine. *J. Biol. Chem.* **238**, 3115.

Werb, Z., and Cohn, Z. A. (1972). Plasma membrane synthesis in the macrophage following phagocytosis of polystyrene latex particles. *J. Biol. Chem.* **247**, 2439.

Wesch, H., Zimmerer, J., Wayss, K., and Volm, M. (1973). Unterschungen uber das Verhalten Essentieller Spurenelemente Wahrend des Wachstums von Impftumoren der Ratte. *Z. Krebsforsch.* **79**, 19.

Wesser, U., Rupp, H., Donay, F., Linnemann, F., and Boelter, W. (1973). Characterization of Cd, Zn-thionein (Metallo-thionein) isolated from rat and chicken liver. *Eur. J. Biochem.* **39**, 127.

Weston, P. G., and Johnston, P. V. (1978). Cerebral prostaglandin synthesis during the dietary and pathological stresses of essential fatty acid deficiency and experimental allergic en-cophalomyelitis. *Lipids* **13**, 308.

Weston, W. L., Huff, J. C., Humbert, J. R., Hambidge, M., Neldner, K. H., and Walravens, P. A. (1977). Zinc correction of defection chemotaxis in acrodermatitis enteropathica. *Arch. Dermatol.* **113**, 422.

Weyman, C., Morgan, S. J., Belin, J., and Smith, A. (1977). Phytohemagglutinin stimulation of human lymphocytes. Effect of fatty acids on uridine uptake and phosphoglyceride fatty acid profile. *Biochim. Biophys. Acta* **496**, 155.

Wharton, B. A. (1970). Hypoglycemia in children with kwashiorkor. *Lancet* **1**, 171.

Wharton, B. A., Howells, G., and Phillips, I. (1968). Diarrhoea in kwashiorkor. *Br. Med. J.* **4**, 608.

White, G., Bradley, D., and White, A. (1972). "Drawers of Water: Domestic Use in East Africa." Univ. of Chicago Press, Chicago, Illinois.

White, H. S. (1976). Zinc content and the zinc-to-calorie ratio of weighed diets. *J. Am. Diet. Assoc.* **68**, 243.

Whitehead, R. G. (1977a). Infection and the development of kwashiorkor and marasmus in Africa. *Am. J. Clin. Nutr.* **30**, 1281.

Whitehead, R. G. (1977b). Protein and energy requirements of young children living in the developing countries to allow for catch-up growth after infections. *Am. J. Clin. Nutr.* **30**, 1545.

Whitehead, R. G. (1977c). Some quantitative considerations of importance to the improvement of the nutritional status of rural children. *Proc. R. Soc. London, Ser. B* **199**, 49.

Whitehead, R. G. (1981). p. 15 Huber, Bern.

Whitehead, R. G., and Alleyne, G. A. O. (1972). Pathophysiological factors of importance in protein-calorie malnutrition. *Br. Med. Bull.* **28**, 72.

Whitehead, R. G., and Harland, P. S. (1966). Blood glucose, lactate and pyruvate in kwashiorkor. *Br. J. Nutr.* **20**, 825.

Whittle, H. C., Mee, J., Werblinska, J., Yakubu, A., Onuoura, C., and Gomwalk, N. (1980). Immunity to measles and malnourished children. *Clin. Exp. Immunol.* **42**, 144.

Willett, W. C., and Macmahon, B. (1984). Diet and cancer—an overview. *N. Engl. J. Med.* **310**, 633.

Williams, E. A. J., Gross, R. L., and Newberne, P. M. (1975). Effect of folate deficiency on the cell-mediated immune response in rats. *Nutr. Rep. Int.* **12**, 137.

Williams, E. A. J., Gebhardt, B. M., Morton, B., and Newberne, P. M. (1979). Effects of early marginal methionine-choline deprivation on the development of the immune system in the rat. *Am. J. Clin. Nutr.* **32**, 1214.

Williams, R. B., Russel, R. M., Dutta, L. K., and Giovetti, A. C. (1979). Alcoholic pancreatitis: Patients at high risk of acute zinc deficiency. *Am. J. Med.* **66**, 889.

Willis, R. A. (1934). Experimental study of possible influence of injury in genesis of tumours of gonads. *Br. J. Exp. Pathol.* **15**, 234.

Wilson, L. D., Onstad, G. R., Williams, R. C., and Carey, J. R. (1968). Selective immunoglobulin A deficiency in two patients with alcoholic cirrhosis. *Gastroenterology* **2**, 253.

Wilson, I. D., Onstad, G. R., and Williams, R. C. (1969). Serum immunoglobulin concentrations in patients with alcoholic liver disease. *Gastroenterology* **57**, 59.

Winberg, J., and Wessner, G. (1971). Does breast milk protect against septicemia in the newborn? *Lancet* **1**, 1091.

Winick, M., and Rosso, P. (1969). Head circumference and cellular growth of the hrain in normal and marasmic children. *J. Pediatr.* **74**, 774.

Work, T. H., Ifekwunigwe, A., Jelliffe, D. B., Jelliffe, P., and Neumann, C. G. (1973). Tropical problems in nutrition. *Ann. Intern. Med.* **79**, 701.

World Bank (1976). "Village Water Supply." World Bank, Washington, D.C.

Woster, A. D., Failla, M. L., and Taylor, M. W. (1975). Zinc suppression in the initiation of sarcoma 180 growth. *J. Natl. Cancer Inst. (U.S.)* **54**, 1001.

Wright, E. B., and Dormandy, T. L. (1973). Liver zinc in carcinoma. *Nature (London)* **237**, 166.

Wyatt, R. G., Garcia, B., Caceres, A., and Mata, L. J. (1973). Immunoglobulins and antibodies in colostrum and milk of Guatemalan mayan women. *Arch. Latinoam. Nutr.* **21**, 629.

Yamada, H., Kumagi, H., Kawasaki, H., Matsui, H., and Ogata, K. (1967). Crystallization and properties of diamine oxidase from pig kidney. *Biochem. Biophys. Res. Commun.* **29**, 723.

Yamamoto, K., and Takahashi, M. (1975). Inhibition of the terminal stage of complement-mediated lysis (reactive lysis) by zinc and copper ions. *Int. Arch. Allergy Appl. Immunol.* **48**, 653.

Yamane, Y., and Sakai, K. (1973). Suppressive effect of concurrent administration of metal salts on carcinogenesis by 3-Methyl-4-(Dimethylamino) Azobenzene, and The effect of these metals on aminoazo dye metabolism during carcinogenesis. *Gann* **64**, 563.

Yamane, Y., Sakai, K., and Kojima, S. (1976). Mechanism of suppressive effect of basic cupric acetate on rat liver carcinogenesis by ethionine. *Gann* **67,** 295.

Young, C. M. (1979). Overnutrition. *In* "Nutrition: World Food Problem," p. 195. Karger, Basel.

Yuen, P., Lin, H. J., and Hutchison, J. H. (1979). Copper deficiency in a low birthweight infant. *Arch. Dis. Child.* **43,** 553.

Zaslavsky, V. (1979). Inhibition of vaccinia virus growth in zinc ions. Effect on early RNA and thymidine kinase synthesis. *J. Virol.* **29,** 405.

Zerfas, A. J. (1975). The insertion tape: A new circumference tape for use in nutritional assessment. *Amer. J. Clin. Nutr.* **28,** 782.

Zidenberg-Cherr, S., Keen, C. L., Lonnerdal, B., and Hurley, L. S. (1983). Superoxide dismutase activity and lipid peroxidation in the rat. Developmental correlations affected by manganese deficiency. *J. Nutr.* **113,** 2498.

Ziegler, H. D., and Ziegler, P. B. (1975). Depression of tuberculin reaction in mild and moderate protein-calorie malnourished children following BCG vaccination. *Johns Hopkins Med. J.* **137,** 59.

Zook, E. G., Green, F. E., and Morris, E. R. (1973). Nutrient composition of selected wheats and wheat products. 6. Distribution of manganese, copper, nickel, zinc, magnesium, lead, tin, cadmium, chromium and selenium determined by atomic absorption spectroscopy and colorimetry. *Cereal Chem.* **47,** 720.

Zoppi, G., Zamboni, G., Siviero, M., Bellini, P., and Cancellieri, M. L. (1978). γ-globulin level and dietary protein intake during the first year of life. *Pediatrics* **62,** 1010.

Zurier, R. B., Damjanov, I., Sayadoff, D. M., and Rothfield, N. F. (1977). Prostaglandin E₁ treatment of NZB/NZE F₁ hybrid mice. II. Prevention of glomerulonephritis. *Arthritis Rheum.* **20,** 1449.

Zwickl, C. M., and Fraker, P. J. (1980). Restoration of the antibody mediated response of zinc/calorie deficient neonatal mice. *Immunol. Commun.* **9,** 611.

Index

A

Acrodermatitis enteropathica, 123, 207, 212
Acute immunodeficiency syndrome (AIDS), 357
Acute-phase reactants, 3
ADCC, *see* Antibody-dependent cellular cytotoxicity
ADLMC, *see* Antibody-dependent lympho-cyte-mediated cytotoxicity
Adrenalectomy, 166
Agammaglobulinemia, 9, 15, 20
AIDS, *see* Acute immunodeficiency syndrome
Albumin, 47, 70, 74, 82–83, 285, 288
Alcohol, 305–323
  animal studies of, 308–311
  and cell-mediated immunity, 317–323
  and humoral immunity, 311–317
  and infectious disease, 306–311
Alcoholism, *see* Alcohol
Allergic encephalomyelitis, experimental, 279–281
Allergy, 105
  food, 304
Allograft rejection, 10–11, 16, 23
  and dietary lipids, 271–275
  in protein deficiency, 175
Alopecia, 204
Amino acids
  and autoimmune disease, 328–333
  in breast milk, 288
  deficiency of, 156–157, 183–189
  metabolism in protein-energy malnutri-tion, 71

requirement for
  of adults, 292
  of infants, 291–292
  therapeutic administration of, 183–184
AN, *see* Anorexia nervosa
Anamnestic response, 24
Anemia, 45, 59, 221
  pernicious, 248, 252–253
Anergy, 26, 80, 82
Angioneurotic edema, hereditary, 42
Angular stomatitis, 77
Anorexia, 4, 305
Anorexia nervosa (AN), 129–130, 138–146
Anthropometry, 43–44, 46, 50–59
Antibody, formation of, 9, 14
Antibody affinity, 94
Antibody-dependent cellular cytotoxicity (ADCC)
  in protein-energy malnutrition, 88
  and vitamin E, 247
Antibody-dependent, lymphocyte-mediated cytotoxicity (ADLMC), 22
Antibody response, and dietary lipids, 275–277
Antigen
  thymic-dependent, 10, 15, 173
  thymic-independent, 10, 15
Antigenic competition, 26–27
Arachidic acid, 267
Arachidonic acid, 261–269, 338, 351
Arginine, 184
Arm circumference, 48, 51, 53–57
Arm muscle area, 52
Arsenic, 224–227
Arthus reaction, 17, 235